ESSENTIALS OF

Orthodontics

Diagnosis and Treatment

ESSENTIALS OF
Orthodontics
Diagnosis and Treatment

Robert N. Staley D.D.S., M.A., M.S.
Professor

And

Neil T. Reske B.A., M.A.
Instructional Resource Associate

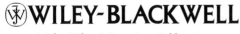
WILEY-BLACKWELL

A John Wiley & Sons, Inc., Publication

Blackwell Publishing was acquired by John Wiley & Sons in February 2007. Blackwell's publishing program has been merged with Wiley's global Scientific, Technical and Medical business to form Wiley-Blackwell.

Registered office: John Wiley & Sons Ltd, The Atrium, Southern Gate, Chichester, West Sussex, PO19 8SQ, UK

Editorial offices: 2121 State Avenue, Ames, Iowa 50014-8300, USA
9600 Garsington Road, Oxford, OX4 2DQ, UK

For details of our global editorial offices, for customer services and for information about how to apply for permission to reuse the copyright material in this book please see our website at www.wiley.com/wiley-blackwell.

Library of Congress Cataloging-in-Publication Data

Staley, Robert N.
  Essentials of orthodontics : diagnosis and treatment / Robert N. Staley and Neil T. Reske.
    p. ; cm.
  Includes bibliographical references and index.
  ISBN 978-0-8138-0868-0 (pbk. : alk. paper)
  1. Orthodontics. I. Reske, Neil T. II. Title.
  [DNLM: 1. Orthodontics–methods. 2. Malocclusion–diagnosis. 3. Malocclusion–
therapy. 4. Orthodontic Appliances. WU 440]
  RK521.S73 2011
  617.6′43–dc22
      2010028089

A catalogue record for this book is available from the British Library.

This book is published in the following electronic formats: eBook 9780470958414; ePub 9780470958476
Set in 10/12 pt Sabon by Toppan Best-set Premedia Limited
Printed and bound in Singapore by Markono Print Media Pte Ltd

Disclaimer

1 2011

Dedication

To: Kathleen H. Staley and Janet L. Reske

Epigraph

We can't have full knowledge all at once. We must start by believing; then afterwards, we may be led on to master the evidence for ourselves.

Thomas Aquinas

Table of Contents

Preface

This book is focused on teaching dental students, orthodontic and pediatric dentistry residents, and dentists the basic concepts and procedures of orthodontic diagnosis and treatment of patients who have simple malocclusion problems. The book is an outgrowth of our experiences in teaching dental students and specialty residents how to diagnose and treat malocclusions that require simple tooth movements. Many patients with the most common problems were followed from the beginning to the end of treatment to illustrate the role of diagnosis and treatment with a variety of appliances. The display of longitudinal records of patients is an important part of the teaching of beginners. The limitations of removable and simple fixed appliances and the problems best treated with one or the other appliance were discussed. We also attempted to help beginners differentiate patients who need simple tooth movements from those who appear to be simple but actually require more complex treatment.

Included are prescriptions and illustrations of the construction of orthodontic appliances used in the treatment of patients with simple tooth movement problems. This knowledge can be useful to laboratory personnel who construct appliances. The connection between fabrication and clinical use of appliances can be helpful to laboratory technicians and clinicians.

Patients with the following malocclusions are not considered as candidates for simple treatment: Class II, Class III, and Class I patients with complications involving severe crowding or extraction of teeth, excessive generalized spacing, severe openbites, deep overbites, and crossbites. The diagnosis and treatment of these patients are beyond the scope of this book.

This book is introductory to orthodontic diagnosis and treatment and is not a definitive source of information. We refer the beginner to the many excellent and more comprehensive books in print and the periodical literature that present in greater depth the concepts of orthodontic diagnosis and treatment.

Our foremost concern is for the welfare of the patient. This concern requires careful consideration before starting orthodontic treatment. Before clinicians move teeth, they must recognize malocclusions and their severity, gain the knowledge to correctly diagnose a malocclusion, and develop the skills to carry out the treatment of a patient.

Acknowledgments

We wish to express our appreciation to several persons who contributed to the preparation of this book. Robert Staley thanks orthodontic laboratory technician Mr. James P. Vance for providing valuable information about laboratory procedures. Neil Reske appreciates the guidance of mentor and friend Mr. Harold Gregorich and teacher Mr. Fred Ulmer, who were instrumental in building a foundation for his laboratory techniques. Mr. James D. Herd, Ms. Patricia J. Conrad, Mr. Ron Irvin, and Mr. Tom Weinsel drew illustrations for the book. Mrs. JoAnne B. Montgomery scanned and adjusted slides for most of the illustrations. We thank Mr. Richard A. Tack for his technical support. Mr. Eric M. Corbin took photographs of appliance construction. We thank Dr. Michael L. Swartz for permission to use orthoclipart illustrations used in Chapters 1 and 13. Dr. George F. Andreasen, former head of the Orthodontic Department, provided helpful suggestions for the discussions involving biomechanics. We thank numerous orthodontic and pediatric dentistry residents who participated in the treatment of several patients described herein. The following faculty of the Orthodontic Department provided radiographs or photographs of patients: Drs. Harold F. Bigelow, Samir E. Bishara, John S. Casko, Theresa L. Juhlin, Karin A. Southard, and Thomas E. Southard. We thank Dr. Thomas E. Southard, head of the Department of Orthodontics, for his support and encouragement of this publication. The following adjunct faculty of the Department of Orthodontics provided invaluable discussions on retention philosophy and laboratory appliance design: Drs. Charles C. Collins, Phillip M. Doster, Paul C. Hermanson, David D. Kinser, and Carney D. Loucks. We thank Dr. Tom M. Graber, who read an earlier edition of the book and provided helpful suggestions for revision. Robert Staley is grateful to Drs. John J. Cunat and Larry J. Green, who introduced him to the specialty of orthodontics at the State University of New York at Buffalo, and Dr. Albert A. Dahlberg, who encouraged him in the study of the biology of the human dentition at the University of Chicago. Dr. Christopher P. Evans proofread the text.

The authors accept full responsibility for the contents of this book.

Introduction

The gathering of information from the patient and steps leading to the development of a diagnosis are discussed in Chapters 1 through 5. Foremost in this section is the recognition of malocclusion, a chair-side skill that is essential for every dentist. Study casts are an important record that will sometime in the near future be obtained digitally from impressions. Dental cast analysis in adults and norms for overbite and overjet are discussed. Prediction of tooth size in the mixed dentition is discussed in Chapter 4. Radiographic and cephalometric analyses are presented in Chapter 5. Cephalometric norms are given for children and adults.

The diagnosis and treatment of commonly observed simple malocclusion problems are described in Chapters 6 through 10. Treatment with lingual arches and the construction of a lower loop lingual arch are included in Chapter 6. The management of anterior cross bites is described in Chapter 7. The construction of an appliance used to close a diastema and correct a crossbite is shown in this chapter. The management of patients with posterior crossbites is discussed and illustrated in Chapter 8. The construction of a removable expander is described in this chapter. The diagnosis and treatment of incisor diastemas are discussed in Chapter 9. The diagnosis and treatment involved with molar up righting and regaining of arch length are presented in Chapter 10. The chapter includes treatment of children and adults with these problems.

The guidelines for differentiating patients who need simple tooth movement from those who need comprehensive treatment are given in Chapter 11. This is a difficult skill to master. The guidelines will help a beginner to successfully choose those patients who have malocclusions appropriate for simple tooth movement.

Chapter 12 is an introduction to biomechanics. Chapter 13 describes the modern edgewise appliance that evolved from its original invention by Dr. Edward H. Angle. Chapter 14 illustrates the construction of removable appliances and retainers. Chapter 15 is a brief summary of materials used in orthodontic treatment.

ESSENTIALS OF
Orthodontics
Diagnosis and Treatment

Orthodontic Diagnosis and Treatment Planning

1

Normal and Ideal Occlusion

To recognize a malocclusion, a clinician needs to understand ideal and normal occlusions. People with **ideal occlusions** have all 32 adult teeth in superb relationships in all three planes of space. The tip of the mesiobuccal cusp of the upper first molar fits into the buccal groove of the lower first molar, and the tip of the upper canine crown fits into the embrasure between the lower canine and first premolar (Fig. 1.1, Class I ideal occlusion). **Overbite**, the extent that the upper central incisors overlap the lower central incisors in the vertical plane, is approximately 20%. **Overjet**, the distance along the anteroposterior plane between the labial surfaces of the lower central incisors and the labial surfaces of the upper central incisors, is approximately 1 to 2 mm. Teeth, moreover, are normally angled in the mesiodistal plane, normally inclined in the buccolingual plane, and aligned without being spaced, rotated, or crowded along the crests of the alveolar processes (Andrews 1972). Ideal occlusions are rare in the United States.

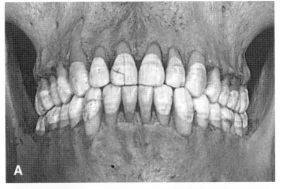
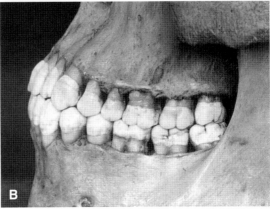

Figure 1.1. A, B, Ideal occlusion in the skeletal remains of a human adult. (Skull "secretum apertum," courtesy of Dr. Richard Summa.)

Essentials of Orthodontics: Diagnosis and Treatment by Robert N. Staley and Neil T. Reske © 2011 Blackwell Publishing Ltd.

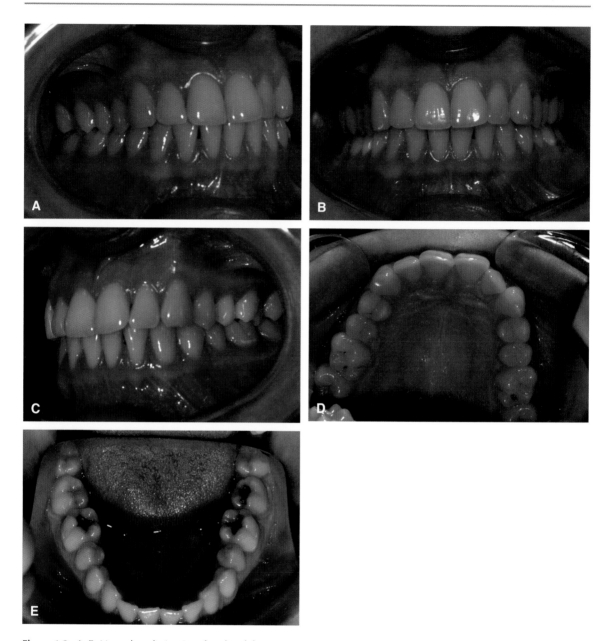

Figure 1.2. A–E, Normal occlusion in a female adult.

Normal occlusions have minimal rotations, crowding, and/or spacing of the teeth. More variability is observed in overbite and overjet in normal occlusions (Fig. 1.2). Normal occlusions are much more frequently observed in the United States than are ideal occlusions.

Normal Occlusion in the Primary Dentition

As a child approaches the age when the normal primary dentition transitions into the mixed dentition, spaces develop between the incisors in

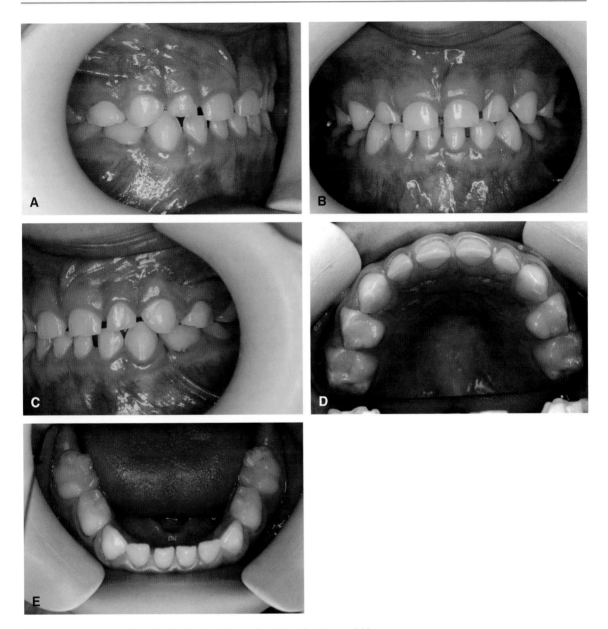

Figure 1.3. A–E, Normal occlusion in the primary dentition of a 5-year-old boy.

both arches with growth of the maxilla and mandible (Fig. 1.3). The spacing of primary incisors is needed to accommodate the erupting permanent incisors that are much larger than their primary counterparts.

Centric Occlusion and Centric Relation

Occlusion is observed and classified when the teeth are in **maximum intercuspation**, the definition for **centric occlusion.** Centric relation is defined as the most retruded occlusal position of the mandible from which opening and lateral movements can be performed (Moyers 1973). Centric occlusion deviated on average 0.7 mm from centric relation in 18 Class I normal occlusion subjects, with a maximum of 2.5 mm; however, in 28 Class II patients, the discrepancy averaged 1.2 mm, with a maximum of 4 mm (Williamson, Caves, Edenfield, and Morse 1978).

Angle Classification of Malocclusion

Angle classified malocclusions on the basis of the **anteroposterior** relationships of the upper and lower teeth (Angle 1899). He concentrated on

the relationships between the upper and lower first molars and canines. His observations on the different classes remain valid and useful today. His classification system also enhances communication between clinicians.

Angle Class I Malocclusion

Class I malocclusions have mostly normal anteroposterior tooth relations combined with a discrepancy between tooth size and dental arch length (Fig. 1.4). The discrepancy is usually crowding and less often excessive spacing between the teeth. Patients with Class I crowded malocclusions have larger-than-normal teeth,

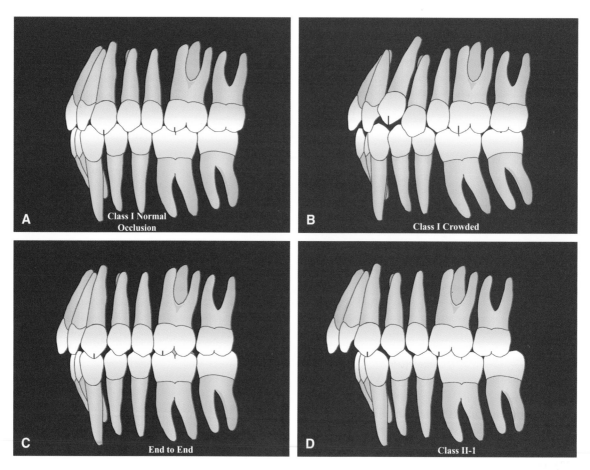

Figure 1.4. A–D, Schemata of Class I normal occlusion and Class I crowded, end-to-end, and Class II division 1 malocclusions.

smaller-than-normal arch lengths, and smaller-than-normal arch widths (Kuntz et al. 2008). Overbite and overjet vary in Class I malocclusions. Anterior and posterior crossbites appear in this type of malocclusion.

Class I Malocclusions in the Primary and Mixed Dentitions

Primary second molars are considered to be Class I normal if a **mesial step** is present between the distal surfaces of the upper and lower molar crowns when viewed from the buccal surfaces (Fig. 1.5). A **mesial step** occurs when the distal surface of the lower primary second molar is mesial to the distal surface of the upper primary second molar.

Crowding problems are rarely found in the primary dentition. If no spacing is seen between the primary incisors, dental crowding can be expected. Crowding is first apparent in the mixed dentition when the permanent incisors begin to erupt. In a crowded dentition, incisors can erupt lingual and labial to the line of arch. The **line of arch** is located along the crest of an alveolar process where the anatomic contact points of the teeth should be located ideally on a given alveolar process. Rotated and displaced incisors are commonly seen in the developing crowded malocclusion.

Angle Class II Division 1 Malocclusion

In Class II-1 malocclusions, the lower teeth are distal to the upper teeth, usually resulting in larger-than-normal overjet. The upper incisors often have increased labial inclination, making the incisor crowns susceptible to accidental fractures. The distobuccal cusp of the upper first molar occludes with the buccal groove of the lower first molar (Fig. 1.4, Class II-1). The maxillary canine crown tip is located near the mesial surface of the mandibular canine (Fig. 1.4, Class II-1). Patients with these malocclusions may or may not have crowded arches and vary in the degree of overbite from openbite to deep

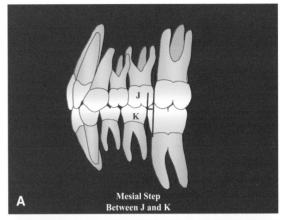

A   Mesial Step
Between J and K

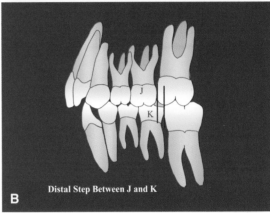

Distal Step Between J and K

B

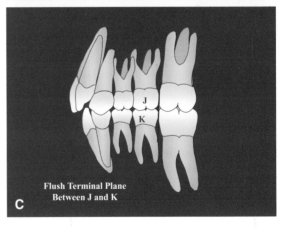

Flush Terminal Plane
Between J and K

C

Figure 1.5. A–C, Schemata of the mixed dentition showing second primary molars with mesial step, distal step, and flush terminal plane occlusions.

overbite. On average, maxillary arch widths are narrower in Class II-1 patients than in persons with normal occlusion (Staley, Stuntz, and Peterson 1985).

Angle Class II Division 2 Malocclusion

In Class II-2 malocclusions, the upper incisor crowns, especially those of the upper central incisors, are inclined to the lingual, in contrast to the excessive labial inclination observed in many Class II-1 malocclusions (Fig. 1.6). The number of maxillary incisors with lingual inclination varies from one to four. The lingual inclination of the upper central incisors results in small to moderate overjet measurements. Overbite is often deeper than normal, because of the lingual inclination of the upper incisors. The **collum angle** between the long axis of the crown and the long axis of the root in maxillary central incisors has been shown to be larger in a sample of Class II-2 patients compared with other occlusion groups. Class II-2 patients with large collum angles are predisposed to larger-than-normal overbites (Delivanis and Kuftinec 1980). The maxillary arches of patients with this malocclusion are narrower than normal but significantly larger than the widths observed in Class II-1 patients (Huth et al. 2007). Few of these patients have posterior crossbites.

Class II Malocclusions in the Primary and Mixed Dentitions

Primary second molar crowns are considered Class II when a **distal step** is observed between the distal surfaces of the upper and lower second primary molar crowns (Fig. 1.5). In this situation, the distal surface of the lower second primary molar is positioned distal to the distal surface of the upper second molar crown.

End-to-End Occlusion

When molars and canines are positioned between Class I and Class II, the relationship is considered

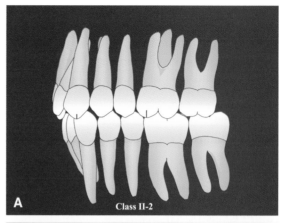
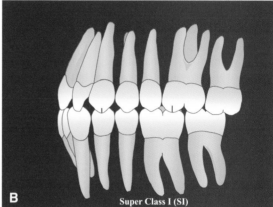
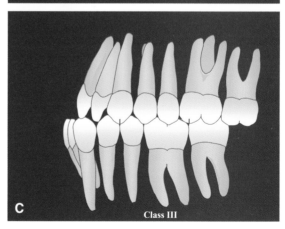

Figure 1.6. A–C, Schemata of Class II division 2, Super Class I, and Class III malocclusions.

to be end to end. These Class II malocclusions are less severe versions of the full Class II occlusion (Fig. 1.4) and are considered Class II malocclusions when assigning Angle Classification. End-to-end occlusions appear in both Class II-1 and Class II-2 types.

In the primary molars, the end-to-end relationship is expressed by what is called a **flush terminal plane** (Fig. 1.5). In a flush terminal plane, the distal surfaces of the upper and lower primary second molars are vertically coincident.

Angle Class III Malocclusion

In this class of malocclusion, the lower teeth are mesial to the upper teeth, usually resulting in anterior crossbite (Fig. 1.6). The mesiobuccal cusp of the upper first molar occludes with the embrasure between the lower first and second molars. Overbite varies from openbite to deep overbite. Alignment of the teeth in the arch varies from good to severe crowding, with the upper arch being more prone to crowding than the lower arch. On average, the maxillary arch widths of these patients are narrower than those in normal occlusions (Kuntz et al. 2008). The narrowness of the upper arch and the anteroposterior displacement of the arches are often associated with posterior crossbites.

Class III Malocclusions in Primary and Mixed Dentitions

Class III malocclusion in the primary dentition is expressed in an exaggerated mesial step between the distal surfaces of the upper and lower second molars. Often, in younger patients, a Class III occlusion is less severe than it will eventually become, because the mandible usually grows forward for a longer time than the maxilla.

Super Class I Malocclusions

When the mesiobuccal cusp tip of the upper first molar occludes distally to the buccal groove of the lower first molar in a position between Class I and full Class III, the malocclusion is termed Super Class I (Fig. 1.6). A Super Class I malocclusion is a mild version of Class III malocclusion and is considered a Class III malocclusion when assigning an Angle Classification to the patient.

Super Class II and Super Class III Malocclusions

These are more severe versions of Class II and Class III malocclusions and are seen only rarely. They can occur in patients who have lost teeth through extraction that permitted first molars to spontaneously move through the alveolus mesially or distally. Excessive or diminutive growth of the mandible can also result in these severe malocclusions.

Subdivision Malocclusions

Class II Subdivision Malocclusions

Class II subdivision malocclusions occur when the first molar relationship is Class II on one side of the arches and Class I on the other side. A Class II-1 subdivision is written as follows: Class II division 1 subdivision right when the Class II molar relation is on the right side of the arches and Class II-1 subdivision left when the molar relation is Class II on the left side of the arches.

The written form for Class II-2 subdivision malocclusions follows the same pattern as given earlier.

Class III Subdivision Malocclusions

Class III subdivision malocclusions occur when the first molar relationship is Class III on one side of the arches and Class I on the other side. Class III subdivision malocclusions are written as Class III subdivision right or left to indicate the Class III side.

Class II-III Subdivision Malocclusions

When the first molar relation is Class II on one side and Class III on the other side, the malocclusion is classified as a Class II-III subdivision right or left to indicate the class that appears on each side of the arch. For example, a malocclusion is defined as Class II R, Class III L. These malocclusions are rare and usually caused by the loss of posterior teeth and resultant shifting of teeth into extraction sites. Angle did not include Class II-III malocclusions in his classification system. This addition to the classification system includes patients with this rare malocclusion.

Incisor Dental Compensations in Class II and Class III Malocclusions

The tendency for the upper and lower incisors to remain near one another as the maxilla and mandible diverge in the anteroposterior plane during growth is called **dental compensation**. As the anteroposterior discrepancy between the upper and lower arches increases, the inclination of the incisors in both arches compensates for the discrepancy. In the Class II patient, compensation is expressed as increased lingual inclination of the upper incisors and increased labial inclination of the lower incisors. In the Class III patient, the compensation is expressed by increased labial inclination of the upper incisors and increased lingual inclination of the lower incisors.

Iowa Notation System for Angle Classification

Clinicians record the Angle relationships of the first molars and canines with an abbreviated notation. For example, a Class I malocclusion is written from the patient's right side to left side as I, I, I, I. A Class II malocclusion is written as II, II, II, II, and a Class III malocclusion is written as III, III, III, III. The term "end-to-end" is used for molar and canine relationships that are intermediate between Class I and Class II. The symbol

E is used for end-to-end in the notation. The symbol E is equivalent to Class II when classifying the malocclusion. The term "Super I" (SI) is used to describe molar and canine relationships falling between Class I and III. The symbol SI is equivalent to Class III when classifying the malocclusion. When a canine or molar cannot be classified because it is missing or not erupted, a dash is put into the notation. The notation system alerts the clinician to the presence of asymmetries in the dentition.

When the distobuccal cusp of the upper first molar occludes somewhere mesial to the buccal groove of the lower first molar or the crown tip of the upper canine is located mesial to the lower canine, the Class II occlusion is exaggerated. The term "Super II" (SII) is used to describe this exaggeration. When the mesiobuccal cusp of the upper molar is located distal to the embrasure between the lower first and second molars or when the tip of the upper canine occludes distal to the embrasure between lower first and second premolars, the Class III malocclusion is exaggerated. The term "Super III" (SIII) is used to describe this exaggeration.

Rules for Assigning Angle Classification

Examples of classifications are given next for molar and canine relations that are either the same or similar:

1. I, I, I, I = Class I
2. II, II, II, II = Class II, division 1 or 2
3. II, E, E, II = Class II, division 1 or 2
4. E, E, E, E = Class II, division 1 or 2
5. III, III, III, III = Class III
6. III, SI, SI, III = Class III

Examples of classifications are given next for three similar molar and canine relations. The Angle Classification is based on the most frequent notation, **with molar relationships taking precedence over canine relationships.**

1. I, II, SII, II = Class II, subdivision left
2. I, I, E, I, = Class I

3. E, E, E, I = Class II, subdivision right
4. III, I, III, III = Class III
5. I, I, I, II = Class II, subdivision left
6. I, I, I, III = Class III, subdivision left

Examples of classification are given next for combinations of two similar notations, of which some are Class I and others are Class II or Class III. Molar relationships take precedence over canine relationships in the assignment of Angle Classification.

1. I, E, E, I = Class I
2. I, II, II, I = Class I
3. I, SI, SI, I = Class I
4. E, I, I, E = Class II
5. SI, I, I, SI = Class III
6. I, I, II, II = Class II, subdivision left
7. SIII, SIII, I, I = Class III, subdivision right
8. I, II, I, II = Class II, subdivision left
9. I, III, I, III = Class III, subdivision left

The following principles are useful guides in assigning Angle Classification:

1. The notation E is equivalent to II.
2. The notation SI is equivalent to III.
3. Neither E nor SI is equivalent to I.
4. Normal occlusion must be differentiated from Class I malocclusion.

Rating the Severity of a Malocclusion

The severity of a malocclusion is related to the number of problems observed within the dental arches and to the relationship of the malocclusion with the face. Within the arches, problems can occur in all three planes of space: anteroposterior, transverse, and vertical (Akerman and Proffit 1969). The severity of a malocclusion increases when it involves two or three of the planes of space. Malocclusion also increases in severity as the maxilla and mandible become more involved in anteroposterior, transverse, and vertical skeletal deviations from normal. An accurate assessment of severity will be beneficial to the patient and clinician as the treatment is planned (Proffit and Akerman 1973).

Orthodontic Records

The data collected from the patient prior to treatment provide essential information on which the treatment plan, treatment, and retention plan are based. The care taken in collecting records will be reflected in the diagnosis and treatment of the patient. Records are essential for the medicolegal protection of the dental clinician.

Records taken at the initial appointment of a patient with a minor malocclusion problem include a clinical examination of the face and oral cavity, impressions for plaster casts of the teeth, facial and intraoral photographs, and a panoramic radiograph. In the mixed-dentition patient, periapical radiographs of the premolars and canines are needed for the mixed-dentition tooth size–arch length analysis. A cephalometric radiograph may be needed in some patients to determine whether the malocclusion problem is minor or complex. Patients with a suspected facial growth problem, such as a mixed-dentition patient with an anterior crossbite, may need a cephalogram to determine whether the mandible has a normal relationship to the maxilla. The cephalogram of the patient with a Class III pattern of growth can be used to assess future facial growth.

After treatment begins, a written chronologic record of treatment becomes an essential part of the patient's records. Oral hygiene practices of the patient and other compliance issues are recorded. Periodically during treatment, additional records may be gathered to assess the progress of treatment. Photographs are often taken to describe important stages and appliances used in the treatment of the patient. When appliances are removed at the end of active treatment, records also are taken. These records establish what was accomplished by the treatment. Post-treatment or retention records may be taken to evaluate the stability of the treatment and the success of the retention plan.

Records are the primary means by which a clinician can understand how the appliance corrected the malocclusion and how facial and dental growth affected the treatment outcome.

Records should be maintained for a reasonable time after treatment to help the patient during the time that retainers are worn and to protect the clinician in the event questions arise about the treatment.

Clinical Examination

A form is used to record the findings of a chairside clinical examination (Figs. 1.7, 1.8, and 1.9). Forms such as these can be digitized for paperless record keeping. In addition to demographic information, the patient is asked to describe his chief concern for seeking orthodontic treatment. A medical history is taken, including an examination of nasal airway competence. A dental history is taken. Habits involving the teeth are recorded. Habits commonly seen are thumb sucking, tongue thrusting during swallowing, and lip biting and sucking. The patient is asked if he has had previous orthodontic treatment.

A temporomandibular joint (TMJ) examination is undertaken to record any abnormal symptoms during mandibular movements and to obtain the history of any abnormal symptoms. Although orthodontic treatment has not been shown to be the cause of TMJ symptoms, these symptoms or lack thereof must be elicited and recorded at the initial examination. If significant symptoms are discovered, refer the patient to a TMJ disorder (TMD) specialist. TMDs can prevent orthodontic patients from wearing elastics or chin cups during treatment.

In viewing the face from the front, a clinician evaluates facial height and bilateral symmetry. Face height in normal adults is divided into three approximately equal parts: (1) *upper,* hairline to radix nasi [root of nose] (2) *middle,* radix nasi to basis nasi [base of nose], and (3) *lower,* basis nasi to base of chin (Fig. 1.10). Children have a smaller lower face height that gradually lengthens to adult proportions during growth. Patients with bilateral facial asymmetry usually have a noticeable deviation of the chin to the right or left of the facial midline. These patients need to be treated by a specialist. Lip position at rest is noted. The presence of a gummy smile can be evidence of excess vertical growth of the face, a shorter-than-normal upper lip length, or vertically short teeth. Face profiles fall into three types: (1) straight, (2) convex, and (3) concave. Convex profiles are often associated with Angle Class II malocclusions, whereas concave profiles are often associated with Angle Class III malocclusions (Fig. 1.10).

The dentition is then examined. The stage of development of the dentition is recorded. Early mixed dentitions have only the permanent first molars and/or incisors erupted. In the late mixed dentition, at least one permanent canine or premolar has erupted. Interceptive orthodontic procedures are initiated in the primary, mixed, and early permanent dentitions.

Periodontal status is important in all adult patients. Periodontal disease must be treated before orthodontic treatment can proceed. Adequate attached (keratinized) gingiva is needed on the buccal and labial surfaces of teeth that are planned to be moved in those directions during treatment. Gingival recession prior to treatment requires a periodontal consult before starting orthodontic treatment. Abnormal maxillary frenum attachments may be associated with a diastema between the upper central incisors. Restorative status must be assessed. Untreated nonvital teeth must receive endodontic treatment before initiation of orthodontic treatment. Prosthetic restorations have an important impact on the choice of an orthodontic appliance and its ability to move teeth. Oral hygiene status is extremely important and should be excellent before starting orthodontic treatment. All caries must be treated before beginning orthodontic treatment.

Anteroposterior relationships include the Angle Classification for molars and canines, overjet, and anterior crossbites. Vertical relationships of the upper and lower teeth are recorded. Patients with anterior and posterior openbites and deep overbites are not good candidates for minor orthodontic treatment. Transverse relationships include dental midline discrepancies with the face, posterior crossbites, and asymmetry in the

ORTHODONTIC EXAMINATION, DIAGNOSIS AND TREATMENT PLAN

Date of Examination _____

Patient's Name _____ Birthdate_____ Gender_____
(last)   (first)   (initial)

1. **Chief Concern** _____

2. **Medical History and Airway Exam**
   a. General health_____
   b. Significant conditions (e.g. requiring antibiotic premedication)_____
   c. Prescribed drugs _____
   d. Tonsils and adenoids   normal _____ enlarged _____
   e. Nasal airway: open _____ obstructed _____ mouth breathing_____

3. **Dental History**
   a. Habits: finger _____tongue _____lip _____
      Bruxism _____ musical instruments_____
   b. Trauma to face and teeth: _____
   c. Previous orthodontic treatment _____

4. **TEMPEROMANDIBULAR JOINT EXAM:** symptoms _____
   pain _____ history _____

5. **Facial Form**
   a. <u>Frontal:</u>
      1) Vertical: Face height: normal _____ long _____ short _____
      2) Bilateral: symmetry _____asymmetry _____
      3) Lips: Position at rest: touching_____ apart (mm) _____
      4) Gummy Smile: Yes_____ No_____
   b. <u>Profile:</u> straight _____convex _____concave_____

6. **Dentition**
   A. **Stage of Dentition:** Deciduous _____Mixed (Early) _____ (Late)_____ Permanent _____
   B. **Periodontal status:** (All adults **must have** recent periodontal probings). _____
      Gingival Recession _____Abnormal Frenum _____
   C. **Restorative Status:** Caries_____ Endodontics _____
      Prosthetic restorations_____
   D. **Oral Hygiene:** Good _____ Poor _____ White Spots_____
   E. **Vertical**
      1. Overbite (%) _____Anterior Open bite (mm) _____Posterior Open bite (mm) _____

Figure 1.7. Page 1 of an orthodontic clinic record form.

F. **Transverse**
1. <u>Dental midlines to face (mm):</u>   Upper _____   Lower _____
2. <u>Posterior Crossbite:</u> Unilateral _____   Bilateral _____

     U/L Molar inclination: Lingual_____ Buccal_____Intermolar width difference (mm) _____
3. Asymmetry in dental arches _____

G. **Anteroposterior**
1. Right Molar _____ Right Canine _____Left Canine _____Left Molar_____

     Choices: III, SI [Super I], I, E, II)

     <u>Angle Classification:</u> Class I _____Class II-1 _____Class II-2 _____ Class III _____
2. <u>Incisor Overjet:</u>(mm) _____   Edge to Edge_____   Anterior Crossbite_____

H. **Functional Shifts on Closure:** Anteroposterior _____Transverse _____

Premature loss of deciduous teeth: _____

Toothsize/Arch Size: Excess Space   Adequate   Crowding

    Maxilla   _____   _____   _____

    Mandible   _____   _____   _____

K. **Radiographic Analysis:**

    Ectopic Eruption _____   Short Roots _____

    Missing Teeth _____   Supernumerary Teeth _____

    Impacted Teeth _____   Root Resorption _____

    Root Dilaceration _____   Periapical Pathology _____

    Alveolar Bone Height _____   Ankylosis_____

    Caries _____   Other _____

Summary of Diagnostic Findings and Problem List

1. **Chief Concern** _____
2. **Medical History** _____
3. **Dental History** _____
4. **Facial Form** _____
5. **Dentition:**
   a. **Perio status** _____
   b. **Restorative status** _____
   c. **Oral Hygiene** _____
   d. **Angle Class:** _____; **RM**_____   **RC**_____   **LC**_____   **LM**_____
   e. **Overbite (%)**_____   **Overjet (mm)** _____
   f. **Crossbites (anterior)**_____   **(posterior)** _____
   g. **Functional Shifts**_____
   h. **Crowding/Spacing (mm) U____ L ____   Molar Width Difference (mm)_____
   i. **Radiograph Findings**_____
6. **Diagnosis:**
   1. Anter-oposterior
   2. Transverse
   3. Vertical
   4. TSALD

Figure 1.8. Page 2 of an orthodontic clinic record form.

TREATMENT PLAN

1. Goals (in response to problem list):

2. Anchorage Source(s):

3. Complicating Factors:

APPLIANCE PLAN

1. Draw Picture Of Removable Appliance:

2. Describe Fixed Appliance:

RETENTION PLAN

1. Describe Appliance:

2. Recommendation To Patient Regarding Wear Time For Retainer(s):

EVALUATION OF TREATMENT

COMMENTS:

Figure 1.9. Page 3 of an orthodontic clinic record form.

upper and lower arches. The presence or absence of a functional shift on closure is important information for all patients who have anterior and posterior crossbites.

Premature loss of primary teeth can lead to mesial drifting of the permanent first molars and impaction of second premolars. Intercepting this problem before it occurs with use of a space

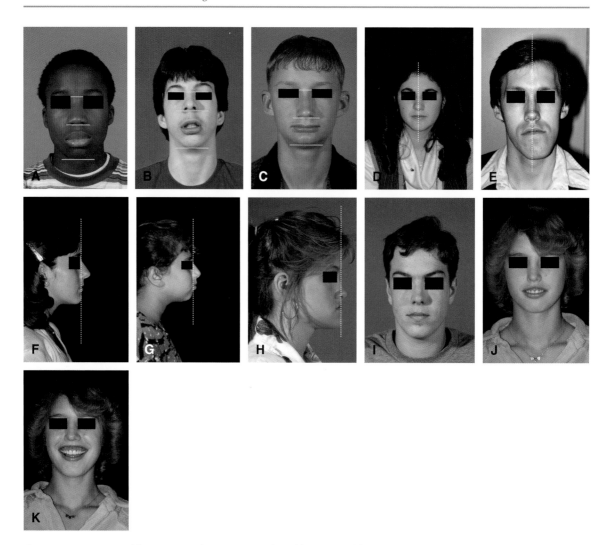

Figure 1.10. A–K, Facial form in vertical, transverse, and profile views and lip postures. **A,** Vertically normal face. **B,** Vertically long face. **C,** Vertically short face. **D,** Bilateral symmetry. **E,** Bilateral asymmetry. **F,** Straight facial profile. **G,** Convex facial profile. **H,** Concave facial profile. **I,** Normal relaxed lip position. **J,** Lips apart at rest. **K,** Gummy smile.

maintainer or with an orthodontic appliance after a premolar has been impacted is an important service to the patient.

Tooth size–arch length relations are recorded. Detailed analysis requires measurements on the dental casts.

Radiographic findings are recorded after images are examined. Several important findings are listed in the clinical examination form.

Summary of Findings, Problem List, and Diagnosis

After the clinical examination, important findings are summarized by the clinician. From this information, a diagnostic summary is developed (Fig. 1.8). The Diagnostic Summary is divided into four sections: (1) anteroposterior findings, (2) vertical findings, (3) transverse findings, and (4) tooth size–arch length discrepancy [TSALD].

A treatment plan is based on the diagnosis and problem list (Ackerman and Proffit, 1969). The treatment plan addresses the problems (Fig. 1.9). Some problems, such as compromised nasal breathing, require referral to a physician. Appliance and retention plans are also developed for the patient. Alternative appliance plans can be formulated, to fully inform and educate the patient about how the malocclusion problem can be corrected. This preparation enables the clinician to meet with the patient to describe his malocclusion problem and reach an agreement with the patient on the best treatment plan and appliance for him based on informed consent.

Consultation with Patient and/or Parent

After the treatment and appliance plans are developed, the next step in the process is to meet with the patient and parents of a minor to discuss the diagnosis and plans for treatment, the appliance(s), and retention phase. The records serve as tools to educate the patient about his malocclusion problem. Informed consent must be obtained from the patient and/or parent before starting treatment.

The patient must be informed about the risks of orthodontic treatment. Hazards that must be mentioned are **root resorption** and **enamel demineralization.** Apical root resorption usually involves a small loss of root structure in one or more of the teeth. Teeth rotate around the center of resistance located approximately at the junction of the middle and coronal thirds of the root. Take a ballpoint pen and hold it with two fingers at the "center of resistance of the root" and rotate it to show how movement of the "crown" causes a great deal of movement of the "end of the root." This will illustrate the vulnerability of the root apex to attack by osteoclasts that remodel alveolar bone but can also resorb part of the root. In 12 studies published since 1970, orthodontic patients experiencing root resorp-

tion ranged from 0% to 100%, with a mean of 44.8% for the 12 studies (Brezniak and Wasserstein 1993). Resorption ceases when the orthodontic appliance is removed from the teeth. A very small percentage of patients experience abnormally large amounts of root resorption during orthodontic treatment. If a patient exhibits root resorption on pretreatment radiographs, this is a strong indicator that root resorption will occur during orthodontic treatment. A routine mid-treatment panoramic radiograph will identify patients who are susceptible to excessive root resorption. In these patients, orthodontic treatment is completed as quickly as possible to arrest the resorption process. Root resorption caused by orthodontic treatment does not require endodontic treatment, unless the teeth are diagnosed as nonvital. Root resorption of 2 or 3 mm caused by orthodontic treatment is not thought to compromise the longevity of the involved tooth.

Enamel demineralization can occur in patients treated with a fixed orthodontic appliance who do not follow good oral hygiene and healthy dietary practices. Increase in the frequency of white spot lesions of 25.6% has been reported for patients who received orthodontic treatment (Gorelick, Geiger, and Gwinnett 1982). Cooperative patients do not usually experience demineralization. A clinician must give the patient hygiene and dietary recommendations at the consultation appointment before the beginning of treatment, and at any later time during treatment when poor oral hygiene is observed. Careful brushing after eating, the use of fluoridated toothpaste and rinses, floss, and water irrigation devices all will help the cooperative patient avoid enamel demineralization. Bonding brackets with resin-modified glass ionomer cement may reduce demineralization of the enamel surrounding the bracket (Schmit et al. 2002).

Patients who present for treatment with poor oral hygiene, active caries, and fillings are associated with white spot development during treatment (Lenius et al. 2009). Topically applied fluoride varnishes and sealants should be used in patients who present with these factors to prevent or at least reduce the impact of poor hygiene practices (Buren, Staley, Wefel, and Qian, 2008). After the appliances are removed and white spots are observed in a patient, the patient's use of low fluoride–containing toothpastes and products that deliver calcium, phosphorous, and fluoride (in low concentration) have the best potential to remineralize the white spots.

The ankylosis of a tooth root to the alveolar bone is a rare occurrence that may become apparent when an orthodontic appliance cannot move a tooth. This risk should be emphasized before the treatment of nonerupted and partially erupted teeth.

Finally, successful orthodontic treatment requires an obedient patient who will follow the instructions given by the clinician. The patient must come to appointments on time and at regular intervals to receive orthodontic treatment in a timely manner. Failures in patient or parent compliance can lead to a request by the clinician for consent to remove the orthodontic appliance.

At the consultation appointment, agreement on the treatment plan is required before proceeding with the treatment. An informed consent document should be given to the patient and/or parent to read and sign before orthodontic treatment begins.

REFERENCES

Ackerman, J. L., and Proffit, W. R. 1969. The characteristics of malocclusion. A modern approach to classification and diagnosis. Am. J. Orthod. 56:443–454.

Andrews, L. F. 1972. The six keys to normal occlusion. Am. J. Orthod. 62:296–309.

Angle, E. H. 1899. Classification of malocclusion. Dental Cosmos. 41:248–264.

Brezniak, N., and Wasserstein, A. 1993. Root resorption after orthodontic treatment. Part I. Literature review. Am. J. Orthod. Dentofac. Orthop. 103:62–66.

Buren, J. L., Staley, R. N., Wefel, J., and Qian, F. 2008. Inhibition of enamel demineralization by an enamel sealant, Pro Seal™: an in vitro study. Am. J. Orthod. Dentofac. Orthop. 133:S88–S94.

Delivanis, H. P., and Kuftinec, M. M. 1980. Variation in morphology of the maxillary central incisors found in Class II division 2 malocclusion. Am. J. Orthod. 78:438–443.

Gorelick, L., Geiger A. M., and Gwinnett, A. J. 1982. Incidence of white spot formation after bonding and banding. Am. J. Orthod. 81:93–98.

Huth, J. B., Staley, R. N., Jacobs, R. M., Bigelow, H. F., and Jakobsen, J. R. 2007. Arch widths in Class II-2 adults compared to adults with Class II-1 and normal occlusion. Angle Orthod. 77:837–844.

Kuntz, T. R., Staley, R. N., Bigelow, H. F., Kremenak, C. R., Kohout, F. J., and Jakobsen, J. R. 2008. Arch widths in adults with Class I crowded and Class III malocclusions compared with normal occlusions. Angle Orthod. 78:597–603.

Lenius, J., Staley, R. N., Qian, F., McQuistan, M., Marshall, T. A., and Wefel, J. S. 2009. Factors associated with white spot lesion occurrence in orthodontic patients. J. Dent. Res. 88(Spec Issue A).

Moyers, R. E. 1973. Handbook of orthodontics for the student and general practitioner. Chicago: Year-Book Medical Publishers.

Proffit, W. R., and Ackerman, J. L. 1973. Rating the characteristics of malocclusion: a systematic approach for planning treatment. Am. J. Orthod. 64:258–269.

Schmit, J. L., Staley, R. N., Wefel, J. S., Kanellis, M., and Jakobsen J. 2002. Effect of fluoride varnish on demineralization adjacent to brackets bonded with RMGI cement. Am. J. Orthod. Dentofac. Orthop. 122:125–134.

Staley, R. N., Stuntz, W. R., and Peterson, L. C. 1985. A comparison of arch widths in adults with normal occlusion and adults with Class II Division 1 malocclusion. Am. J. Orthod. 88:163–169.

Williamson, E. H., Caves, S. A., Edenfield, R. J., and Morse, P. K. 1978. Cephalometric analysis: comparison between maximum intercuspation and centric relation. Am. J. Orthod. 74:672–677.

Dental Impressions and Study Cast Trimming

2

Study Casts

Study casts accurately represent the teeth, their supporting tissues, and the relationship between upper and lower teeth in centric occlusion. They contribute greatly to diagnosis and treatment planning and are valuable instructional and illustrative aids during a consultation with patients. Even if you are observing a young patient prior to the onset of treatment, study casts are useful three-dimensional records for a growing and changing patient. Study casts are among the most important records taken prior to, during, and after orthodontic treatment. For treatment planning, casts are indispensable. You *must* study the positions of the maloccluded teeth, to plan how and where the teeth need to be moved during treatment. After treatment, study casts will show the changes that occurred during treatment. You need high-quality working casts for appliance fabrication.

Digital Casts

With advances in digital model technology, dentists will eventually no longer take impressions

and trim plaster diagnostic casts as described in this chapter. Even the laboratory fabrication of orthodontic appliances will be accomplished through digital technology. Several companies are selling equipment designed to capture digital images of individual teeth and arches for restorative dentistry (Helvey 2009). This technology is reducing errors commonly made in recording margins for crowns made in dental laboratories (Shannon, Qian, Tan, and Gratton 2007). Services and equipment that digitize orthodontic casts and alginate impressions are being marketed to orthodontists. A clinician can send plaster casts or impressions to a company for digitizing. Cone beam computed tomography machines can create digital casts. Digitized casts can be forwarded electronically to another clinician when patients transfer from one office to another. Through CAD/CAM (computer-aided design/computer-aided manufacturing) procedures, a three-dimensional cast can be created from a digital model.

The accuracy of measurements taken from digital models has been reported in several publications. The reports agree that the accuracy of currently available digital models is very good and quite acceptable for use in orthodontic diagnosis and treatment. With further hardware and software developments, improved accuracy will be available. One study compared tooth width

Essentials of Orthodontics: Diagnosis and Treatment
by Robert N. Staley and Neil T. Reske
© 2011 Blackwell Publishing Ltd.

measurements on digital and plaster models and found some statistically significant differences, but the differences were clinically acceptable (Stevens et al. 2006); a second study found no significant differences in tooth widths (Mullen, Martin, Ngan, and Gladwin 2007); and a third study found only significant differences for canine tooth widths, recommending a smaller rotational angle during scanning in the canine region to improve accuracy (Nouri et al. 2009). One study compared digital and plaster cast measurements of arch length and reported significant differences that were clinically acceptable (Mullen et al. 2007). One study compared space analysis in digital and plaster casts and found no difference in the mandibular arch but a significant difference in the maxillary arch that was considered clinically acceptable (Leifert, Leifert, Efstratiadis, and Cangialosi 2009); a second study of space analysis reported no difference in the maxillary arch for four segment and six segment arch lengths and found no difference for six segment arch lengths in the mandibular arch, but found a difference in the lower arch when using four segment arch lengths (Goonewardene et al. 2008). Arch widths were compared in digital and plaster casts, with one study finding no differences (Gracco, Buranello, Cozzani, and Siciliani, 2007) and another study reported no differences in lower intercanine widths but significant differences in intermolar widths (Asquith, Gillgrass, and Mossey 2007). Two studies found that digital measurements were more quickly taken than manual measurements with calipers (Gracco et al. 2007; Mullen et al. 2007).

Alginate Impressions

To obtain high-quality casts, you *must* obtain high-quality impressions. The objectives in making impressions for orthodontic study casts are somewhat different from the objectives in making impressions for restorative and prosthetic patients. We want accurate impressions of the teeth and much more coverage of the surrounding anatomic structures of both upper and lower arches. The impressions should record as much of the upper and lower arch as possible. This is accomplished by displacing the soft tissue upward and outward beyond the mucobuccal folds in the upper impression and downward and outward in the lower impression. Use **perforated trays** of the proper size for each arch. Trays need to be large enough to extend at least ¼ inch beyond the most distal tooth in each arch and wide enough so that teeth do not come into contact with any part of the impression tray. Add soft wax strips to extend the tray flanges into the mucobuccal fold and to act as stops to keep the tray from contacting teeth. Wax is sometimes added to the palatal surface of an upper tray to obtain a satisfactory impression of a high palatal vault. The goal is a good impression of both the teeth and the supporting structures with no voids. If the tray is seated far enough to contact teeth, a clicking sound is heard as the incisal edges or cusps of teeth hit the bottom of the tray. This will result in a poor impression and poor casts because the impression will be perforated at the places the teeth contact the tray.

Any good alginate impression material will produce a good impression if you are familiar with the working properties of the impression material. Always mix the material according to the manufacturer's directions. After the impression material is mixed, it is placed in the tray and should be smoothed with wet fingers. The patient's teeth should be clean, and the patient should rinse his mouth thoroughly before an impression is made. Before seating the filled impression tray, you can smear alginate on the occlusal and lingual surfaces of the teeth and the palate with your finger to reduce the occurrence of saliva bubbles on these surfaces.

Mandibular Impression

Because patients usually tolerate lower arch impressions better than they do upper arch impressions, you should take the lower impressions first. Seat the patient upright in the chair.

Stand in front of the patient. Ask the patient to roll back his tongue as you put the lower arch impression tray into the mouth and ask him to move his tongue forward above the impression tray after you seat the tray fully. This prevents the tongue from getting trapped beneath the impression tray and allows the tongue to mold the lingual alginate. As you seat the impression tray, center the tray handle in line with the nose and keep the tray level with the occlusal plane. The patient may be instructed to hold his head forward and down slightly; this will help the patient breathe and, if necessary, to drool his saliva onto the napkin while the tray is in the mouth. When the leftover alginate in the mixing bowl is set, the impression can be removed from the mouth. Grasp the tray by its handle and roll it back and forth gently to break the seal. In order to overcome the suction that holds the alginate impression in the arch, you may need to place your finger under the buccal rim on one side of the tray to forcibly pull it upward. If taken properly, the impression should have no large voids and the alginate should not have pulled away from the tray (Graber and Swain 1985, Monetti 1993).

After removing the impression from the mouth, rinse it thoroughly with cool tap water to wash out saliva and debris. Shake or blow out excess water from the impression and inspect the impression for voids. Determine if all desirable anatomic parts of the impressed arch have been duplicated accurately. Follow proper disinfecting procedures and place the impression into a plastic bag for transport to the laboratory for pouring of the cast. **If the impression must sit for more than 15 minutes after removing it from the mouth, it must be placed in an airtight container to keep it from drying out, which causes distortion of the impression.**

Maxillary Impression

Put only enough alginate in the upper tray to make a good impression. If you overload the tray and place the tray over the anterior teeth first, the excess alginate will flow down the soft palate as you seat the tray over the posterior teeth. Most patients gag when alginate flows freely down the surface of the soft palate. Stand behind the patient and bring the tray to the upper arch so that the alginate contacts the occlusal surfaces of all the teeth. Center the tray handle on the nose. Hold the tray level with the occlusal plane. Position the tray so that the alginate can flow evenly upward into the mucobuccal fold area. When a patient has flared upper incisors, position the impression in the molar region first to achieve an adequate flow of alginate into the anterior mucobuccal fold. Pull the upper lip of the patient over the tray flanges to keep the lip from becoming trapped beneath the tray. Ask the patient to breathe through his nose when you take the impression. This makes the procedure more comfortable and takes the patient's mind off gagging. Always ask the patient if he can breathe through his nose before you take an upper arch impression. Patients who have nasal airway blockage are poor candidates for upper arch impressions. Have the patient close his mouth lightly by saying, "You may close your mouth until your lower teeth lightly touch my fingers." Closing the mouth slightly allows the muscles of mastication to relax, making the patient more comfortable (Graber and Swain 1985; Monetti 1993).

Remove the tray after the alginate has set by following the procedures described earlier for the mandibular arch.

Record of Centric Occlusion

After the impressions are taken, ask the patient to bite into a piece of wax to record the relationship of the teeth in centric occlusion (maximum intercuspation). The patient must bite through the wax into full tooth contact. The wax bite registration serves as a guide in the cast trimming process. Rinse the wax bite with cool water, disinfect it, and place it into the plastic bag with the upper and lower impressions.

Pouring of Plaster Study Casts

Casts should be poured shortly after the impressions are taken. In pouring a cast, two pitfalls must be avoided: (1) lack of proper density of gypsum material and (2) voids or bubbles within the gypsum. Proper density is obtained by mixing the correct amount of plaster with the correct amount of water as prescribed by the manufacturer. Normal-size upper and lower impressions for study casts will require about 600 grams of powdered gypsum. Plaster can be weighed and stored in bags, so that it can be quickly mixed with the appropriate volume of water. Mix enough plaster for both impressions in a metal mixing bowl. Bubbles can be minimized by incorporating the gypsum powder into the water with a hand spatula, followed by 25 or 30 seconds of mixing with a vacuum power mixing machine. After mixing, remove the vacuum hose. Vibrate the mixing bowl and remove the mixing blade from the metal bowl, and vibrate the mixed plaster from the blades into the bowl.

Remove the alginate impressions from the plastic bag and rinse them under cool running water to remove disinfectant and debris. Shake out excess water. The surface of the impression should be shiny without puddles of water evident in tooth areas.

Vibrate the mixed plaster into the impressions. Begin by putting a small drop of plaster on one side of the impression at the most posterior molar. Keep adding successive amounts of plaster as you rotate the impression, while watching the plaster flow around to the opposite side of the impression and out of the distal end of the impression. Take care not to trap air beneath the plaster. Fill the impression from the bottom up. When all the crown impressions have been filled, tip the impression so that the plaster tends to run out the other side. This will remove any excess water from the impression and uncover any trapped air bubbles that have been overlooked. Then, add large quantities of mixed plaster to fill up the impression until it reaches the top. Set this impression aside and fill the other impression in the same fashion. Fill base former molds of

appropriate size with the remaining plaster mix. If the plaster-to-water ratio adheres to the manufacturer's recommendations, you may invert the filled impression trays and place them into the filled base formers to complete the pour-up. If the plaster mix is too thin—that is, watery—the inverted tray will sink into the base former mold or the tray handle will tip downward. Voids will appear in the tooth regions of the cast when the thin plaster mix flows downward and away from the alginate impression material. For the beginner, it is best to pour the impressions first with about a 300-gram mix and allow the plaster to reach an initial set. Then make another 300-gram mix to fill the base formers with the appropriately mixed plaster and invert the filled impression trays over the bases. Keep the impression trays level with the bottom of the base former and the tray handle pointed directly toward the front of the base former. If the tongue space in the lower impression is not filled with wax or alginate, the excess plaster in this area can be removed with a finger or spatula before the plaster hardens.

Clean the mixing bowl, blade, and spatulas. Save the wax bite for the cast trimming steps. Allow the plaster to set for 1 hour before removing impressions. **If you leave the impressions filled with plaster overnight, the alginate will dry out, making separation of the impression difficult.** If this should occur, soak the dried alginate in water for a few minutes before carefully removing the impression from the plaster casts.

Study Cast Trimming

Casts may be trimmed after a 1-hour set; however, we recommend waiting a few hours until the plaster becomes harder. The plaster's maximum hardness will develop in 24 hours. Casts may be dried more quickly by placing them in a low-temperature oven, such as a toaster oven set below 212°F. Overheating or overdrying casts will crack and break them. Before trimming, soak the dry casts a short time in water to prevent

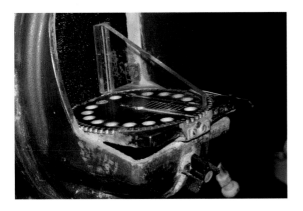

Figure 2.1. Check for 90-degree angle.

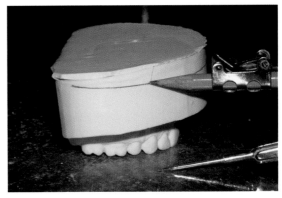

Figure 2.2. Upper cast base marked parallel to occlusal plane.

them from sticking to the model trimmer table during trimming.

A model trimmer equipped with a movable protracting table is ideal for trimming the proper angles on the **art bases** of orthodontic casts. The table should be equipped with a **vertisquare** and **sliding T-square**. Before trimming, make sure the table of the trimmer is perpendicular to the trimming wheel (Fig. 2.1). Make certain that when you put the T-square in the slot, the table is set at 0 degrees, and the T-square is parallel to the wheel. A pencil, a compass with a pencil, a lab knife, and a ruler are essential tools (American Board of Orthodontics 1999; Tweed 1966).

When trimming casts, it is best to trim the upper cast first, because the curve of Spee is usually less pronounced in the upper arch and the midpalatal raphe is a reference for establishing symmetric casts. Place the upper cast on a flat bench top with the teeth in contact with the flat surface. Set the compass at 1½ inch, and check this setting with the ruler. Place the pointed end of the compass against the bench top, and scribe a line parallel to the occlusal plane of the upper arch around the cast (Fig. 2.2). Turn the model trimmer on and make sure there is a small stream of water to wet and clean the wheel while trimming. Slide the vertisquare into the table slot. Hold the occlusal surface of the teeth against the foam pad of the vertisquare while keeping the backside of the cast slightly off the trimmer table

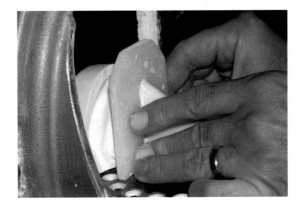

Figure 2.3. Trimming upper cast base.

(Fig. 2.3). Push the cast and vertisquare toward the trimmer wheel and slowly trim the top side of the upper cast.

While trimming, check to make sure the surface you are trimming is parallel to the pencil line. Continue until the cast is trimmed to the pencil line. The top surface of the upper cast should now be parallel to the occlusal plane of the teeth. Look at the palate of the cast and scribe a pencil line on the midpalatal raphe of the cast (Fig. 2.4). When we trim the backside of the cast, we want it to be perpendicular to the midpalatal raphe and perpendicular to the top surface of the cast (Fig. 2.5). Remove the vertisquare from the

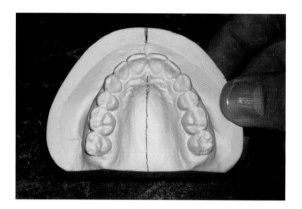

Figure 2.4. Upper cast backside trimmed perpendicular to palatal midline.

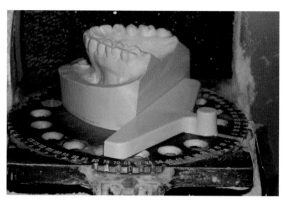

Figure 2.6. Cut left side 65 degrees with T-square guide.

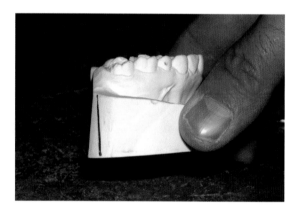

Figure 2.5. Mark backside of upper cast for 90-degree cut to base.

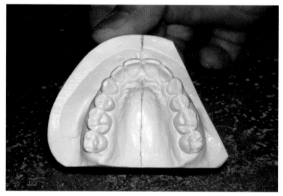

Figure 2.7. After 65-degree cut of left side.

trimming table. Place the top surface of the cast down onto the trimmer table and trim the backside to the hamular notch or ¼ inch from the most posterior teeth, keeping the backside perpendicular to the midpalatal raphe. Check the cast for squareness. Next, slide the T-square into the table slot. Turn the table protractor to 65 degrees to trim one side of the cast. The number "65°" should line up at the front of the protracting table (Fig. 2.6). Place the backside of the cast against the T-square. Push the cast and T-square toward the wheel, and trim the side of the cast no closer than ¼ inch from the teeth (Fig. 2.7). Rotate the protractor table to 65 degrees on the

other side. Then place the backside of the cast against the T-square to trim the other side of the cast no closer than ¼ inch from any tooth (Fig. 2.8). The cast should now have both sides trimmed 65 degrees to the backside (Fig. 2.9). Now set the protractor table to 25 degrees, and with the backside still against the T-square, trim the front side of the cast from midline to middle of the canine (Fig. 2.10). Trim no closer than ¼ inch from any tooth. Rotate the cast and place the trimmed 25-degree angled front of the cast against the T-square; trim the opposite backside of the cast (Fig. 2.11). This will give a 130-degree angle off the back of the cast (Fig. 2.12).

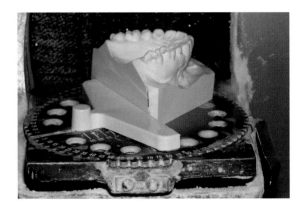

Figure 2.8. Cut right side 65 degrees.

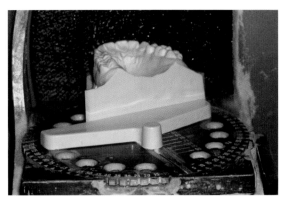

Figure 2.10. Cut left front side 25 degrees.

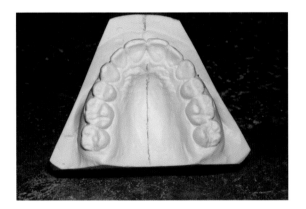

Figure 2.9. After 65-degree cut on both sides.

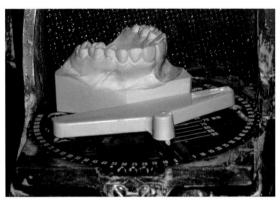

Figure 2.11. Cast rotated to cut right back corner 130 degrees.

Now rotate the table to 25 degrees to trim the other front side of the cast (Fig. 2.13). The front point of the cast should be in line with the midline of the palate (Fig. 2.14). On an ideal cast, the midpoint to canine length on each side should measure the same distance. Now rotate the cast and place the second trimmed 25-degree-angled front side against the T-square and trim the opposite backside (Fig. 2.15). An ideal upper cast is symmetric (Fig. 2.16). The length of the line from canine to the front of the back corner should be similar on each side. The back corners should also be the same length.

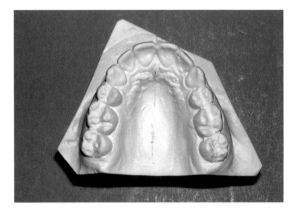

Figure 2.12. After left front and right back corner cuts.

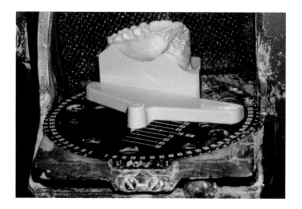

Figure 2.13. Cut right front side 25 degrees.

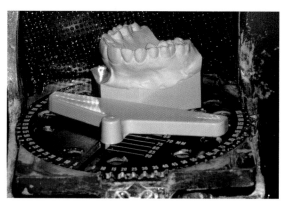

Figure 2.15. Cast rotated to cut left back corner 130 degrees.

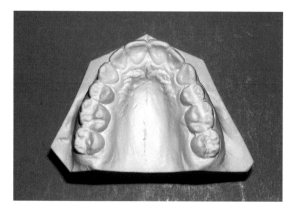

Figure 2.14. Front point of 25-degree cuts coincides with palatal midline.

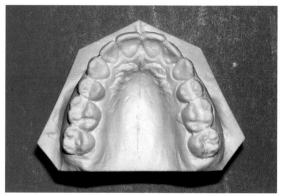

Figure 2.16. Upper cast is trimmed.

With a lab knife, remove any plaster bubbles from the occlusal surfaces of the teeth on both the upper and lower casts to ensure maximum intercuspation in centric occlusion. The wax bite helps to determine centric occlusion. With the casts together and the top of the upper cast on a bench top, scribe a line with the compass set at 3 inches (Fig. 2.17). Insert the vertisquare into the table, and trim the bottom side of the lower cast to the scribed line, which should be parallel to the occlusal plane and the top of the upper cast (Fig. 2.18). Remove the vertisquare. Then,

with the upper and lower casts in occlusion, trim the back of the lower cast flush with the back of the upper cast (Fig. 2.19). Set the upper cast aside. Install the T-square and set the protractor table to 65 degrees. Trim one side of the lower cast with the backside against the T-square to no closer than ¼ inch from any tooth (Fig. 2.20). Rotate the table to 65 degrees on the other side and trim the opposite side of the lower cast (Fig. 2.21). With a pencil, mark the anterior portion of the lower cast using the mucobuccal fold as a guide (Fig. 2.22). Trim the anterior in a smooth

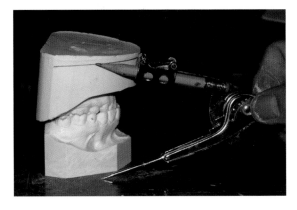

Figure 2.17. Marking base of lower cast parallel to base of upper cast. Bases are about 3 inches (7.6 cm) apart.

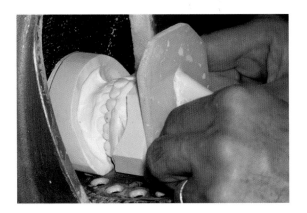

Figure 2.18. Trimming lower cast base.

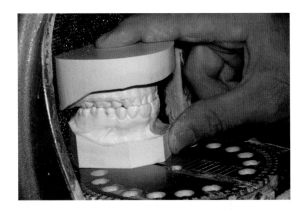

Figure 2.19. Trimming lower cast backside in same plane as backside of upper cast.

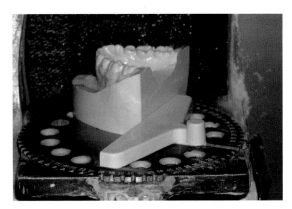

Figure 2.20. Right side is cut 65 degrees.

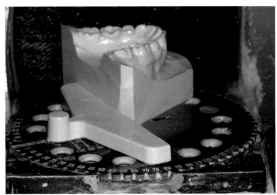

Figure 2.21. Left side is cut 65 degrees.

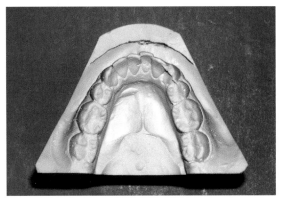

Figure 2.22. Lower cast marked for rounded anterior trim.

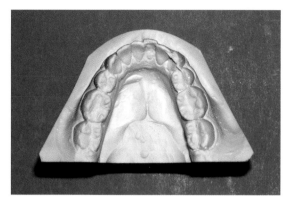

Figure 2.23. After rounded cut of lower cast front side.

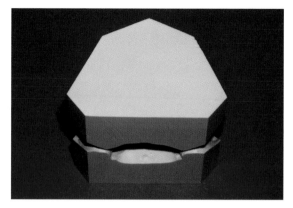

Figure 2.26. After back corners are trimmed flush.

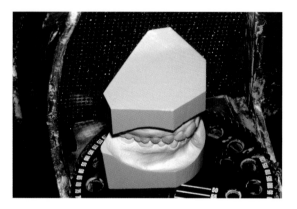

Figure 2.24. Trimming lower left back corner flush with upper cast.

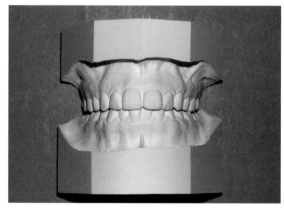

Figure 2.27. Casts rest on backsides in centric occlusion.

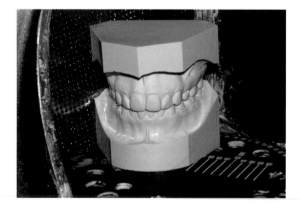

Figure 2.25. Trimming lower right back corner flush with upper cast.

arc from the middle of the canine on one side to the middle of the canine on the other side (Fig. 2.23). Hold the upper and lower casts together in centric occlusion, and trim the back corner of the lower cast flush with the back corner of the upper cast (Fig. 2.24). Trim the opposite corner (Fig. 2.25). Both casts should be symmetric (Fig. 2.26). When the casts are put together in centric occlusion, all lines should be vertical (Fig. 2.27).

Cast **art bases** are wet sanded with 600 grit sandpaper. The backsides of the casts are sanded

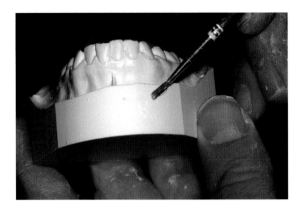

Figure 2.28. Apply wet plaster to fill voids in cast.

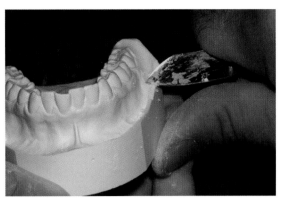

Figure 2.29. Carve cast tissue borders with knife.

while holding them together in centric occlusion. **The finished casts must be in centric occlusion when placed on their backsides on a flat surface.** The back corners may also be sanded while holding the casts together. All other trimmed surfaces must be sanded, but keep the surfaces flat, except for the rounded front of the lower cast. Do not blur or round the edges where different sides meet.

A void in the cast should be filled with plaster. Dip a small brush in water and then into dry plaster to pick up a small ball of plaster, and dab it into the void to fill and smooth (Fig. 2.28). Teeth may also be repaired with this method, but care must be taken to ensure tooth dimensions are not altered. Use a plaster knife to trim away all bubbles caused by impression voids in the vestibule areas. Trim away undesirable areas between mucobuccal folds and the art base of the cast (Fig. 2.29). On the lower cast, trim the tongue area flat, but leave the tongue attachment intact. With a small piece of sandpaper, sand the tongue area. **Avoid sanding teeth or tissue areas** (Fig. 2.30).

Let the casts dry for 24 hours for maximum hardness. Place casts in a model soap solution for 15 minutes. Rinse casts under running water, dry, and polish with a 2 × 2 gauze sponge for a high luster. Soaping of the casts in soap solution

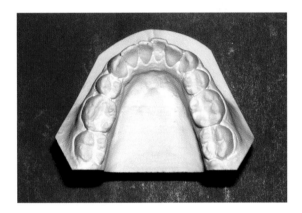

Figure 2.30. Tongue space flattened and smooth on lower cast.

keeps them clean while handling, makes subsequent cleanings easier, and strengthens the plaster.

A model trimming technique guide is illustrated in Figure 2.31. The trimming of plaster casts as described here is very similar to instructions given in a textbook of orthodontia written by a former professor and head of the Department of Orthodontia at the University of Iowa (Rose 1935).

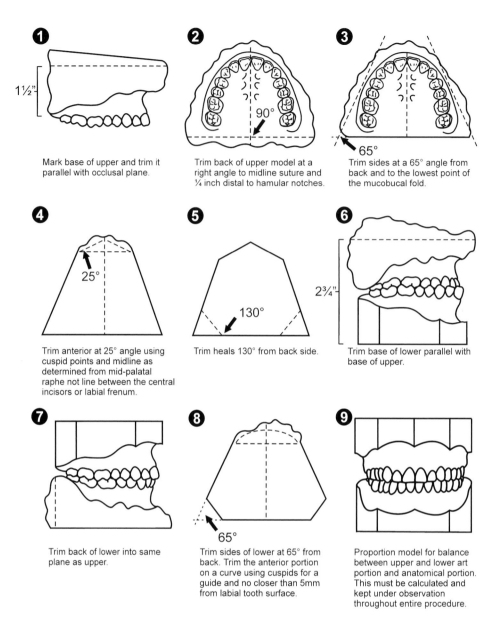

**① ** Mark base of upper and trim it parallel with occlusal plane.

$1\frac{1}{2}$"

**② ** Trim back of upper model at a right angle to midline suture and ¼ inch distal to hamular notches.

90°

**③ ** Trim sides at a 65° angle from back and to the lowest point of the mucobucal fold.

65°

**④ ** Trim anterior at 25° angle using cuspid points and midline as determined from mid-palatal raphe not line between the central incisors or labial frenum.

25°

**⑤ ** Trim heals 130° from back side.

130°

**⑥ ** Trim base of lower parallel with base of upper.

$2\frac{3}{4}$"

**⑦ ** Trim back of lower into same plane as upper.

**⑧ ** Trim sides of lower at 65° from back. Trim the anterior portion on a curve using cuspids for a guide and no closer than 5mm from labial tooth surface.

65°

**⑨ ** Proportion model for balance between upper and lower art portion and anatomical portion. This must be calculated and kept under observation throughout entire procedure.

Figure 2.31. *1–9,* Iowa technique for cast trimming and finishing.
Finishing suggestions:
- Sand art portion of model with 600 grit wet/dry sandpaper. Do not sand anatomic parts.
- Remove bubbles and other artifacts with plaster carving tools.
- Patch air bubbles in models where needed.
- Flatten tongue area and remove remaining rough spots with fine sandpaper.
- Allow models to thoroughly dry (at least 24 hours) and soak 10 to 15 minutes in warm concentrated soap solution. Rinse completely.
- Permit models to dry and rub with gauze sponge or damp paper towel until glossy.

REFERENCES

American Board of Orthodontics. 1999. Specific instructions for candidates. St. Louis: Author.

Asquith, J., Gillgrass, T., and Mossey, P. 2007. Three dimensional imaging of orthodontic models: a pilot study. Eur. J. Orthod. 29:517–522.

Goonewardene, R. W., Goonewardene, M. S., Razza, J. M., and Murray, K. 2008. Accuracy and validity of space analysis and irregularity index measurements using digital models. Aust. Orthod. J. 24:83–90.

Graber, T. M., and Swain, B. F. 1985. Orthodontics: current principles and techniques. St. Louis: CV Mosby.

Gracco, A., Buranello, M., Cozzani, M., and Siciliani, G. 2007. Digital and plaster models: a comparison of measurements and time. Prog. Orthod. 8:252–259.

Helvey, G. A. 2009. The current state of digital impressions. Inside Dentistry October:86–89.

Leifert, M. F., Leifert, M. M., Efstratiadis, S. S., and Cangialosi, T. J. 2009. Comparison of space analysis evaluations with digital models and plaster casts. Am. J. Orthod. Dentofac. Orthop. 136:16.

Monetti, L. 1993. Making a good dental impression. Dental Teamwork. 6:31–32.

Mullen, S. R., Martin, C. A., Ngan, P., and Gladwin, M. 2007. Accuracy of space analysis with emodels and plaster models. Am. J. Orthod. Dentofac. Orthop. 132:346–352.

Nouri, M., Massudi, R., Bagheban, A. A., Azimi, S., and Fereidooni, F. 2009. The accuracy of a 3-D Laser scanner for crown width measurements. Aust. Orthod. J. 25:41–47.

Rose, J. E. 1935. A textbook of orthodontia. Ann Arbor, MI: Edwards Brothers.

Shannon, A. J., Qian, F., Tan, P., and Gratton, D. 2007. In vitro vertical marginal gap comparison of CAD/CAM zirconium copings. J. Dent. Res. 86(Spec Issue A):No. 0828.

Stevens, D. R., Flores-Mir, C., Nebbe, B., Raboud, D. W., Heo, G., and Major, P. W. 2006. Validity, reliability and reproducibility of plaster vs digital study models: comparison of peer assessment rating and Bolton analysis and their constituent measurements. Am. J. Orthod. Dentofac. Orthop. 129:794–803.

Tweed, C. H. 1966. Clinical orthodontics. St. Louis: CV Mosby.

Dental Cast Analysis in Adults

3

Tooth Size–Arch Length Analysis

The measurement of tooth widths, arch lengths, and arch widths and computation of tooth size–arch length discrepancies (TSALDs) are important ways to practice evidence-based orthodontics. Taking these measurements will demonstrate how a patient differs from a representative sample of persons with normal occlusion. A tooth size–arch length analysis is needed for patients who have crowded or spaced teeth in one or both arches. This analysis quantifies the amount of crowding or spacing. An accurate measurement of crowding or spacing is key for any proposed orthodontic treatment. In the assessment of a crowded permanent dentition, **the lower arch has primacy over the upper arch,** because the smaller size of the anterior mandibular alveolar structure limits the possibility for movement of anterior teeth. In adults, forward movement of crowded incisors can result in the loss of gingiva and bone labial to the teeth. For these reasons, an analysis of arch length and assessment of alveolar and gingival tissues are more critical in the mandibular arch than in the maxillary arch.

Essentials of Orthodontics: Diagnosis and Treatment by Robert N. Staley and Neil T. Reske © 2011 Blackwell Publishing Ltd.

Measurement of Tooth Size and Arch Length

To determine the amount of crowding or spacing in an arch, subtract the sum of widths of the teeth mesial to the first molars from the sum of arch lengths mesial to the first molars. A crowded arch has a negative remainder, and the arch with spaces has a positive remainder. The acronym *TSALD* describes both crowding and spacing. *UTSALD* is used to describe upper arch discrepancies, and *LTSALD* is used to describe lower arch discrepancies.

The teeth measured for determining the TSALD are the incisors, canines, and premolars. The size of a tooth is measured as the width between its mesial and distal **anatomic** contact points. When a tooth is rotated, its width is measured between the anatomic contact points, not between the actual contact points. Usually the measurement is taken from the buccal or labial surface of the tooth. When a tooth is rotated, the best approach is to measure its width from the incisal or occlusal surface of the tooth's crown.

Arch length is measured from the mesial surface of the first molar on the right side around the arch to the mesial surface of the first molar on the left side in six segments (Fig. 3.1). The line of arch consists of a line along the crest of an alveolar ridge that represents where the

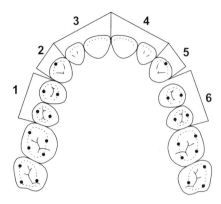

Figure 3.1. Segmental arch length measurements in an adult upper arch.

anatomic contact points of the teeth should be located ideally on a given alveolar ridge. Arch length measurements are an estimate of the length of the true line of arch mesial to the first molars in an arch. Hovda (1987) compared five different methods for measuring arch length on casts: (1) dial calipers, (2) brass wire method, (3) Brader Arch Forms method, (4) an F-curve ruler, and (5) the Reflex Metrograph (Ross Instruments Ltd., Salisbury, Wiltshire, England), a research instrument acting as the control. He found that measuring six segments around an arch with a dial calipers was the most reliable and repeatable method for measuring arch length. On the basis of these findings, we recommend using calipers or a Boley gauge, with sharpened measuring arm tips.

The six segments around the upper arch are illustrated in Figure 3.1. The tips of the measurement instrument are placed between the teeth below the contact points at the height or peak of the gingival papillae on the buccal and labial sides of the arches. Typical segments include (1) from the papilla between the first molar and second premolar to the papilla between the canine and first premolar, (2) from the papilla between the first premolar and the canine to the papilla between the canine and lateral incisor, and (3) from the papilla between the canine and lateral incisor to the papilla midway between the central incisors. The segments should not overlap or have gaps between them. Because many measurements are taken, repeating a measurement can help assure an accurate result. Practicing measurement techniques on a well-aligned arch, in which the goal is zero crowding, would be a helpful exercise for a beginner.

A form for collecting tooth size and arch length measurements is shown in Figure 3.2.

Factors Influencing a Tooth Size–Arch Length Analysis

A TSALD must be considered one part of a larger diagnosis. A number of other important factors associated with TSALDs are discussed next. In addition to these factors, treatment procedures such as rapid palatal expansion increase arch perimeter (arch length) in an upper arch (Adkins, Nanda, and Currier 1990).

Curve of Spee

When the upper and lower teeth are observed in occlusion from the side, the teeth usually conform, in the anteroposterior plane, to a curve known as the curve of Spee. The curve of Spee is leveled during orthodontic treatment. During leveling of the lower arch, the incisors move labially (Fig. 3.3). Figure 3.3 does not represent the tooth movements and forces that occur in the leveling of a lower arch. Figure 3.3 illustrates that the leveled arch will be longer in its anteroposterior length than the curved arch, if prior to treatment no spaces are found between the teeth or the teeth are crowded and if the width of the lower arch is maintained during treatment. If prior to treatment the lower incisors are either in a satisfactory anteroposterior position or inclined too far labially, leveling the curve of Spee may move the incisors too far in the labial direction. If sufficient excess arch length exists in an arch, incisors can be leveled without moving them too far labially as the curve of Spee is leveled.

Baldridge (1969) studied 30 patients who had exaggerated curves of Spee in their mandibular

TOOTH SIZE AND ARCH LENGTH ANALYSIS

Patient: _____   Date: _____

MESIODISTAL WIDTHS OF PERMANENT TEETH

	MAXILLA				MANDIBLE		
LEFT		RIGHT	BOTH	LEFT		RIGHT	BOTH
____	I^1	____		____	I_1	____	
____	I^2	____	TOTAL(UA)	____	I_2	____	TOTAL(LA)
____	C	____	_____	____	C	____	_____
____	PM^1	____		____	PM_1	____	
____	PM^2	____		____	PM_2	____	
TOTAL(1)* ____	TOTAL(1)* ____			TOTAL(1)* ____	TOTAL (1)* ____		
____	M^1	____	TOTAL(U)	____	M_1	____	TOTAL(L)
TOTAL(UL) ____	TOTAL(UR) ____		_____	TOTAL(LL) ____	TOTAL(LR) ____		_____

*TOTAL(1) is used in the arch length discrepancy analysis; TOTALS UA, U, LA, and L are used in the Bolton analysis.

ARCH LENGTH MEASUREMENTS

		MAXILLA		MANDIBLE	
		Left	Right	Left	Right
1.	Anterior[1]	____	____	____	____
2.	Canine Region[2]	____	____	____	____
3.	Posterior[3]	____	____	____	____
4.	Total Arch Length (1+2+3)	____	____	____	____
5.	Tooth Size (Total 1)	____	____	____	____
6.	Discrepancy (4 minus 5)	____	____	____	____
Total Arch Length Discrepancy[4]		____		____	

1. Distance between distal of lateral incisor and midpoint between central incisors.
2. Distance across the canine.
3. Distance between mesial of first molar and distal of canine.
4. + = spacing; - = crowding

Figure 3.2. Form to collect tooth size and arch length measurements.

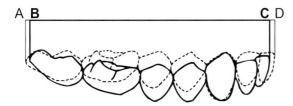

Figure 3.3. Leveling of the curve of Spee. Arch length before leveling (**B–C**). Arch length after leveling (**A–D**).

arches with all the permanent teeth erupted, except the third molars. He found the mean additional arch length required in the lower arch for leveling without labial tipping of the incisors was 3.54 ± 0.14 mm, with a minimum of 2.3 and a maximum of 5.2 mm. As the curve of Spee becomes more exaggerated, arch length deficiency increases. Baldridge developed a method for predicting the additional arch length required for leveling a particular arch without moving the incisors too far labially in the permanent dentition. From a flat plane between the incisors and second molars, measure the greatest depth of the curve connecting the incisors and most distal molars on both sides of the lower arch. Divide the sum of these two measurements by 2 and add the sum of 0.5 mm to obtain an estimation of the required additional arch length.

Incisor Inclination and Anteroposterior Position

The inclination and anteroposterior position of the incisors influence an arch length analysis. As the incisors incline lingually, crowding in an arch usually increases; however, orthodontic movement of lingually inclined incisors in a labial direction will increase arch length, perhaps enough to eliminate crowding in an arch. In contrast, the orthodontic movement of labially positioned incisors in a lingual direction will require additional arch length.

Incisor inclination and position are observed in oral and cast examinations; however, accurate assessment requires a cephalometric radiograph (see Chapter 5). Family dentists are not expected to take cephalograms; therefore, they should refer patients with significant crowding of teeth to a specialist. If a cephalometric assessment leads you to expect that incisor position and inclination will contribute to either more or less crowding, state this on the TSALD form. Your conclusion does not need to be stated in a specific number of millimeters.

On a cephalometric radiograph, the inclination of upper incisors is often described by the angle between the long axis of the central incisor and the sella-nasion plane. The inclination of the lower incisors is described by the angle between the long axis of the central incisor and the Frankfort horizontal plane (see Chapter 5). Tweed (1954) recommended that for each degree of desired change in lower incisor inclination, 0.8 mm of arch length be either added to or subtracted from the arch length on each side of the arch.

The anteroposterior position of the maxillary central incisor is estimated by measuring the distance from the incisal edge of the most labially positioned central incisor along a perpendicular to the A-pogonion line (see Chapter 5). The anteroposterior position of the mandibular incisors is estimated by measuring the distance from the incisal edge of the most labially positioned central incisor along a perpendicular to the line between nasion and point B (see Chapter 5).

Second and Third Molar Evaluation

Thus far, the tooth size–arch length relation has focused on the teeth mesial to the permanent first molars. The relationship in the second and third molar regions of the arches must also be assessed. Some second molars, particularly lower second molars, are or become impacted. Impaction of a lower second molar usually stems from a posterior arch length deficiency. Sometimes a lower third molar is impacted against the distal surface of a second molar. Removal (extraction) of the impacted third molar may be necessary in order to bring the second molar into occlusion. This treatment should be referred to a specialist.

Comparison of TSALD Analysis and the Irregularity Index

These two methods of measuring incisor crowding may confuse clinicians. An excellent study compared the two methods (Harris, Vaden, and Williams 1987). The authors found that a TSALD analysis is more attuned to displacements of teeth, whereas the Irregularity Index (Little, 1975) is more susceptible to rotations of the teeth. The Spearman rank correlation between the methods was positive at 0.53, statistically significant but of little clinical value. The basic purpose of a space analysis is to estimate the discrepancy between the size of the teeth and the size of the alveolar bone support. It appears that the TSALD method presented in this chapter more directly attempts to assess this relationship than the Irregularity Index.

Arch Width Measurements

Arch width measurements are useful for determining the severity of a posterior crossbite and for choosing the appropriate appliance to treat the crossbite. If a crossbite requires an expansion of the upper molars from 1 to 5 mm, then the expansion can be accomplished with a removable appliance, with simple fixed appliances such as a W-spring and with arch-wires in the fixed edgewise appliance. If the molars must be expanded beyond 5 mm, the best appliances are the fixed W-spring and rapid maxillary expander.

To make this clinical decision, take the measurements illustrated in Figure 3.4. Compare the arch width measurements of your patient with norms shown in Figure 3.5. These data are taken from Iowa adults of northwest European origin who had normal occlusion (Huth et al. 2007). To estimate the amount of expansion needed to correct the crossbite, subtract the mandibular

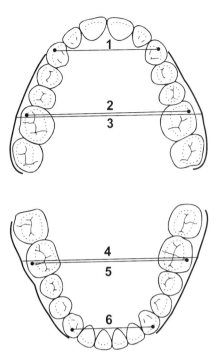

Figure 3.4. Measurement of arch widths: (*1*) maxillary intercanine, (*2*) maxillary intermolar, (*3*) maxillary alveolar, (*4*) mandibular alveolar, (*5*) mandibular intermolar, and (*6*) mandibular intercanine.

intermolar width from the maxillary intermolar width and calculate the absolute sum of the patient's intermolar difference and the mean intermolar difference of either the male or female normal occlusions (Fig. 3.5). The estimate will enable the clinician to choose the correct expander device and jackscrew capacity.

Another important factor to consider is the inclination of the lower molars. If the lower posterior teeth are inclined too far lingually, their buccal movement during treatment to normal inclination will require buccal expansion of the upper posterior teeth to accommodate the wider lower arch. In these patients, treatment to move the lower molar crowns bucally should be done in conjunction with expansion of the upper arch, to coordinate the widths of the two arches.

Patient _____
Case Number_____
Malocclusion: I, II-1, II-2, III (circle)

Arch Widths in Class I Normal Occlusion (mm)[1]

Width	Males (n = 18)				Females (n = 16)				Date	Date	Date	Date	Date
	Mean	S.D.	Min.	Max.	Mean	S.D.	Min.	Max					
Max Intercanine Width	36.1	2.3	32.9	41.9	33.1	1.3	31.3	35.4					
Max Intermolar Width	54.5	2.1	51.4	58.0	49.9	1.8	46.6	53.1					
Max Alveolar Width (at first molars)	61.6	3.0	57.2	67.9	56.4	2.3	53.2	60.4					
Mand Intercanine Width	26.3	1.9	23.3	31.0	25.1	2.2	22.6	27.6					
Mand Intermolar Width	53.0	1.6	50.2	56.0	48.7	1.6	46.4	52.2					
Mand Alveolar Width (at first molars)	58.3	1.7	55.3	61.6	53.8	1.3	51.5	56.2					
Max minus Mand Intermolar Widths	1.5	1.5	-0.5	4.3	1.2	1.2	-1.3	4.3					

[1]Huth J B, et al. Angle Orthodontist 2007;77:837-844.
Expansion Estimate = Absolute sum patient Mx-Mn M.W. + mean Mx-Mn M.W. of Class 1 Normals   _____

Measurement of arch and alveolar widths

1. **Maxillary intercanine width** – between cusp tips.
2. **Maxillary intermolar width** – between the mesiobuccal cusp tips of the first molars.
3. **Maxillary alveolar width** – widest points on attached gingiva above the mesiobuccal cusp tips of the maxillary first molars.
4. **Mandibular alveolar width** – widest points on attached gingiva below the buccal grooves of the mandibular first molars.
5. **Mandibular intermolar width** – between points on the buccal grooves located at the middle of the buccal surfaces.
6. **Mandibular intercanine width** – between the cusp tips.

Figure 3.5. Form to record arch widths with norms for white Americans.

Diagnostic Setup

Size interrelationships between the upper and lower teeth are important for a good occlusion. To predict the occlusion of the teeth after treatment, some teeth are removed from plaster duplicates of the pretreatment casts and arranged in wax into an occlusion resembling the occlusion after treatment. This procedure is called a **diagnostic setup** (Kesling 1956). When performing a diagnostic setup, the teeth should be arranged in the arches in conformity with the patient's alveolar support and not in positions that cannot be attained during orthodontic treatment.

Bolton Analysis

The diagnostic setup is time consuming, and this motivated Bolton to develop a tooth size analysis that predicts the occlusion of the upper and lower teeth if the goal of treatment is Class I occlusion without extraction of premolars at the end of treatment. Bolton (1958) measured the mesiodistal widths of the upper and lower teeth of 55 persons who had excellent occlusions. He took the sums of the widths of 12 upper and 12 lower teeth and computed a ratio by dividing the mandibular sum by the maxillary sum. He computed another ratio for the six anterior teeth. He developed a chart to help clinicians determine whether the teeth of a patient will fit together well in a Class I occlusion (Fig. 3.6). The analysis can be programmed into a computer for quick calculations.

When the upper and lower teeth do not fit together well, the Bolton analysis will predict either a maxillary or mandibular tooth size excess. Maxillary tooth size excess results in an excessive over jet after the teeth are aligned in

Bolton Analysis of Tooth Size Discrepancies
Overall Ratio

Sum mandibular 12 _____mm

_____ = _____ x 100 _____%

Sum maxillary 12 _____mm   Overall Ratio

Mean 91.3 ± 1.9%
Range 87.5-94.8 %

Maxillary 12	Mandibular 12	Maxillary 12	Mandibular 12	Maxillary 12	Mandibular 12
85	77.6	94	85.8	103	94
86	78.5	95	86.7	104	95
87	79.4	96	87.6	105	95.9
88	80.3	97	88.6	106	96.8
89	81.3	98	89.5	107	97.8
90	82.1	99	90.4	108	98.6
91	83.1	100	91.3	109	99.5
92	84.0	101	92.2	110	100.4
93	84.9	102	93.1		

Patient Analysis

If the overall ratio exceeds 91.3, the discrepancy is excessive mandibular tooth size. In the above chart locate the patient's maxillary 12 measurement and opposite it is the correct mandibular measurement. The difference between the actual and correct mandibular measurements is the excess mandibular tooth size.

_____ – _____ = _____

    Actual Mandibular 12   Correct Mandibular 12   Excess Mandibular 12

If the ratio is less than 91.3:

_____ – _____ = _____

    Actual Maxillary 12   Correct Maxillary 12   Excess Maxillary 12

Anterior Ratio

Sum mandibular 6 _____mm

_____ = _____x 100 = _____%

Sum maxillary 6 _____ mm   Anterior Ratio

Mean 77.2 ± 1.65 %
Range 74.5-80.4%

Maxillary 6	Mandibular 6	Maxillary 6	Mandibular 6	Maxillary 6	Mandibular 6
40	30.9	45.5	35.1	50.5	39
40.5	31.3	46	35.5	51.0	39.4
41	31.7	46.5	35.9	51.5	39.8
41.5	32.0	47	36.3	52	40.1
42	32.4	47.5	36.7	52.5	40.5
42.5	32.8	48	37.1	53	40.9
43	33.2	48.5	37.4	53.5	41.3
43.5	33.6	49	37.8	54	41.7
44	34	49.5	38.2	54.5	42.1
44.5	34.4	50	38.6	55	42.5
45	34.7				

Patient Analysis

If anterior ratio exceeds 77.2:

_____ – _____ = _____

    Actual Mandibular 6   Correct Mandibular 6   Excess Mandibular 6

If the anterior ratio is less than 77.2:

_____ – _____ = _____

    Actual Maxillary 6   Correct Maxillary 6   Excess Maxillary 6

Figure 3.6. Bolton analysis chart.

Class I occlusion and the curve of Spee is leveled during orthodontic treatment. Mandibular tooth size excess results in spacing between the maxillary teeth after they are aligned in Class I occlusion during orthodontic treatment. The Bolton analysis gives useful information prior to treatment to both the clinician and patient. If, for example, a mandibular excess is predicted by the Bolton analysis, the patient should be informed before treatment starts that cosmetic composite resin buildups of upper incisors will probably be needed to close diastemas between the upper anterior teeth after orthodontic treatment.

The diagnostic setup and the Bolton Analysis are very useful diagnostic tools.

Overbite and Overjet Measurements

Overbite, openbite, overjet, and anterior crossbite are measured as illustrated in Figure 3.7. Overbite is the percentage of a lower central

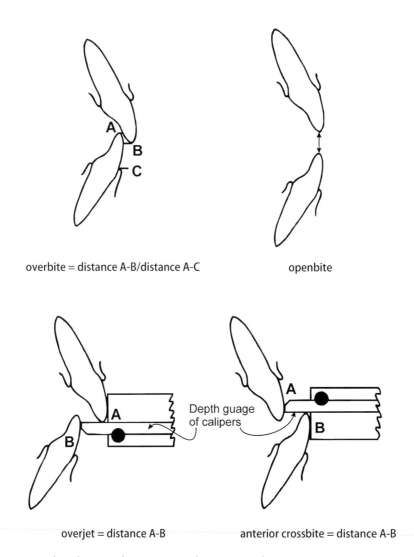

Figure 3.7. Measurement of overbite, openbite, overjet, and anterior crossbite.

Table 3.1. Overbite, Overjet, and Mandibular Crowding in Subjects with Normal Occlusion

Gender	Overbite %					
	N	Mean	SD.	Minimum	Maximum	Normal ± 1 SD.
Female	20	35.9	14.6	15.0	64.0	21.3 ± 50.5
Male	20	37.8	14.9	13.9	73.8	22.9 ± 52.7
	Over jet (mm)					
Female	20	3.0	1.1	1.4	5.1	1.9 ± 4.1
Male	20	2.5	0.7	1.1	3.3	1.8 ± 3.2
	Mandibular Crowding [−] or Spacing [+] (mm)					
Female	20	0.3	1.0	−1.4	2.3	−0.7 ± +1.3
Male	20	0.2	0.9	−1.6	2.4	−0.7 ± +1.1

From Kuntz, T. R. 1993. An anthropometric comparison of cephalometric and dental arch measurements in Class I normals, Class I crowded, and Class III individuals. Master's thesis, University of Iowa.

Table 3.2. Tooth Widths in Normal Occlusion

Tooth #	Males			Females		
	N	Mean(SD)	Range	N	Mean SD	Range
2*	17	10.3 (0.6)	9.4–11.7	16	9.9 (0.5)	8.8–10.9
3	19	10.6 (0.5)	9.6–11.4	19	10.4 (0.5)	9.6–11.2
4	19	6.9 (0.5)	6.0–7.8	19	6.7 (0.4)	6.1–7.6
5	19	7.1 (0.5)	6.4–8.0	19	6.9 (0.4)	6.3–7.5
6*	19	8.0 (0.4)	7.5–8.8	19	7.8 (0.4)	7.0–8.3
7	19	6.8 (0.4)	6.1–7.5	19	6.6 (0.6)	5.4–7.8
8	19	8.8 (0.5)	7.9–9.7	19	8.6 (0.7)	7.5–10.5
9	19	8.7 (0.6)	7.9–9.8	19	8.6 (0.7)	7.6–10.4
10	19	6.9 (0.6)	6.3–8.8	19	6.5 (0.6)	5.2–7.6
11	19	7.9 (0.4)	7.2–8.6	19	7.7 (0.3)	7.3–8.5
12	19	7.1 (0.5)	6.4–8.4	19	7.0 (0.5)	6.4–8.0
13	19	6.9 (0.5)	5.9–8.1	19	6.7 (0.34	6.0–7.2
14*	19	10.6 (0.5)	9.5–11.4	19	10.3 (0.4)	9.5–11.0
15†	18	10.3 (0.6)	9.1–11.5	17	9.8 (0.5)	9.0–10.6
18†	18	10.7 (0.5)	9.9–11.8	15	10.4 (0.5)	9.6–11.7
19	19	11.0 (0.9)	9.0–12.3	19	10.7 (0.7)	9.0–11.7
20	19	7.4 (0.7)	6.5–9.9	19	7.1 (0.4)	6.6–8.0
21	19	7.0 (0.4)	6.5–8.0	19	7.0 (0.3)	6.7–7.6
22*	19	6.9 (0.3)	6.4–7.6	19	6.6 (0.3)	6.2–7.4
23	19	6.0 (0.4)	5.3–6.8	19	5.9 (0.4)	5.3–6.9
24	19	5.5 (0.5)	4.7–7.0	19	5.4 (0.4)	4.5–6.1
25	19	5.6 (0.6)	4.8–7.3	19	5.3 (0.4)	4.6–6.2
26	19	6.0 (0.4)	5.3–6.9	19	5.8 (0.4)	5.2–7.0
27	19	6.9 (0.3)	6.2–7.6	19	6.7 (0.4)	6.3–7.5
28	19	7.1 (0.4)	6.5–8.0	19	7.0 (0.3)	6.6–7.8
29	19	7.2 (0.5)	6.3–8.0	19	7.0 (0.3)	6.6–7.6
30*	19	11.1 (0.7)	9.9–12.3	19	10.5 (0.9)	9.0–11.5
31	18	10.7 (0.5)	9.9–11.9	14	10.4 (0.6)	9.3–11.6

* Signif. $p < 0.05$ t-test
†Signif. $p < 0.05$ Wilcoxon Rank sum
From R. N. Staley, T. L. Juhlin, and C. Kummet, 2009, unpublished data.

incisor crown that is overlapped vertically by an upper central incisor crown. Percentages for normal overbite are listed in Table 3.1.

Openbite is the vertical distance in millimeters between the incisal edges of the upper and lower central incisors (Fig. 3.7) measured with a ruler.

Overjet is the horizontal distance in millimeters between the labial surface of the lower central incisor crown to the labial surface of the upper central incisor crown (Fig. 3.7). Overjet can also be measured with a ruler. Norms for overjet are listed in Table 3.1.

Anterior crossbite is the horizontal distance between the labial surface of the upper central incisor crown and the labial surface of the lower central incisor crown. It is measured as shown in Figure 3.7 or with a ruler.

Measurement of these vertical and horizontal relationships can be done on casts or directly in the mouth when the teeth are in centric occlusion and/or centric relation.

Mandibular Crowding

The TSALDs in the mandibular arches of a sample of normal occlusions from the Iowa Facial Growth Study (Kuntz 1993) are listed in Table 3.1. If you have an adult patient with crowding or spacing beyond the maximum and minimum values of the normal sample, consider referring the patient to a specialist for treatment.

Tooth Widths in Normal Occlusion

The widths of the permanent teeth, excluding third molars, in normal Class I males and females who participated in the Iowa Facial Growth Study are listed in Table 3.2. Tooth widths were measured in 19 males and 19 females (R. N. Staley and T. L. Juhlin, 2000, unpublished data.) If a clinician needs to know the average size of an upper lateral incisor versus the average size of

a central incisor, and the normal ratio between the sizes of these teeth for aesthetic dentistry purposes or prosthetic reconstructions, this table provides norm values for reference. Normal values for individual teeth are measurements that fall within 1 standard deviation of the mean. These tooth size norms can help a clinician understand the etiology and diagnosis of a patient's malocclusion.

REFERENCES

Adkins, M. D., Nanda, R. M., and Currier, G. F. 1990. Arch perimeter changes on rapid palatal expansion. Am. J. Orthod. Dentofacial Orthop. 97:194–199.

Baldridge, D. W. 1969. Leveling the curve of Spee: its effects on mandibular arch length. J. Pract. Orthod. 3:26–41.

Bolton, W. A. 1958. Disharmony in tooth size and its relation to the analysis and treatment of malocclusion. Angle Orthod. 28:113–130.

Harris, E. F., Vaden, J. L., and Williams, R. A. 1987. Lower incisor space analysis: a contrast of methods. Am. J. Orthod. Dentofac. Orthop. 92:375–380.

Hovda, R. A. "A comparison of five methods used to determine the dental arch perimeter length." Master's Thesis, University of Iowa, 1987.

Huth, J. B., Staley, R. N., Jacobs, R., Bigelow, H., and Jakobsen, J. 2007. Arch widths in Class II-2 adults compared to adults with Class II-1 and normal occlusion. Angle Orthod. 77:837–844.

Kesling, H. D. 1956. The diagnostic setup with consideration of the third dimension. Am. J. Orthod. 42:740–748.

Kuntz, T. R. An anthropometric comparison of cephalometric and dental arch measurements in Class I normals, Class I crowded, and Class III individuals. Master's thesis, University of Iowa, 1993.

Little, R. M. 1975. The irregularity index: a quantitative score of mandibular anterior alignment. Am. J. Orthod. 68:554–563.

Tweed, C. H. 1954. The Frankfurt mandibular incisor angle in orthodontic diagnosis, treatment planning, and prognosis. Angle Orthod. 24:121–169.

Dental Cast Analysis in the Mixed Dentition

4

Tooth Size–Arch Length Analysis

Why do we need to do a tooth size–arch length analysis in a mixed-dentition patient? Incisor crowding is common in the mixed dentition, because the erupting permanent incisors have larger crowns than the primary incisors [**incisor liability**] (Moorrees and Chadha 1965). In the posterior segments of the arches, the erupting permanent canines and premolars usually have smaller crowns than the primary canines and molars [**leeway space**] (Moorrees and Chadha 1965). **The main purpose of the mixed dentition space analysis is to differentiate patients with severely crowded arches from those who have up to as much as 4 mm of incisor crowding but who still have enough room in the entire arch, as a result of leeway space, for successful eruption of the permanent premolars and canines and proper alignment of the incisors.** The patients just described are excellent candidates for a lower lingual arch or palatal holding arch. Treatment of these patients with a lingual or palatal arch

provides them with an **important and beneficial service.** Intervention with these two preventive appliances can eliminate the need for future orthodontic treatment or simplify future orthodontic treatment.

Patients predicted to have crowding of 5 or more mm in an arch should be referred to the orthodontist. This is also an important service to patients and their parents. Arch length deficiencies occur in the mixed dentition for two reasons: (1) the arch length is too small to accommodate the size of the teeth and (2) arch length is lost because of local causes. When the deficiency results from an imbalance between the size of the teeth and the arch, primary canines are prematurely exfoliated by the erupting incisors and the distances between the distal surfaces of the permanent lateral incisors and mesial surfaces of the primary first molars are small or nonexistent. In crowded dentitions, erupting permanent incisors may erupt outside the line of arch on the lingual and labial sides of the arches. Incisors that erupt too far labially may show recession of the labial gingival tissue.

Local causes that reduce the arch length of a patient include loss of primary teeth through trauma and caries. Caries and restorations that

Essentials of Orthodontics: Diagnosis and Treatment by Robert N. Staley and Neil T. Reske © 2011 Blackwell Publishing Ltd.

do not restore a carious tooth to its original mesial-distal size contribute to loss of arch length. Ankylosis of a primary second molar can allow the mesial tipping of a permanent first molar, thereby shortening arch length. Permanent canines that erupt ectopically lingual or labial to the line of arch and are impacted are often associated with the loss of arch length.

Prediction of the Widths of Nonerupted Canines and Premolars

In the **early mixed dentition**, the permanent incisors and first molars are erupted (Fig. 4.1). The permanent canines and premolars have not erupted. Their mesial-distal widths can be measured on periapical radiographs, but the images are enlarged in comparison to the true widths of the teeth. Orthodontists have devised several methods of predicting the size of the nonerupted canines and premolars. The prediction methods use three basic predictor variables: (1) only erupted teeth, (2) only measurements from radiographs, and (3) a combination of variables 1 and 2. All methods of prediction involve error. The error of a prediction method is called its **standard error of estimate**. The smaller the standard error of estimate, the more accurate is the prediction method. The lowest standard errors are associated with equations based on multiple regression

analysis that used a combination of radiographic and cast predictor variables (Staley and Hoag 1978; Staley, Hu, Hoag, and Shelly, 1983; Staley, Shelly, and Martin 1979). Upper arch multiple regression equations had a range of standard errors from 0.25 mm to 0.4 mm, and lower arch equations had a range from 0.17 mm to 0.28 mm. Multiple regression equations must be calculated for each individual patient and do not have one prediction graph. For convenience, it is more practical to use predictions and graphs based on simple regression analysis.

The standard errors of estimate for several prediction methods based on simple regression analysis are listed in Table 4.1. The prediction methods that use the mesial-distal widths of the erupted permanent teeth have the highest standard errors (Moyers 1988; Tanaka and Johnston 1974). The advantage of these methods is that measurements of predictor variables can be taken in the mouth at the time of a clinical examination and do not require periapical radiographs. A complete mixed-dentition space analysis should include a panoramic radiograph.

The Hixon and Oldfather prediction method was based on data from white Americans who participated in the Iowa Facial Growth Study at the University of Iowa. The original prediction method published in 1958 was found to systematically underpredict the size of the canines and premolars (Staley and Kerber 1980). The Hixon-

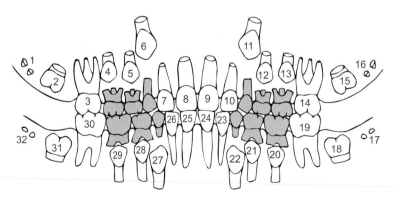

Figure 4.1. Schema of the early mixed dentition. The primary canines and molars are shaded.

Table 4.1. Comparison of Standard Errors of Estimate of Several Prediction Methods

Arch	Prediction Method	Standard Error (mm)*
Upper	Iowa, 1984	0.48
Upper	Tanaka and Johnston, 1974	0.86
Upper	Moyers, 1988	1.0
Lower	Revised Hixon-Oldfather, 1980	0.44
Lower	Iowa, 1984	0.48
Lower	Hixon and Oldfather, 1958	0.57
Lower	Tanaka and Johnston, 1974	0.85
Lower	Moyers, 1988	1.1

*Standard error of estimate for one side of the arch.

Oldfather prediction method and its revised version are good predictors, because they use the radiographic widths of the patient's nonerupted premolars, the most efficient predictor variables. The prediction methods that use radiographic images of the nonerupted canines and premolars as predictor variables are more accurate in predicting tooth size in non-Caucasian populations than are prediction methods that use only erupted teeth as predictor variables (Sorbero and Brown-Bryant 2003).

Because the revised Hixon-Oldfather method only predicts the size of lower canines and premolars, a similar method based on data from the Iowa Facial Growth Study was developed for both upper and lower arches (Staley et al. 1984). This method is known as the Iowa Prediction Method. The revised Hixon-Oldfather and Iowa prediction methods have low standard errors of estimate and were successfully validated in a sample of 53 orthodontic patients.

Radiographic Enlargement of Nonerupted Canines and Premolars

We conducted a pilot study to determine image enlargement of an analog periapical radiograph of a lower canine and first premolar in a dry mandible. The radiograph was taken with an 18-inch cylindrical cone angled at +30 degrees at 65 KVP and 10 amperes. The mesiodistal width of the canine was enlarged 7.8% on the radiograph, and the width of the first premolar was enlarged 5.1% (R. N. Staley, 1986, unpublished study). The correction of this enlargement is the primary purpose of the prediction methods described in this chapter. The emerging technology of cone beam computed tomography (CBCT) has reduced image enlargement to about 1% (Pinsky et al. 2006; Williams et al. 2010). CBCT images of nonerupted teeth in mixed-dentition patients will not become frequent in the near future. More likely, clinicians will increasingly take digital periapical images as analog radiography becomes less common. Williams et al. (2010) found similar enlargement of tooth images in digital and analog periapical radiographs. When CBCT images become commonplace, the prediction methods described in this chapter will become obsolete. The CBCT images of the nonerupted canines and premolars can then be directly measured for use in a mixed-dentition space analysis.

Revised Hixon-Oldfather Prediction Method

Records needed to perform the prediction and arch length analysis include (1) periapical radiographs of the unerupted lower premolars taken with a long cone paralleling or right angle technique and (2) a lower study cast. The following steps are taken to complete the prediction of canine and premolar widths and to complete the arch length analysis:

1. The mesial-distal widths of the lower incisors are measured on the cast and entered into the chart (Fig. 4.2).
2. The mesial-distal widths of the lower first and second premolars are measured on the periapical radiographs and entered into the chart.

Revised Hixon-Oldfather Mixed-Dentition
Tooth Size-Arch Length Analysis
Lower Arch (millimeters)

Patient_____

Date_____

	Left	Right	Both Sides
Posterior Arch			
1. Cast widths of central incisors	____	____	
2. Cast widths of lateral incisors	____	____	
3. Radiograph widths of lower first premolars	____	____	
4. Radiograph widths of lower second premolars	____	____	
5. Sum of incisor and premolar widths	____	____	
6. Predicted sum of premolar and canine widths	____	____	
7. Add standard error of estimate	0.44	0.44	
8. Posterior tooth width sum (add lines 6 + 7)	____	____	
9. Posterior arch length (molar to lateral)	____	____	
10. Arch length excess (+) or deficit (-) [line 9 – 8]	____	____	____
Anterior Arch			
11. Sum of cast widths of incisors	____	____	
12. Anterior arch length	____	____	
13. Arch length excess (+) or deficit (-) [line 12- 11]	____	____	____
Total Arch			
14. Arch length excess (+) or deficit (-) [lines 10 + 13]			____
Adjustments			
15. Antero-posterior position of incisors			____
16. Other adjustments (curve of Spee), etc.			____
17. Adjusted total arch length excess (+) or deficit (-)			____

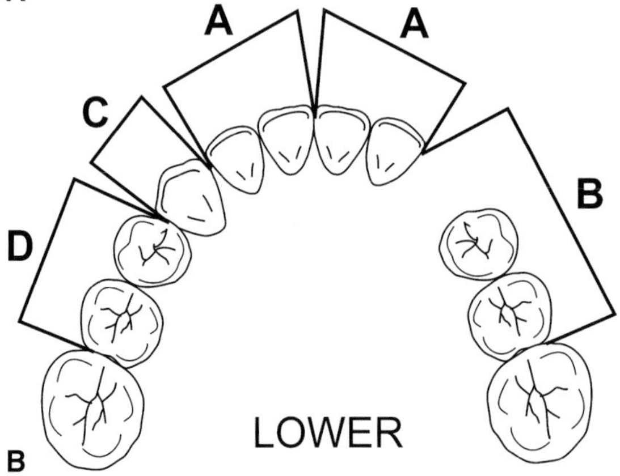

Figure 4.2. A, B, Hixon-Oldfather mixed-dentition analysis chart.

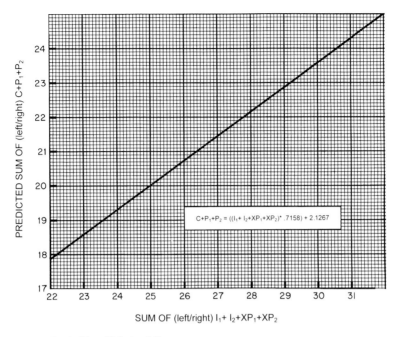

Standard Error of Estimate = 0.44 mm

Figure 4.3. Hixon-Oldfather prediction graph.

3. The sum of these four measurements on each side of the arch is used to predict the sum of the widths of the nonerupted canine and premolars on each side of the arch. The sum of the predictor measurements for each side is entered at the bottom of the prediction graph (Fig. 4.3). The predicted sum of the widths of the canine and premolars on each side is read on the left side of the graph at the horizontal line that intersects the diagonal prediction line where the vertical line from the predictor measurements intersects the prediction line.

4. A standard error of estimate is added to the predicted sum of canine and premolar widths.

5. Posterior arch lengths from the mesial surfaces of the permanent first molars to the distal surfaces of the lateral incisors at the level of the gingival papillae are measured and entered into the chart.

6. Posterior tooth widths are subtracted from the arch lengths to determine the amount of spacing (+) or crowding (−). The two sides are added for a total of posterior spacing or crowding.

7. The sum of the incisor widths is entered into the chart.

8. Anterior arch lengths from the distal of the lateral incisors to the midline are entered into the chart.

9. Anterior tooth widths are subtracted from the arch lengths to determine the amount of spacing or crowding. The two sides are added for a total of anterior spacing or crowding.

10. Total arch spacing or crowding is determined by adding the totals for the posterior and anterior arches.

11. A mixed-dentition space analysis must include additional diagnostic information. Adjustments involve assessment of incisor position on a cephalogram and measurement of curve of Spee. For the family dentist, cephalometric adjustments are optional.

Iowa Prediction Method for Both Arches

The records needed to perform the prediction and arch length analysis include (1) periapical radiographs taken with a long cone or paralleling technique of the nonerupted upper second premolars and canines and the nonerupted lower premolars and (2) upper and lower study casts.

Upper Arch

The following steps are taken to predict the mesial-distal widths of nonerupted upper canines and premolars and to complete the arch length analysis:

1. The radiograph widths of the upper canines and second premolars are entered into the chart (Fig. 4.4).
2. The sums of the radiograph widths for both sides of the arch are entered into the bottom of the prediction graph (Fig. 4.5). The predicted sum of the nonerupted canine and premolar widths for each side is read at the horizontal line that intersects the **middle** diagonal prediction line where the vertical line from the sum of predictor variables intersects the diagonal prediction line.
3. A standard error of estimate is added to the predicted widths.
4. Posterior arch lengths from the mesial surfaces of the permanent first molars to the distal surfaces of the permanent lateral incisors are entered for both sides of the arch.
5. The sum of predicted tooth widths is subtracted from the sum of the arch length on each side to determine how much crowding (−) or spacing (+) is predicted in the posterior parts of the arch.
6. The cast widths of the incisors are entered into the chart and summed for each side.
7. The anterior arch lengths from the distal of the permanent lateral incisors to a point between the central incisors are entered for each side.
8. The sum of the incisor widths is subtracted from the arch length on each side to determine the amount of crowding (−) or spacing (+).
9. The posterior and anterior arch discrepancies between tooth size and arch length are added to obtain a total for the whole arch.
10. Adjustments are not all quantified, but the influence of these factors in a tooth size–arch length analysis is important in all patients.

Lower Arch

The steps taken on the chart for the lower arch are similar to those described for the upper arch (Fig. 4.6). The sums of radiographic widths of the lower first and second premolars are taken to the lower prediction graph (Fig. 4.7) to estimate the widths of the nonerupted premolars and canines.

Standard Error of Estimate

The standard error of estimate for the lower arch prediction equation of the Iowa Mixed Dentition Analysis is 0.47 mm. The meaning of this statistic is illustrated in Figure 4.8. For all possible patients having a sum of lower first and second premolar widths from periapical radiographs of 14.0 mm and a predicted sum of widths of lower canine and premolars of 19.9 mm, approximately 68% of the patients will have a true sum of canine and premolar widths in the range of values from 1 standard error above and below the mean estimate of 19.9 mm, ranging from 19.43 mm to 20.37 mm. In 95.4% of all these patients, the true sum of canine and premolar widths will fall in a range of values from 2 standard errors of estimate above and below the mean, ranging from 18.96 mm to 20.85 mm.

Iowa Mixed-Dentition Tooth Size-Arch Length Analysis
Upper Arch (millimeters)

Patient_____

Date_____

	Left	Right	Both Sides
Posterior Arch			
1. Radiograph widths of upper canines	____	____	
2. Radiograph widths of upper second premolars	____	____	
3. Sum of radiograph widths	____	____	
4. Predicted sum of canine and premolar widths	____	____	
5. Add standard error of estimate	0.48	0.48	
6. Posterior tooth width sum (add lines 4 + 5)	____	____	
7. Posterior arch length (molar to lateral)	____	____	
8. Arch length excess (+) or deficit (-) [line 7 – 6]	____	____	____
Anterior Arch			
9. Cast widths of upper central incisors	____	____	
10. Cast widths of upper lateral incisors	____	____	
11. Sum of incisor widths	____	____	
12. Anterior arch length	____	____	
13. Arch length excess (+) or deficit (-) [line 12 – 11]	____	____	____
Total Arch			
14. Arch length excess (+) or deficit (-) [lines 8 + 13]			____
Adjustments			
15. Antero-posterior position of incisors			____
16. Other adjustments (curve of Spee), etc.			____
17. Adjusted total arch length excess (+) or deficit (-)			____

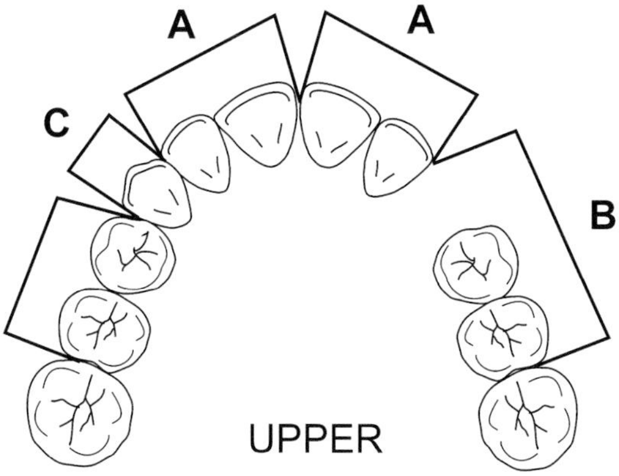

Figure 4.4. A, B, Iowa mixed-dentition analysis chart for the upper arch.

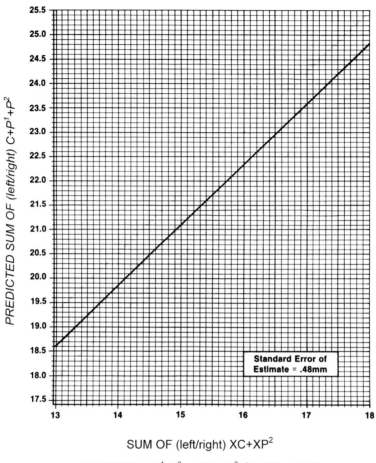

Figure 4.5. Iowa prediction graph for the upper arch.

The mean estimate at the 50th percentile is larger than the true sum of widths for half of all possible patients and smaller than the true sum of widths for half of all patients. To be sure that the estimate for tooth size is larger than the true size in 84% of all possible patients, 1 standard error of estimate is added to the mean estimate for both the revised Hixon-Oldfather and Iowa prediction equations. The addition of 1 standard error of estimate to the mean estimate protects against underestimation of the size of the teeth.

Iowa Mixed-Dentition Tooth Size-Arch Length Analysis
Lower Arch (millimeters)

Patient_____
Date_____

	Left	Right	Both Sides
Posterior Arch			
1. Radiograph widths of lower first premolars	____	____	
2. Radiograph widths of lower second premolars	____	____	
3. Sum of radiograph widths	____	____	
4. Predicted sum of canine and premolar widths	____	____	
5. Add standard error of estimate	0.47	0.47	
6. Posterior tooth width sum (add lines 4 + 5)	____	____	
7. Posterior arch length (molar to lateral)	____	____	
8. Arch length excess (+) or deficit (-) [line 7 – 6]	____	____	____
Anterior Arch			
9. Cast widths of lower central incisors	____	____	
10. Cast widths of lower lateral incisors	____	____	
11. Sum of incisor widths	____	____	
12. Anterior arch length	____	____	
13. Arch length excess (+) or deficit (-) [line 12 – 11]	____	____	____
Total Arch			
14. Arch length excess (+) or deficit (-) [lines 8 + 13]			____
Adjustments			
15. Antero-posterior position of incisors			____
16. Other adjustments (curve of Spee), etc.			____
17. Adjusted total arch length excess (+) or deficit (-)			____

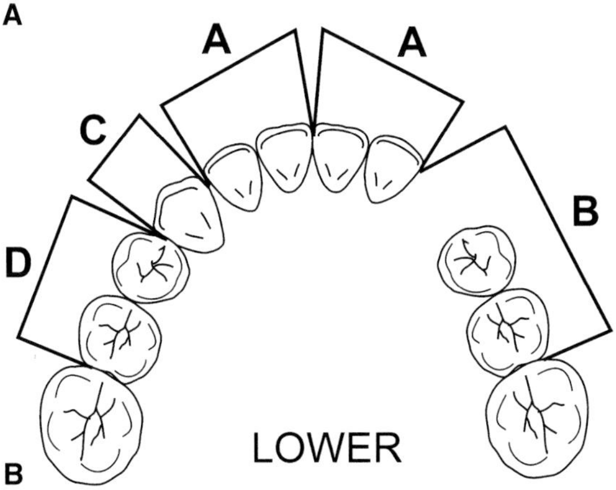

Figure 4.6. A, B, Iowa mixed-dentition analysis chart for the lower arch.

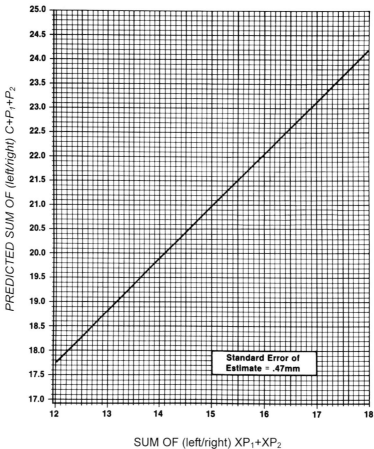

**IOWA PREDICTION GRAPH FOR
LOWER CANINE AND PREMOLAR WIDTHS
(Millimeters)**

PREDICTED SUM OF (left/right) $C+P_1+P_2$

Standard Error of
Estimate = .47mm

SUM OF (left/right) XP_1+XP_2

EQUATION: $C+P_1+P_2 = ((XP_1+XP_2) * 1.07) + 4.923$

Figure 4.7. Iowa prediction graph for the lower arch.

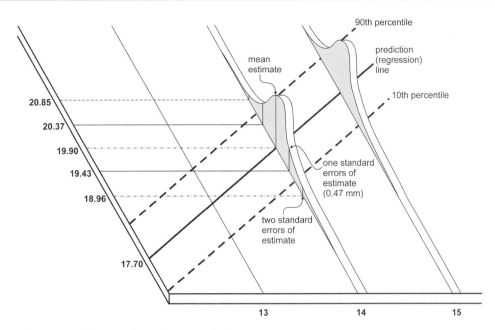

Figure 4.8. Illustration of the error of a prediction method.

Radiograph Image Problems

The nonerupted teeth should not appear rotated on the radiograph. If a premolar or canine is rotated on the radiograph, use the measurement for its nonrotated antimere tooth on the opposite side of the arch for both sides. If both antimeres are rotated, measure the one with the least rotation. Right and left antimere teeth have a high degree of bilateral symmetry, and for that reason the substitutions mentioned earlier can be made without affecting the accuracy of the prediction. Some patients do have significant size asymmetry between antimere teeth, and for these patients it is important to measure the nonerupted teeth on both sides of the arch.

Proportional Equation Prediction Method

The **late mixed dentition** starts with the eruption of one of the permanent canines or premolars. At the beginning stages of the late mixed dentition, the revised Hixon-Oldfather and Iowa pre-diction methods can still be used. If most of the canines and premolars are erupted and if the nonerupted tooth or teeth are easily measured on a periapical radiograph, an alternative prediction method can be used. The method corrects the radiographic enlargement of a nonerupted tooth. The mesial-distal widths of the nonerupted tooth and an erupted tooth are measured on the same periapical radiograph. The mesial-distal width of the erupted tooth is measured on a plaster cast. These three measurements provide the elements of a proportion that can be solved to obtain the width of the nonerupted tooth on the cast.

If

$$\frac{\text{Nonerupted tooth width (cast)}^*}{\text{Nonerupted tooth width (radiograph)}} = \frac{\text{Erupted tooth width (cast)}}{\text{Erupted tooth width (radiograph)}}$$

Then

$$\text{Nonerupted tooth width (cast)}^* = \frac{(\text{ETW cast})(\text{NETW radiograph})}{(\text{ETW radiograph})}$$

Table 4.2. Tanaka and Johnston Prediction Method (mm)*

Sum of widths of all four lower incisors													
20.5	21.0	21.5	22.0	22.5	23.0	23.5 Upper	24.0 Arch	24.5	25.0	25.5	26.0	26.5	27.0
Predicted sum of widths of canine PMS													
20.8	21.0	21.3	21.5	21.8	22.1	22.3 Lower	22.6 Arch	22.8	23.1	23.3	23.6	23.8	24.1
Predicted sum of widths of canine PMS													
20.2	20.5	20.7	21.0	21.3	21.5	21.8	22.1	22.3	22.6	22.9	23.1	23.4	23.7

*All predicted tooth sums are for one side of the arch.

where asterisk indicates unknown cast width; ETW, erupted tooth width; and NETW, non-erupted tooth width.

Tanaka and Johnston Prediction Method

Tanaka and Johnston (1974) and Moyers (1988) created nonradiographic prediction methods by correlating the sum of the widths of the lower permanent incisors with the sum of the widths of the lower premolars and canine on one side of the arch. Tanaka and Johnston developed prediction equations for both arches with correlation coefficients of 0.63 and 0.65 for the upper and lower arches, respectively. The standard error of estimate was 0.86 for the upper teeth and 0.85 for the lower teeth on one side of the arch. The genders were combined in this method. The prediction table contains the 50th percentile values that are appropriate for most patients (Table 4.2).

Tanaka and Johnston (1974) and Moyers (1988) developed prediction equations in white Americans. Similar equations have been developed for black Americans by Ferguson, Macko, Sonnenberg, and Shakun (1978) and Asian Americans by Lee-Chan, Jacobson, Chwa, and Jacobson (1998).

Measurement of Arch Lengths on Casts

Always measure arch length segments from the buccal and labial sides of the arch at the peak of

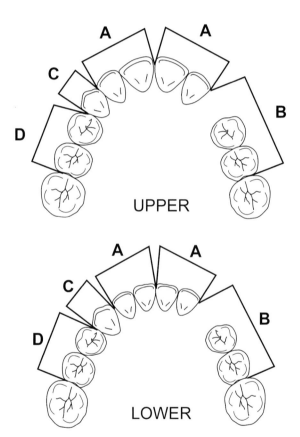

Figure 4.9. Measurement of anterior and posterior arch lengths in the mixed dentition.

the gingival papillae near the contact points between the teeth (Fig. 4.9). The posterior arch lengths are usually measured between the mesial contact point areas of the permanent first molars and the distal surfaces of the permanent lateral incisors. If primary canines are present, posterior measurements can be taken as illustrated in figure 4.9. Anterior arch length measurements are taken between the distal surfaces of the permanent lateral incisors to the midline gingival papilla between the central incisors.

Measurement Instruments and Guidelines

Digital calipers or a Boley gauge is recommended when taking measurements of the teeth on casts. As we move into digital records, the measurements will be taken from digital casts and digital periapical radiographs using computer software. Digital cephalometric radiographs are also measured with computer software.

The width of a tooth is measured between its **anatomic contact points** on the mesial and distal surfaces.

Factors that Influence a Mixed-Dentition Arch Length Analysis

The factors described for the adult dentition in Chapter 3 also apply to the mixed dentition. These factors include (1) incisor inclination and position, (2) curve of Spee, and (3) position of permanent second molars. As stated in Chapter 3, the influence of these factors is recorded as contributing to more or less discrepancy without stating an exact millimeter amount.

Interpretation of a Mixed-Dentition Arch Length Analysis

If the analysis predicts **borderline crowding** of +2 mm to −4 mm in both arches of a **Class I patient**, consider holding arch length with a **palatal (Nance) arch** and a **lower lingual holding arch**. This intervention may prevent the need for future orthodontic treatment, or at least reduce the severity of the malocclusion.

If the analysis predicts **severe crowding** in excess of −6 mm in one or both arches of a **Class I patient**, holding arches are not needed. In patients with crowding, primary canines may be extracted in both upper and lower arches to allow the permanent lateral incisors to erupt and to prevent the erupting incisors from shifting to the right or left of the facial midline. The crowded malocclusion will require comprehensive orthodontic treatment. These patients may benefit from serial extraction treatment.

If the analysis predicts **borderline crowding** between +2 mm and −5 mm in the lower arch of a **Class II patient**, it is important to place a **lower lingual holding arch** to preserve arch length. If the lower holding arch allows the permanent teeth mesial to the first molars to erupt, the eventual treatment of a nonsurgical Class II malocclusion will be simplified. It should be clear that holding lower arch length per se with an appliance will not correct the Class II malocclusion.

If the analysis predicts **severe crowding** in excess of −5 mm in the lower arch of a **Class II patient**, a lingual holding arch may still be appropriate for the nonsurgical malocclusion. These patients have a malocclusion that is very difficult to treat, and they should be referred for comprehensive orthodontic treatment.

If the analysis predicts **borderline crowding** of +2 mm to −5 mm in the upper arch of a **Class III patient**, it is important to place a **palatal holding arch** to preserve arch length. In these patients, extraction of premolars to relieve upper arch crowding complicates orthodontic treatment. Holding upper arch length will not correct the Class III malocclusion but can assist in the eventual treatment of a nonsurgical malocclusion.

If the analysis predicts **severe crowding** in excess of −6 mm in the lower arch of a **Class III patient**, a holding arch may be appropriate. The arch length preserved by the holding arch could enable an orthodontist to retract lower anterior teeth in a nonsurgical Class III malocclusion. These patients should be referred for comprehensive orthodontic treatment.

REFERENCES

Ferguson, F. S., Macko, D. J., Sonnenberg, E. M., and Shakun, M. L. 1978. The use of regression constants in estimating tooth size in a Negro population. Am. J. Orthod. 73:68–72.

Hixon, E. H., and Oldfather, R. E. 1958. Estimation of the sizes of unerupted cuspid and bicuspid teeth. Angle Orthod. 28:236–240.

Lee-Chan, S., Jacobson, B. N., Chwa, K. H., and Jacobson, R. S. 1998. Mixed dentition analysis for Asian-Americans. Am. J. Orthod. Dentofacial Orthop. 113:293–299.

Moorrees, C. F. A., and Chadha, J. M. 1965. Available space for the incisors during dental development. Angle Orthod. 35:12–22.

Moyers, R. E. 1988. Handbook of orthodontics. Chicago: Yearbook Medical Publishers.

Pinsky, H. M., Dyda, S., Pinsky, R. W., and Misch, K. A. 2006. Accuracy of three-dimensional measurements using cone-beam CT. Dentomaxillofac. Radiol. 35:410–416.

Sorbero, C. L., and Brown-Bryant, J. D. 2003. The Moyers and Hixon Oldfather's mixed dentition analyses in African-American patients. J. Dent. Res. 82(Spec Issue A):1175.

Staley, R. N., and Hoag, J. F. 1978. Prediction of the mesiodistal widths of maxillary permanent canines and premolars. Am. J. Orthod. 73:169–177.

Staley, R. N., Hu, P., Hoag, J. F., and Shelly, T. H. 1983. Prediction of the combined right and left canine and premolar widths in both arches of the mixed dentition. Pediatr. Dent. 5:57–60.

Staley, R. N., and Kerber, P. E. 1980. A revision of the Hixon and Oldfather mixed dentition prediction method. Am. J. Orthod. 78:296–302.

Staley, R. N., O'Gorman, T. W., Hoag, J. F., and Shelly, T. H. 1984. Prediction of the widths of unerupted canines and premolars. J. Am. Dent. Assoc. 108:185–190.

Staley, R. N., Shelly, T. H., and Martin, J. F. 1979. Prediction of lower canine and premolar widths in the mixed dentition. Am. J. Orthod. 76:300–309.

Tanaka, M. M., and Johnston, L. E. 1974. The prediction of the size of unerupted canines and premolars in a contemporary orthodontic population. J. Am. Dent. Assoc. 88:798–801.

Williams, A., Staley, R., Qian, F., Vela, K., Alareddy, V. T., and Uribe, L. M. 2010. Validating tooth measurements using CBCT, digital and analog periapical radiography. J. Dent. Res. 89 Spec. Issue A.

Radiographic Analysis

5

Periapical Survey

Periapical radiographs give useful information about caries, periodontal condition, periapical pathology, shape of the roots, size of the teeth, position of impacted teeth, and spatial location of teeth not yet erupted. Measurements of the mesial-distal widths of the periapical images of nonerupted premolars and upper canines are essential for the prediction of tooth size in the Hixon-Oldfather and Iowa mixed-dentition space analyses. A periapical survey of a patient in the early mixed dentition is illustrated in Figure 5.1. These radiographs give an accurate image of the roots that serve as a pretreatment baseline for the posttreatment assessment of root resorption. The pretreatment radiographs can also show the presence of root resorption before treatment. A 16-inch-long cone paralleling or right angle technique is recommended for taking the periapical radiograph.

During treatment, periapical radiographs are used to monitor the position and movement of nonerupted teeth and the growth of the roots of developing teeth. At the end of active treatment,

Essentials of Orthodontics: Diagnosis and Treatment by Robert N. Staley and Neil T. Reske © 2011 Blackwell Publishing Ltd.

these radiographs can assess the presence and effect of root resorption.

Panoramic Radiograph

The panoramic radiograph gives a complete view of the dentition and supporting bones (White and Pharoah 2004). The stage of development of nonerupted teeth and the dental age of the patient can be determined by rating root development of several teeth. The shape of the condyles of the mandible can be observed, and abnormal or asymmetric shapes of the condyles can be noted and related to patient symptoms. Views of the relationship of nonerupted third molars to second molars and surrounding structures can help shape treatment planning decisions for these teeth.

Several panoramic radiographs illustrate different developmental stages of growth, ankylosis, congenitally missing teeth, and impacted teeth in Figures 5.2 through 5.12. Figure 5.2 shows the erupted primary dentition and all of the developing nonerupted permanent teeth, except for the third molars. The early mixed dentition is shown in Figure 5.3. At this stage of development, the permanent incisors and first molars are erupted. In the late mixed dentition,

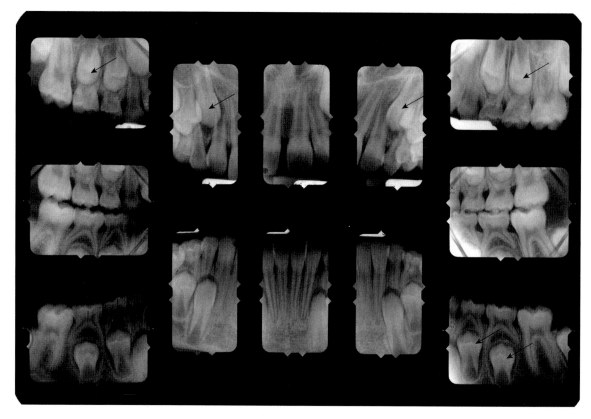

Figure 5.1. Periapical survey of the early mixed dentition. *Arrows* point to the tooth images measured for the revised Hixon-Oldfather and Iowa tooth size prediction methods.

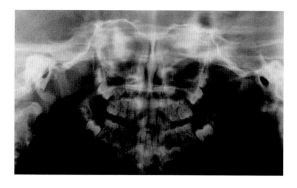

Figure 5.2. Panoramic of the primary dentition. (Courtesy of Dr. Thomas Southard.)

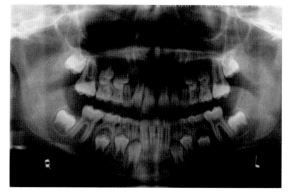

Figure 5.3. Panoramic of the early mixed dentition.

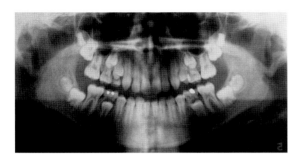

Figure 5.4. Panoramic of the late mixed dentition. (Courtesy of Dr. Harold Bigelow.)

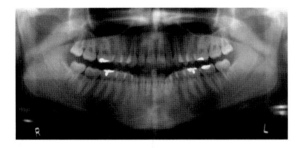

Figure 5.5. Panoramic of an adult dentition including third molars. (Courtesy of Dr. Harold Bigelow.)

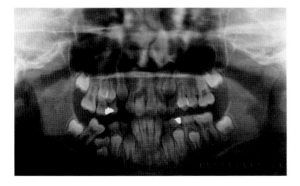

Figure 5.6. Panoramic showing ankylosed tooth T and tipping of tooth #30 that have prevented the eruption of tooth #29.

at least one of the permanent canines or premolars has erupted. Figure 5.4 shows a patient with erupted permanent incisors, canines, first premolars, and first molars. The third molar buds are visible at this stage of development. The permanent teeth of an adult female are shown in Figure 5.5. All the permanent teeth, including the third molars, are in occlusion.

The panoramic radiograph of a patient in the early mixed dentition who had an **ankylosed** mandibular right primary second molar is shown in Figure 5.6. The ankylosed molar sank below the normal teeth on either side of it, as growth of the alveolar bone took the normal teeth farther vertically. By the time a pediatric dentist saw the patient, the mandibular right permanent first molar had tipped forward over the occlusal surface of the akylosed primary molar. The mandibular right permanent second premolar is impacted beneath the ankylosed primary molar. Figure 5.7 is a panoramic radiograph of an early mixed-dentition patient (male) whose developing second premolars are displaced mesial to his primary second molars. Also, all of his erupted primary and permanent molars are prismatic or taurodont. In taurodont teeth, the pulp chamber is elongated and the distance between the bifurcation of the roots and the cementoenamel junction is greater than normal (Kovacs 1971). Normal distances are 4.8 ± 0.76 mm on the mesial side of permanent first molars. The distances on this panoramic film of the first molars are about 9 mm, not corrected for enlargement. Figure 5.8 shows the panoramic radiograph of a patient who had three congenitally missing second premolars—one maxillary and two mandibular. Arrows point to the retained and ankylosed primary second molars associated with the missing premolars. The panoramic radiograph of a patient in the early mixed dentition who lost prematurely a maxillary right primary second molar is shown in Figure 5.9. After the loss of tooth A, the maxillary right permanent first molar tipped mesially into the space formerly occupied by the lost primary second molar and is now blocking eruption of the maxillary right second premolar.

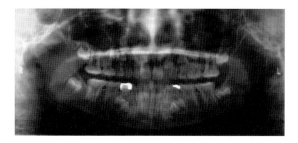

Figure 5.7. Panoramic of a male patient with aberrant second premolars and taurodont molars. (Courtesy of Dr. Cynthia Christensen.)

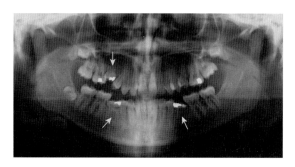

Figure 5.8. Panoramic of a patient congenitally missing an upper right second premolar and both lower second premolars. Primary second molars are retained and ankylosed (*arrows*). (Courtesy of Dr. Theresa Juhlin.)

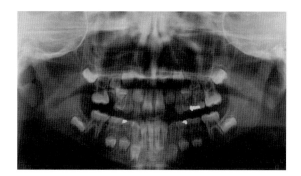

Figure 5.9. Panoramic of a patient who lost tooth A prematurely, which allowed the mesial migration of the upper right first molar that impacted the upper right second premolar.

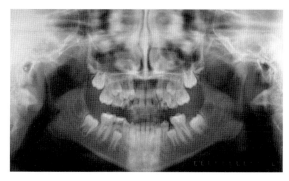

Figure 5.10. Panoramic of a patient who lost tooth K prematurely, which allowed the mesial migration of the lower left first molar that impacted the lower left second premolar.

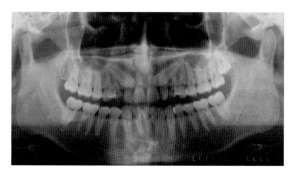

Figure 5.11. Panoramic of a patient with both maxillary canines impacted on the palatal side of the arch. The upper primary canines are retained.

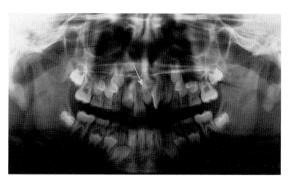

Figure 5.12. Panoramic of an early mixed dentition with a supernumerary tooth (mesiodens) located between the maxillary central incisors (*arrow*). (Courtesy of Dr. Samir Bishara.)

Figure 5.10 illustrates the premature loss of the mandibular left second primary molar in a late mixed-dentition patient. Loss of the primary molar allowed the mandibular left permanent first molar to tip mesially, causing the impaction of the mandibular left second premolar. An adult patient with both permanent maxillary canines impacted on the palatal side of the arch is illustrated in Figure 5.11. Please note that the primary maxillary canines were still retained in the mouth. Figure 5.12 illustrates a mixed dentition patient with a supernumerary tooth called a mesiodens located between the maxillary central incisors. Note the 90-degree rotation of the maxillary left central incisor and the diastema between the central incisors.

Occlusal Radiographs

Maxillary and mandibular occlusal radiographs provide useful supplemental information on the position of impacted teeth, especially canines and premolars (White and Pharoah 2004). A maxillary occlusal radiograph is taken as a pretreatment baseline view of the midpalatal suture whenever a rapid maxillary expander is used in treatment. The radiograph can be repeated during the expansion of the arch to observe whether the midpalatal suture has opened and how much it opened. Figure 5.13 is an occlusal view of the patient illustrated in Figure 5.11. The canines are far forward on the palate, near the roots of the permanent incisors. Also note the image of a supernumerary tooth in the middle of the palate between the canines. The supernumerary tooth is a mesiodens that is undergoing resorption, a fate common to many of these teeth. Figure 5.14 shows impacted maxillary second premolars in an adolescent patient. The teeth are erupting toward the midline suture of the palate. Figure 5.15 illustrates the opening of the mid palatal suture of an adolescent patient treated with a rapid maxillary expander. Note the V-shaped opening of the maxillary suture and the diastema created by the appliance. The mandibular occlusal radiograph of an orthodontic patient with cleidocranial dysostosis is shown in Figure 5.16. Note the presence of several supernumerary teeth and the severely impacted mandibular left permanent canine. The impacted canine was located on the labial side of the alveolus and was brought into the arch through orthodontic treatment.

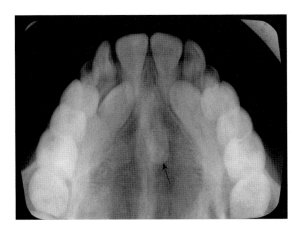

Figure 5.13. View of two impacted canines and a resorbing supernumerary tooth located in the midline of the palate (*arrow*).

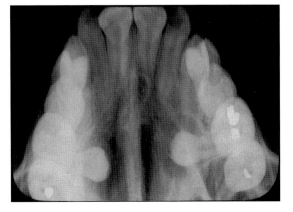

Figure 5.14. View of two ectopic maxillary second premolars.

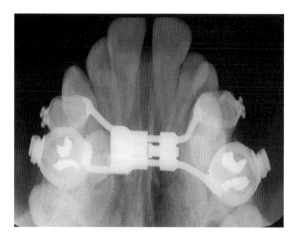

Figure 5.15. View of the midpalatal suture opened by a rapid palatal expander.

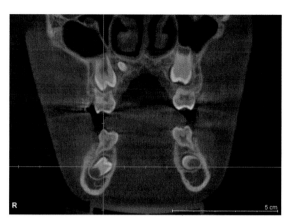

Figure 5.17. Coronal view (cone beam computed tomography) of lower second premolars and supernumerary tooth.

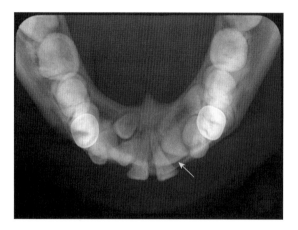

Figure 5.16. View of the mandibular arch of a patient with supernumerary teeth and an impacted mandibular left canine (*arrow*).

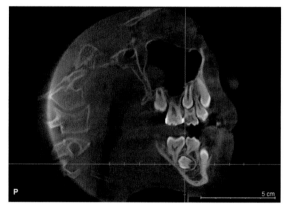

Figure 5.18. Lateral, lingual (cone beam computed tomography) view of the lower left second premolar.

Cone Beam Radiographs

Cone beam radiographs are shown of a patient who had ectopic lower second premolars and a maxillary supernumerary tooth. A conventional panoramic radiograph showed the ectopic teeth through their long axes, not showing where the crowns were located and how long the roots had grown. The supernumerary tooth was located in the upper right palate alongside the canine and premolars. Figure 5.17 is a coronal section through the lower second premolars that gives an excellent view of the developing lower right second premolar and the supernumerary in the upper right palate. Figure 5.18 is a sagittal view of the left mandible illustrating the development of the lower left second premolar. Figure 5.19 is a lingual volumetric view of the lower right second premolar. Figure 5.20 is a lingual volumetric view of the lower left second premolar. Figure 5.21 is an excellent lingual volumetric view of the supernumerary tooth.

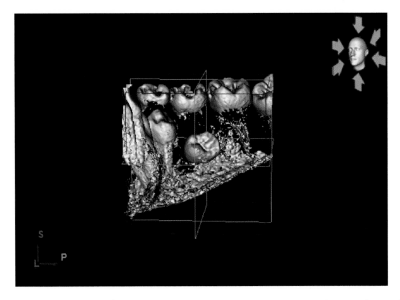

Figure 5.19. Lingual volumetric (cone beam computed tomography) view of the lower right second premolar.

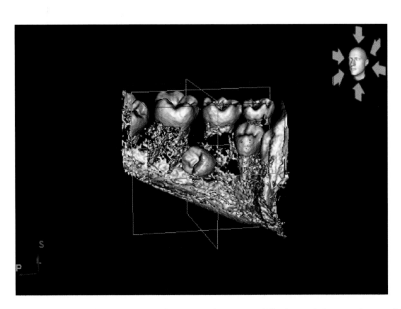

Figure 5.20. Lingual volumetric (cone beam computed tomography) view of the lower left second premolar.

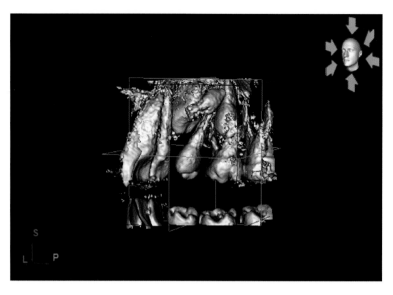

Figure 5.21. Lingual palatal volumetric (cone beam computed tomography) view of the supernumerary tooth in the upper right canine region.

Lateral Cephalometric Radiographs

The lateral cephalometric radiograph is taken in an apparatus that creates a standardized fixed position for the patient, x-ray source, and film, so that future radiographs of the patient taken in the same apparatus can be superimposed to accurately study the effects of growth and orthodontic treatment (Athanasiou 1995). The x-ray source is placed about 5 feet away from the middle of the patient's head to reduce enlargement of the head structures. The film is placed as close to the patient as possible, while still accommodating the largest head, again to reduce enlargement of the image. Enlargement of anatomic structures varies from approximately 10% to 14% depending on the distances chosen for each cephalometric apparatus.

The patient's head is held firmly in an apparatus that orients the Frankfort plane parallel to the floor. This is accomplished by placing the ear rods of the head holder into the external auditory orifices and positioning orbitale, located at the inferior border of the orbit, to a standardized part of the head holder. The central x-ray beam passes through the right and left ear rods whose images should be closely superimposed on the cephalogram. The bilateral facial structures on the right and left sides of the mid-sagittal plane will not be perfectly superimposed.

The focal spot is an area, not a point, from which the roentgen radiation is emitted. Because the rays come from an area, a penumbra effect blurs the image of anatomic structures. The penumbra effect increases as the focal spot becomes larger. The penumbra effect also increases as the distances from the x-ray source to the subject and from the subject to the film increase. A variable white light collimator allows the technician to limit the x-ray beam to the area of the face. The film cassette contains a grid that absorbs secondary radiation and thus reduces another cause of blurring of the image. Intensifying screens within the cassette permit lower radiation exposure. The patient wears a lead shield to protect the body from radiation.

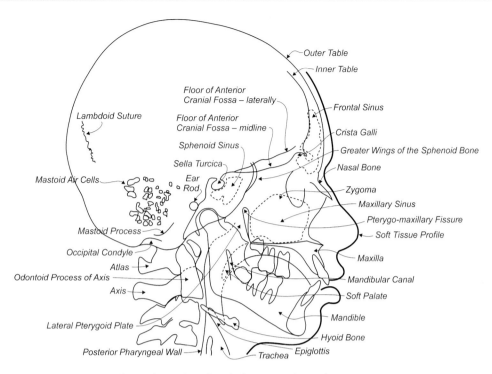

Figure 5.22. Anatomic structures observed on a lateral cephalometric radiograph.

Anatomic Landmarks

Knowledge of craniofacial anatomy is required for the interpretation of a cephalometric radiograph. Structures commonly observed on a lateral cephalogram are illustrated in Figure 5.22. Skeletal structures are often more easily recognized in children and adolescents than in adults, because the more dense bone structure of the adult may obscure details. Structures such as the mastoid process and frontal sinus change during growth. Soft tissues like the pharyngeal wall, adenoidal tissues, tongue, nose, and facial integument are part of the analysis and should be visible on the cephalogram.

Cephalometric Landmarks

In the 1940s, orthodontists began to routinely use cephalograms as an important diagnostic tool. Clinicians use cephalometric landmarks that are relevant in diagnosis (Downs 1948; Reidel 1948; Steiner 1953; Tweed 1962). The landmarks on a two-dimensional lateral cephalogram represent face structures located in three planes of space (Fig. 5.23). The anteroposterior (AP) relationships of interest are (1) the relations of the maxilla and mandible with the anterior cranial base and to one another, (2) the relation of the upper central incisor with the anterior cranial base, and (3) the relation of the lower central incisor with the mandible and Frankfort plane. The vertical relationships of interest are (1) the relation of the lower border of the mandible to the anterior cranial base and Frankfort plane and (2) anterior face height from nasion at the root of the nose to menton at the bottom of the bony chin. Advanced analysis involves numerous additional measurements, including those of the soft tissue profile.

Most landmarks are located on anatomic structures, but two important landmarks are exceptions: (1) sella is in the middle of the bony

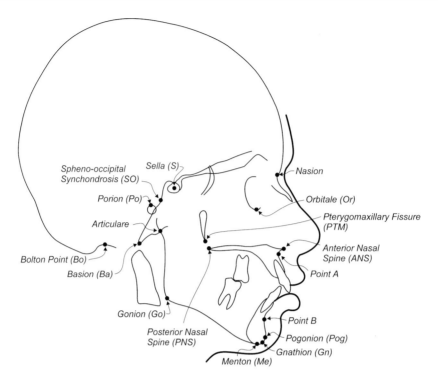

Figure 5.23. Locations of cephalometric points.

outline of the pituitary fossa and (2) porion is located at the most superior point on the ear rod. Some points are more easily and reliably located than others (Baumrind and Frantz 1971a, 1971b). For example, nasion is relatively easy to locate compared to posterior nasal spine. Location of a point may be easier in one plane of space than in the other. The vertical position of the posterior nasal spine is more easily located than its AP position.

In bilaterally symmetric faces, facial structures on the left side, including teeth, are superior and posterior to structures on the right side. Permanent first molars on the left side are usually traced. The images of the right and left sides of the mandible are bisected and traced as one bisection line. Orbitale at the inferior border of the orbit is located between the images of the right and left orbits. The most anterior upper and lower central incisors are traced.

Cephalometric Point Locations

The points described next are illustrated in Figure 5.23 (Athanasiou 1995; Krogman and Sassouni 1957).

Sella (S) is located in the center of the outline of the pituitary fossa. Locating the point before tracing the shadow of the anterior and posterior clinoid processes and floor of the fossa that surround the pituitary gland is probably more accurate than locating the point after tracing the sella turcica.

Nasion (Na) is located at the most inferior, anterior point on the frontal bone adjacent to the frontonasal suture. Again, point location should precede tracing of the bony outlines.

Orbitale (Or) is located on the lowermost point of the bony orbit outline. When both right and left orbital outlines are visible, orbitale is located at the bisection of the two orbit outlines.

Orbitale may be difficult to locate in some subjects.

ANS is located at the tip of the **anterior nasal spine**.

Pterygomaxillary fissure (Ptm) is located at the point at the base of the fissure where the anterior and posterior walls meet.

Point A is located at the most posterior part of the anterior shadow of the maxilla, near the apex of the maxillary central incisor root.

Point B is located at the most posterior point on the shadow of the anterior border of the mandible, near the apex of the central incisor root.

Pogonion (Pog) is located at the most anterior point on the shadow of the chin.

Menton (Me) is located at the most inferior point on the shadow of the chin.

Porion is located at the midpoint of the upper contour of the external auditory canal. Machine porion is located at the most superior point on the shadow of the ear rod. Porion may be difficult to locate in underexposed cephalograms in which neither the external auditory canal nor machine porion can be seen.

Articulare (Ar) is the point of intersection between the shadow of the inferior border of the zygomatic process of the temporal bone and the posterior border of the ramus of the mandible.

Cephalometric Planes

A plane requires three points for definition; however, the cephalometric planes illustrated in Figure 5.24 are lines connecting two points on a two-dimensional surface.

The **Frankfort horizontal plane** is a line passing through the porion and orbitale. Misplacement of the ear rods at the time of exposure will result in inaccurate location of the porion. Careful placement of the ear rods is essential for obtaining a correctly positioned Frankfort plane. **On a cephalometric tracing, the Frankfort plane should be parallel to the top and bottom edges of the tracing sheet.**

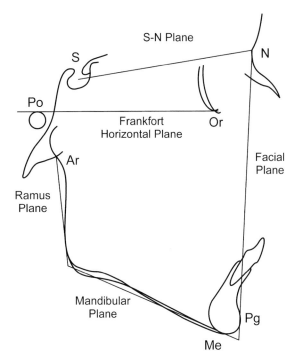

Figure 5.24. Cephalometric planes.

The **sella-nasion plane** is a horizontal line passing through the sella and nasion. All measurements using this plane are affected by its cant or tilt in relation to the Frankfort plane. The sella-nasion plane is usually oriented at 6 to 8 degrees to the Frankfort horizontal plane. As the sella-nasion plane becomes more parallel to the Frankfort plane, angular measurements to vertical lines from the nasion to the maxilla and mandible become larger. As the sella-nasion plane is canted more upward in the area of nasion, angular measurements to vertical lines from nasion to the maxilla and mandible become smaller.

The **facial plane** is a line passing through nasion and pogonion.

The **mandibular plane** is a line passing through menton and tangent to the posterior portion of the lower border of the mandible just as it turns upward to the posterior border of the ramus. The mandibular plane will be accurately positioned only when the patient is in maximal occlusal contact in centric occlusion during exposure to the radiation.

The **ramus plane** is tangent to the averaged inferior, posterior surface of the ramus and passes through articulare.

Cephalometric Angles and Distances

A cephalometric analysis is divided into skeletal and dental components. The **skeletal measurements** relate the maxilla and mandible to the cranium. The **dental measurements** relate the upper and lower incisors to one another, the maxillary incisors to the cranial base, and the mandibular incisors to the cranium and to the lower border of the mandible. Soft tissue profile analysis is available and widely used in orthodontic diagnosis, but will not be discussed in this book.

Skeletal Angles and Distance

Five angles are illustrated in Figure 5.25. The mandibular plane angles are shown in Figure 5.26.

Sella-nasion-pogonion (SNPog) angle describes the AP position of the chin in relation to the anterior cranial base.

Sella-nasion–point A (SNA) angle describes the AP position of the maxilla in relation to the anterior cranial base.

Sella-nasion–point B (SNB) angle describes the AP position of the mandible in relation to the anterior cranial base.

Point A–nasion–point B (ANB) angle describes the AP position of the maxilla as related to the AP position of the mandible. Angle SNB is subtracted from angle SNA to determine ANB. Severe Class II malocclusions have large positive ANB angles, whereas severe Class III malocclusions have large negative ANB angles.

Frankfort horizontal plane–nasion-pogonion (FH-NPog or facial angle) describes the AP position of the chin as related to the Frankfort horizontal plane.

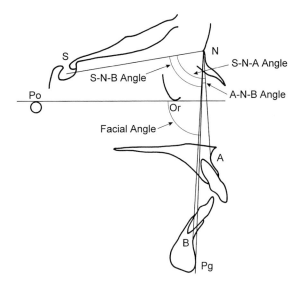

Figure 5.25. Skeletal angles relating the maxilla and mandible to the cranium.

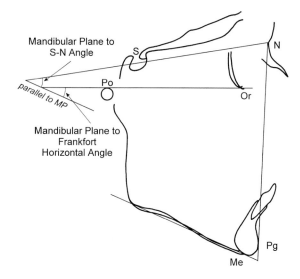

Figure 5.26. Skeletal angles relating the lower border of the mandible to the cranium.

Mandibular plane–sella–nasion plane (MPSN) relates the steepness (cant) of the mandibular plane to a line passing through the anterior cranial base.

Mandibular plane–Frankfort horizontal plane (MPFH or FMA) relates the steepness (cant) of the mandibular plane to a line passing through the anterior cranial base.

Anterior face height is measured from nasion to menton (N:Me). An adjustment for enlargement, averaging about 12% for traditional analog cephalometric radiographs, is made by multiplying any measured distance by 0.88. Digital cephalograms can approximate life size, and distance measurements can be taken directly from the radiograph without needing an adjustment for enlargement.

Dental Angles

Maxillary incisor–to–S-N plane angle relates the axial inclination of the most labial maxillary incisor to a line passing through the anterior cranial base (Fig. 5.27).

Maxillary incisor–to–mandibular incisor angle relates the axial inclination of the maxillary incisor to the axial inclination of the mandibular incisor. As the incisors become more protrusive, the angle decreases, and as the incisors lose inclination, the angle increases (Fig. 5.27).

Frankfort horizontal plane–to–mandibular incisor angle (FMIA) relates the axial inclination of the most labial mandibular incisor to the Frankfort horizontal plane (Fig. 5.27). This angular relationship is a reliable method for assessing the inclination of the lower incisor if porion and orbitale are located accurately.

Mandibular incisor–to–mandibular plane angle (IMPA) relates the axial inclination of the most labial incisor to the mandibular plane (Fig. 5.27). This angle is affected by the morphology of the mandible. As the angle between the mandibular plane and sella-nasion plane decreases, the IMPA angle becomes larger. As the angle between the mandibular plane and sella-nasion plane increases, the IMPA angle decreases. The inverse relationship must be taken into account when using this angle to assess the inclination of the lower incisor.

Distances of Incisors to Anterior Vertical Lines

All distances measured on an analog cephalogram must be corrected for enlargement according to the distances between x-ray source, subject, and film. Enlargement averages about 12%, so multiply the distance by 0.88. The measurements corrected for enlargement can then be compared to the cephalometric norms in Tables 5.1, 5.2, and 5.3. These norms and most cephalometric norms have been corrected for enlargement.

Maxillary incisor–to–line A-Pog distance is measured along a perpendicular line between the incisal edge of the most labial incisor and the A-Pog line (Fig. 5.28). This distance is used to assess the AP position of the maxillary incisor.

Mandibular incisor–to–line Nasion–Point B distance is measured along a perpendicular line between the incisal edge of the most labial incisor and the N-B line (Fig. 5.28). This distance is used to assess the AP position of the mandibular incisor.

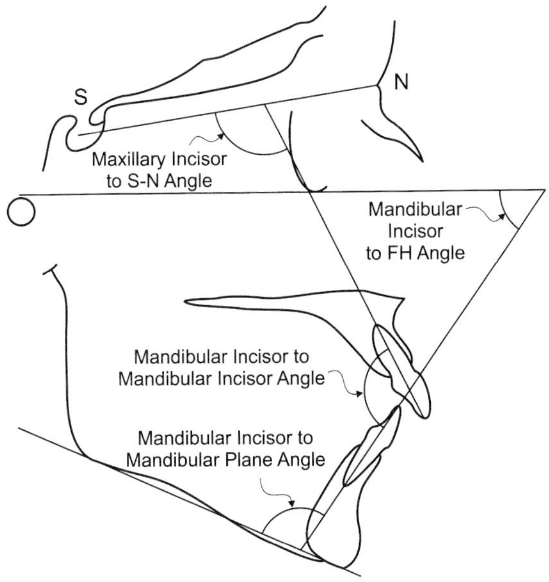

Figure 5.27. Dental angles relating the teeth to one another, the maxillary incisor to the cranial base, and the mandibular incisor to the cranium and lower border of the mandible.

Table 5.1. Cephalometric Standards for Males 5–10 Years and Females 5–12 Years Old

Measurement	Mean	SD	Minimum	Maximum
Skeletal A-P°				
SNA°	80	4.0	74	90
SNB°	76	3.4	70	83
ANB°	4	1.6	1	9
SN:Pog°	76	3.5	68	84
FH:NPog°	83	2.8	76	90
Skeletal vert.				
N-Me mm	99	4.7	89	108
MP:SN°	35	4.6	25	42
MP:FH°	27	4.3	19	36
Dental angular				
UI:LI°	131	7.3	117	143
UI:SN°	101	4.6	93	109
LI:FH°	59	4.7	49	69
LI:MP°	94	5.1	83	104
Dental linear				
UI:APog mm	4	1.6	2	8
LI:NB mm	4	1.2	1	6

From Bishara (1981).

Table 5.3. Cephalometric Standards for Adult Females

Measurement	Mean	SD	Minimum	Maximum
Skeletal A-P°				
SNA°	80	3.8	74	90
SNB°	77	3.3	71	84
ANB°	3	2.1	0	7
SN:Pog°	77	3.3	72	84
FH:NPog°	84	2.5	79	89
Skeletal vert.				
N-Me mm	107	5.0	96	116
MP:SN°	34	4.2	24	39
MP:FH°	28	4.9	19	35
Dental angular				
UI:LI°	129	9.0	111	142
UI:SN°	102	5.4	96	110
LI:FH°	58	6.5	46	65
LI:MP°	95	5.5	86	106
Dental linear				
UI:APog mm	6	1.7	3	9
LI:NB mm	4	2.0	2	8

From Bishara (1981).

Table 5.2. Cephalometric Standards for Adult Males

Measurement	Mean	SD	Minimum	Maximum
Skeletal A-P°				
SNA°	82	3.7	76	89
SNB°	80	3.7	73	86
ANB°	2	2.4	–2	6
SN:Pog°	81	4.2	72	88
FH:NPog°	86	4.5	79	94
Skeletal vert.				
N-Me mm	122	6.0	113	135
MP:SN°	28	7.2	13	43
MP:FH°	23	7.4	7	42
Dental angular				
UI:LI°	134	9.8	115	152
UI:SN°	102	6.3	89	115
LI:FH°	62	10.1	48	85
LI:MP°	96	9.2	78	108
Dental linear				
UI:APog mm	4	1.9	0	7
LI:NB mm	4	2.5	–1	9

From Bishara (1981).

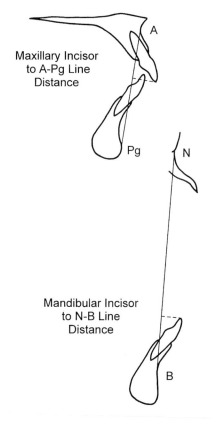

Figure 5.28. Horizontal distances of incisors to anterior vertical lines.

Cephalometric Norms and Treatment Goals

Cephalometric norms are taken from measurements of a representative sample of persons who have normal occlusion and have not undergone orthodontic treatment. Norms have been established for Americans of European, African, and Asian origins. The cephalometric measurements of a patient should be compared to racial peers of a similar age. Norms from the longitudinal Iowa Facial Growth Study are representative of Americans of European origin and include data for growing children and adults (see Tables 5.1 through 5.3) [Bishara 1981]. Some norms used by clinicians were derived from samples of adults only.

The most useful cephalometric normative data should include, for every angle and distance, the mean, the standard deviation, and the minimum and maximum values. The mean value is a mathematic central point derived from measurements taken from many individuals. Only a few subjects of the normal sample will have a particular angular measurement identical to the mean value. Because variability is a basic characteristic of the human body, the likelihood that any one person will have several measurements identical to the mean value of a norm sample is very remote. **On the basis of variability, normal measurements are defined here as those that fall within 1 standard deviation above and below the mean value of the normal sample.** Whereas the mean value is too restrictive for the definition of normal, the range from minimum to maximum is so broad that finding an abnormal measurement in a patient becomes increasingly unlikely.

Although the normal values of cephalometric analysis and orthodontic diagnosis are useful as diagnostic tools, these values should not be used as treatment goals (Koski 1955). Each patient has a unique set of cephalometric measurements and dental relationships. The objective of treatment is to move abnormal dental structures toward the normal mean so that they are in greater harmony with the facial and dental morphology of the individual patient.

Lateral Cephalometric Tracing

The advent of digital cephalometry is quickly making obsolete the tracing of analog cephalometric radiographs discussed next. The digital tracing is done within the constraints of a particular software program, and currently most software is not able to create a tracing fully in conformity with the patient. As digital tracing software develops, it will enable the clinician to create a digital tracing in full conformity with the patient's anatomy. The convenience of digital tracing and the transmission of digital tracings are very useful.

In the United States, the facial profile is customarily placed on the right side of the tracing sheet. The radiograph is attached to an illuminated view box with masking tape. The tracing is made on a sheet of acetate. Begin by marking the cephalometric points with a sharp pencil. Then trace the sella turcica, following it forward onto the plane of the sphenoid bone and continuing forward on the contour of the cribiform plate of the ethmoid bone (Athanasiou 1995). Trace the floor of the anterior cranial base, which is above and lateral to the cribiform plate and the greater wings of the sphenoid bone as they intersect the plane of the sphenoid bone (see Fig. 5.8).

Trace along the anterior surfaces of the frontal and nasal bones. Trace the maxilla from the anterior nasal spine along the floor of the nasal cavity back to the posterior nasal spine. Trace the pterygomaxillary fissure whose inferior end points toward the posterior nasal spine. Trace from the posterior nasal spine along the roof of the palate to the lingual alveolar process around the incisors. Trace the anterior surface of the maxilla from the anterior nasal spine to the alveolar process labial to the incisors. Trace the most anterior central incisor and the maxillary left first molar. Check the molar relationship on the casts before tracing the outlines of the molars. If the molar relationship differs between the right to left sides, indicate that on the tracing.

Trace the most labial lower central incisor, and outline the lower anterior alveolar bone and the symphysis of the mandible. Trace the lower and

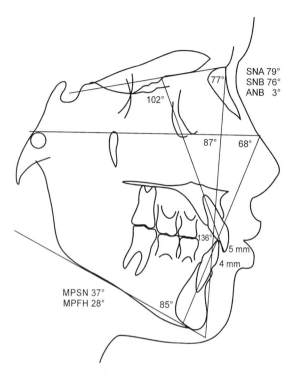

Figure 5.29. Cephalometric tracing of a 9-year 10-month-old white male.

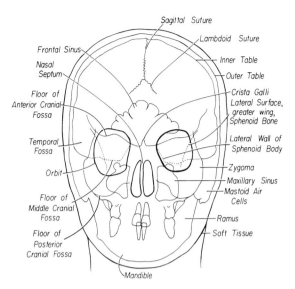

Figure 5.30. Anatomic structures observed on a posteroanterior cephalometric radiograph.

posterior borders of the mandible, taking the tracing up to articulare where the shadow of the inferior border of the zygomatic process of the temporal bone intersects the shadow of the posterior border of the ramus of the mandible (Fig. 5.8). The tracing of the mandible follows a line that bisects the shadows of the right and left sides of the mandible. Trace the shadow of the lower left first molar. Trace both orbital rims, marking orbitale between the two shadows. Trace the ear rod. A completed tracing with selected measurements is shown in Figure 5.29.

Posteroanterior Cephalometric Radiograph

If a facial bilateral asymmetry is observed in an orthodontic patient, a posteroanterior (PA) cephalometric radiograph can be taken to

quantify the severity of the asymmetry. Anatomic landmarks are illustrated in Figure 5.30. The junctions of the lateral walls of the orbits with the floor of the anterior cranial fossa are connected with a horizontal line to establish the horizontal axis of the cranium. The most superior point on Crista Galli helps to establish the vertical axis of the cranium. A perpendicular line drawn through the most superior point on Crista Galli to the line drawn horizontally between the junctions of the lateral walls of the orbits and floor of the anterior cranial fossa creates a vertical cranial axis that divides the face into two lateral halves (Fig. 5.31).

In persons with normal head and dental symmetry, the vertical axis deviates little from the dental and chin midlines. In a patient with marked bilateral asymmetry, the vertical line deviates from the dental and chin midlines (Fig. 5.31) The occlusal cant in the patient illustrated in Figure 5.31 can be estimated by drawing a line between the buccal images of the most distal and buccal molars on both sides of the arch. The angular measurement is taken between the cranial horizontal axis and the radiographic

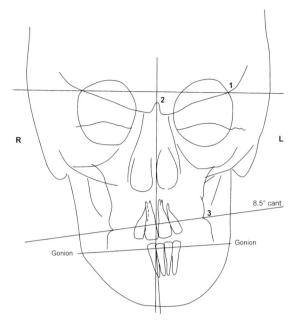

Figure 5.31. Analysis of facial asymmetry using a posteroanterior cephalometric radiograph.

occlusal plane just described. A line drawn through the right and left sides of the mandible at the gonial angles (the greatest dimension across the mandible at the gonial angle) can be drawn to assess the deviation of the lower dental midline from the middle of the chin (Fig. 5.31). The chin midline is estimated by dropping a perpendicular from the midpoint of the line across the gonial regions of the mandible. The patient illustrated in Figure 5.31 should be referred to an orthodontist.

Analog versus Digital Radiography

Digital radiography is an advancement in dentistry that has many advantages and some disadvantages (Kantor 2005). Analog film remains the standard image for radiographic diagnosis; however, digital radiography will eventually replace film technology. Digital radiography is amenable to immediate viewing, standardized image archiving, and image retrieval (Van der

Stelt 2005). Computer image enhancement and interpretation may prove to be advantageous. Software programs are available for cephalometric analysis of digital cephalograms. Clinicians still need to know how to locate anatomic structures and cephalometric points on the digital image in order to accurately use the software. It is clear that radiation dose reduction for digital radiography compared to film radiography is quite limited. Reduction is possible only when the practitioner takes care to select the lowest exposure that still provides a diagnostically useful image (Van der Stelt 2005). Digital radiography requires computers and network infrastructure to get the images to the chair-side. Sensors in the digital apparatus are installed with corresponding software that has a database for archiving images. Because of software changes, digital images taken now may not be viewable in 10 or 20 years (Kantor 2005).

REFERENCES

Athanasiou, A. E. 1995. Orthodontic cephalometry. London: Mosby-Wolfe.

Baumrind, S., and Frantz, R. 1971a. The reliability of head films measurements, 1. Landmark identification. Am. J. Orthod. 60:111–127.

Baumrind, S., and Frantz, R. 1971b. The reliability of head films measurements. 2. Conventional and angular linear measurements. Am. J. Orthod. 60:505–517.

Bishara, S. E. 1981. Longitudinal cephalometric standards from 5 years of age to adulthood. Am. J. Orthod. 79:35–44.

Downs, W. B. 1948. Variation in facial relationships: their significance in treatment and prognosis. Am. J. Orthod. 34:812–840.

Kantor, M. L. 2005. Dental digital radiography, more than a fad, less than a revolution. J. Am. Dent. Assoc. 136: 1358–1362.

Koski, K. 1955. The norm concept in dental orthopedics. Angle Orthod. 25:113–117.

Kovacs, I. 1971. A systematic description of dental roots. In Dental morphology and evolution (pp. 225–230), ed. A. A. Dahlberg. Chicago: University of Chicago Press.

Krogman, W. M., and Sassouni, V. A. 1957. Syllabus in roentgenographic cephalometry. Philadelphia: Philadelphia Center for Research in Child Growth.

Reidel, R. A. 1948. A cephalometric roentgenographic study of the relation of the maxilla and associated parts to the cranial base in normal and malocclusion of the teeth. Master's thesis, Northwestern University.

Steiner, C. C. 1953. Cephalometrics for you and me. Am. J. Orthod. 39:729–755.

Tweed, C. H. 1962. Was the development of the diagnostic facial triangle as an accurate analysis based on facts or fancy? Am. J. Orthod. 48:823–840.

Van der Stelt, P. F. 2005. Filmless imaging, the uses of digital radiography in dental practice. J. Am. Dent. Assoc. 136:1379–1387.

White, S. C., and Pharoah, M. J. 2004. Oral radiology: principles and interpretation. St. Louis: Mosby.

Lingual and Palatal Arches

6

Incisor Liability and Leeway Space

In the mixed dentition, the discrepancy between the mesiodistal widths of the smaller primary and larger permanent incisors averages approximately −7.4 mm in the maxillary arch and −5.1 mm in the mandibular arch (Moorrees and Chadha 1965). This discrepancy, called **incisor liability**, is one of the reasons why mixed-dentition patients experience crowding of the larger permanent incisors as they erupt. The other major reason for crowding is inadequate growth in the size of the alveolar arches in relation to the size of the permanent teeth.

In the posterior segments of the mixed dentition, the discrepancy between the mesiodistal widths of the larger primary canines and molars and the smaller permanent succedaneous canines and premolars, called the **leeway space**, averages approximately 2.4 mm in the upper arch and 4.3 mm in the lower arch (Moorrees and Chadha 1965). The leeway space can be used to align crowded incisors in many patients.

Essentials of Orthodontics: Diagnosis and Treatment
by Robert N. Staley and Neil T. Reske
© 2011 Blackwell Publishing Ltd.

Passive Lower Lingual Holding Arch

A passive lower lingual arch can be placed in mixed-dentition patients who exhibit mild incisor crowding and have adequate leeway space to accommodate the erupting permanent teeth. Passive lingual arch therapy helped resolve up to 5 mm of lower incisor crowding (Brennan and Gianelly 2000). They reported that 60% of 107 patients who have an average of 4.85 mm of incisor crowding finished treatment with adequate arch length. The passive lingual arches lost an average of 0.4 mm of arch length during the course of the entire treatment. Another study found that lower incisor alignment remained stable for 9 years postretention in 76% of a group of mixed-dentition patients treated with a passive lingual arch (Dugoni, Lee, Valera, and Dugoni 1995). The evidence from these studies strongly supports the use of passive lower lingual holding arches as effective interceptive and preventive appliances in mixed-dentition patients who have minimal total arch length deficiencies.

Mixed-dentition analyses like the Iowa or revised Hixon-Oldfather analyses are essential tools that help a clinician identify patients who have minimal total arch length deficiency and who can benefit from the placement of a passive lower lingual arch (see Chapter 5). For example, mixed-dentition patients with mild incisor crowding who are predicted by an analysis to have some excess of total arch length can benefit from passive lingual arch therapy. A patient with mild incisor crowding in the mixed dentition had a predicted total excess of 0.2 mm (Figs. 6.1 and 6.2). A lower lingual holding arch was placed in the patient's mouth; his lower arch is shown in Figure 6.2 after the permanent canines and premolars had erupted. The patient illustrated in Figure 6.1 had a Class I occlusion; however, the same principles apply to patients with Class II and Class III malocclusions.

Prevalence of Incisor Crowding

The U.S. Public Health Service surveyed the incidence of incisor irregularity in a large sample of whites, blacks, and Mexican Americans from 1988 to 1991 (Tables 6.1 and 6.2) (Brunelle, Bhat, and Lipton 1996). About 25% of the sample had excellent incisor irregularity scores (a score of 0). About 20% of U.S. citizens between 8 and 50 years of age had incisor irregularity scores or 5 or greater. The remaining 55% of the population had incisor irregularity scores between 1 and 4. Unfortunately the Incisor Irregularity Index (Little 1975) does not directly correspond to the tooth size–arch length discrepancy (TSALD) measurement; nevertheless, we can probably assume a large number of the children with alignment scores between 1 and 4 can potentially benefit from appropriately timed placement of a lower passive lingual holding arch.

Table 6.2 summarizes the mean Incisor Irregularity Index scores by age, gender, and race in the maxilla and the mandible. Blacks had higher mean Incisor Irregularity Index scores than whites and Mexican Americans in upper and lower arches. In the mandibular arch, females had significantly lower irregularity scores than males.

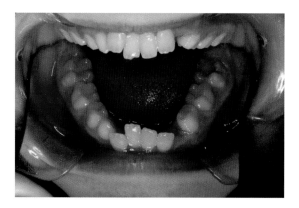

Figure 6.1. Iowa mixed-dentition analysis predicted an excess of 0.2 mm in the lower arch of this patient.

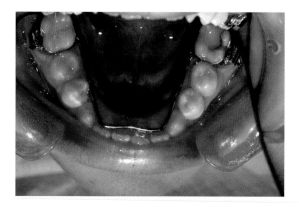

Figure 6.2. Lower lingual arch was placed and is shown after the eruption of the permanent canines and premolars.

Table 6.1. Incisor Irregularity Scores in Americans 8–50 Years Old

	Maxilla			Mandible	
mm	N	Percent	mm	N	Percent
0	1,699	24.6	0	1,718	21.9
1	1,609	23.2	1	1,451	20.5
2	1,095	16.7	2	1,190	16.9
3	702	9.6	3	742	10.9
4	535	8.4	4	586	9.2
5	321	6.0	5	368	5.9
6+	750	11.4	6+	983	14.7

From Brunelle, Bhat, and Lipton (1996).

Table 6.2. Incisor Irregularity Index Scores by Age, Gender, and Race of Americans Ages 8–50 Years Old[1]

		Age Groups (Mean [SE] in mm)		
	All Ages	8–11 Years	12–17 Years	18–50 Years
Maxillary alignment				
All persons*	2.4 (0.08)	1.7 (0.10)	2.4 (0.15)	2.6 (0.10)
Males	2.6 (0.10)	1.5 (0.17)	2.6 (0.18)	2.7 (0.12)
Females	2.3 (0.10)	1.9 (0.15)	2.1 (0.18)	2.4 (0.11)
Race/ethnicity				
Whites	2.5 (0.09)	1.7 (0.12)	2.2 (0.20)	2.6 (0.11)
Blacks	2.1 (0.13)†	1.6 (0.14)	2.2 (0.15)	2.2 (0.14)
Mexican Americans	2.6 (0.10)	1.9 (0.12)	3.0 (0.28)	2.7 (0.12)
Mandibular alignment				
All persons*	2.7 (0.07)	1.6 (0.14)	2.5 (0.15)	2.9 (0.09)
Males	2.9 (0.09)‡	1.5 (0.14)	2.8 (0.16)	3.1 (0.12)
Females	2.6 (0.09)	1.8 (0.19)	2.1 (0.21)	2.8 (0.10)
Race/ethnicity				
Whites	2.8 (0.07)	1.6 (0.17)	2.5 (0.20)	3.0 (0.09)
Blacks	2.2 (0.16)†	1.6 (0.15)	1.8 (0.20)	2.3 (0.17)
Mexican Americans	3.0 (0.11)	1.7 (0.13)	3.1 (0.17)	3.2 (0.13)

*Includes persons of "other" race/ethnicity designations.
†Blacks are different from whites and Mexican Americans, $p \leq 0.01$.
‡Males are different from females, $p < 0.01$.
[1]From Brunelle, Bhat, and Lipton 1996.

Premature Loss of a Primary Molar

Mixed-dentition patients who have crowding due to larger teeth and shorter and narrower arches are more susceptible to premature loss of a primary molar than are those who have adequate arch length and width to accommodate the permanent teeth (Ronnerman and Thilander 1978). Normal eruption may occur in children who lose a primary molar prematurely but who also have adequate arch lengths and widths.

To preserve needed arch length and prevent unnecessary crowding complications in those patients who have minimal to moderate crowding problems, clinicians must insert a passive lingual or palatal holding arch after the premature loss of a primary second molar. Premature loss of a primary first molar in the lower arch should also prompt the placement of a lower lingual arch in these patients (Northway 2000). If the unilateral premature loss of a primary molar is ignored, it may result in a bilateral asymmetry in arch length, leading to an asym-

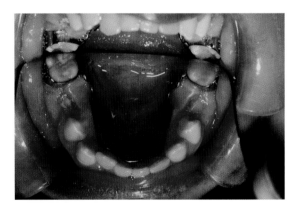

Figure 6.3. Loss of both primary second molars in a patient with minimal arch length deficiency prompted placement of a holding arch.

metric malocclusion in the permanent dentition. Intervention in the mixed dentition with a lingual or palatal holding arch may prevent the need for future orthodontic treatment or reduce the severity of a malocclusion.

A patient who lost his primary lower second molars is shown in Figures 6.3 and 6.4. Shortly

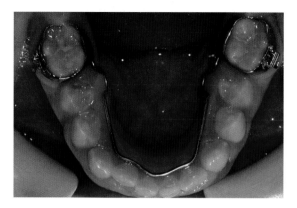

Figure 6.4. Lower arch after eruption of the second premolars.

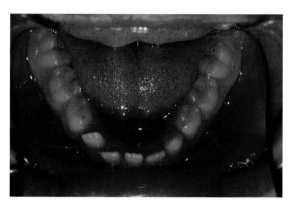

Figure 6.5. Ectopic eruption of the lower right lateral incisor forced the exfoliation of the right primary canine.

after the loss, a lower lingual holding arch was placed (Fig. 6.3). Orderly eruption of the permanent premolars is illustrated in Figure 6.4.

Asymmetric Loss of a Primary Canine

Patients who have an incisor liability and inadequate arch length in the anterior part of their arches often experience the asymmetric loss of a primary canine. As the permanent lateral incisors try to erupt, one of them can stimulate the resorption of the root of a primary canine. The unilateral loss of the canine not only provides arch length for the eruption of the lateral incisor but also causes a shift in the dental midline to the side of the lost canine. Clinicians who observe the early stages of this phenomenon can often prevent the midline shift by extracting the remaining primary canine. Once the dental midline is shifted away from the facial midline, the permanent teeth in the anterior part of the arch will retain this asymmetry. Intervention in the mixed dentition with a fixed appliance can correct the already shifted midline. The retained primary canine must be extracted to accomplish

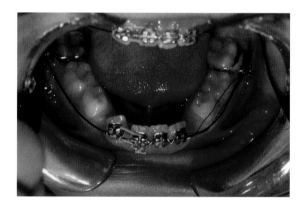

Figure 6.6. After extraction of the left primary canine, the lower incisors were moved leftward and centered on the lower arch.

the treatment. The corrected lower incisors are retained with a passive lower lingual arch that has spurs soldered on the wire to keep the incisors from shifting laterally until the permanent canines erupt. A Hawley retainer with wires on the distal surfaces of the lateral incisors

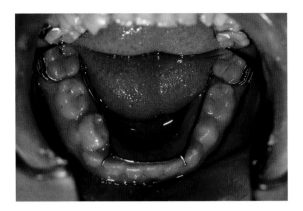

Figure 6.7. Lower lingual arch with spurs to hold the incisors from drifting is viewed when the spurs needed removal and the wire adjusted to allow eruption of the left first premolar.

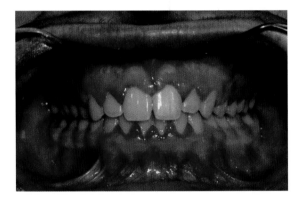

Figure 6.8. Teeth are seen after a fixed appliance, used in phase 2 treatment, was removed. The dental midlines were coincident.

had shifted 2 mm to the right of the facial midline. The maxillary dental midline was 1 mm to the left of the facial midline. His mixed-dentition analysis predicted an excess of 0.9 mm on the lower right side and 5.1 mm on the lower left side. In Figure 6.6, the edgewise fixed appliance used to correct the midline and align the lower incisors is shown. A lower lingual arch with soldered spurs, shown in Figure 6.7, was cemented after the incisors were aligned. Figure 6.8 shows coincident upper and lower dental midlines following phase 2 comprehensive orthodontic treatment of this patient during his adolescent years.

Nance Holding Arch

The Nance or palatal holding arch consists of two bands on the upper first molars connected by a wire with an acrylic pad that rests on the anterior palate. This passive appliance is used to maintain upper arch length when premature loss of a primary molar occurs or when maintenance of arch length is desired in a patient who has borderline arch length deficiency.

A patient who prematurely lost her upper right primary second molar is shown in Figures 6.9 through 6.12. Her upper right first molar drifted mesially into the arch space needed for the upper right second premolar. The mixed dentition analysis predicted a TSALD of −6.2 mm in the upper arch, with −5.8 mm of the discrepancy on the right side of the arch. A periapical radiograph of the upper right quadrant showing the crowding caused by the mesial tipping of the upper right first molar is shown in Figure 6.10. The edgewise fixed appliance used open space on the right side is shown in Figure 6.11. The upper left primary second molar crown spontaneously fractured because of a large restoration and was extracted during the orthodontic treatment. A palatal holding arch was cemented on the upper first molars as a retainer following treatment (Fig. 6.12). A laboratory prescription for a Nance holding arch is shown in Figure 6.13.

is used to retain the corrected incisors in the upper arch.

A patient with an ectopically erupted lower right lateral incisor that exfoliated the lower right primary canine is shown in Figures 6.5 through 6.8. The patient's lower dental midline

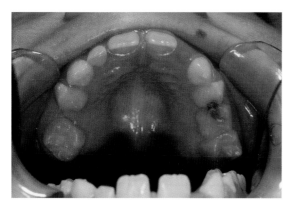

Figure 6.9. Upper right first molar has drifted mesially in response to the loss of the upper right primary second molar.

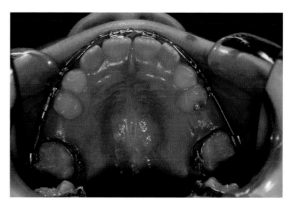

Figure 6.11. Upper right molar has been moved distally with a fixed appliance.

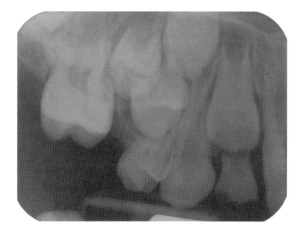

Figure 6.10. Radiograph showing the impaction of the upper right second premolar by the mesially malpositioned first molar.

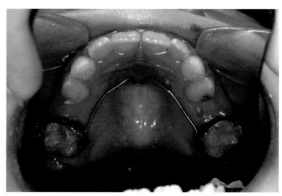

Figure 6.12. Nance palatal holding arch was placed in the upper arch to maintain arch length.

Doctor **A. Able**   No. **712**   Date **9-15-04**

Patient **Anne T. Zane**   No. **60**

Date Needed **9-22-04**   Time **1pm**

Rx

Please fabricate a
Maxillary Nance Holding Arch
with .036 rd wire soldered
to bands on 1st Molars and
a clear acrylic button.

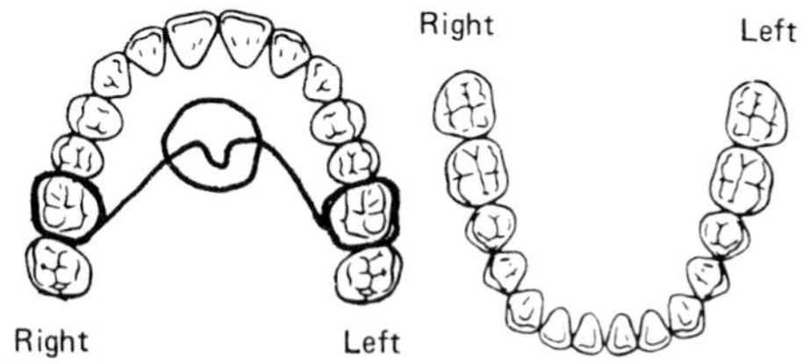

Right   Left

Right   Left

Material   Shade

For Lab Use Only

Instructor

Signature

Figure 6.13. Laboratory prescription for a Nance holding arch.

Trans-palatal Arch

An arch called the trans-palatal arch (TPA) consists of bands on the upper permanent first molars connected by a wire that passes over the palate and is soldered to the bands. When a TPA is used as a passive appliance, it will maintain arch width. The TPA is often used as a retainer following widening of the upper arch by an orthodontic appliance.

In Figure 6.14, a modified rapid maxillary expander is shown after expanding the maxillary arch in the mixed dentition of a male patient. A soldered TPA was cemented to the upper first molars to retain the expansion result for 1 year (Fig. 6.15). A laboratory prescription for a TPA is shown in Figure 6.16.

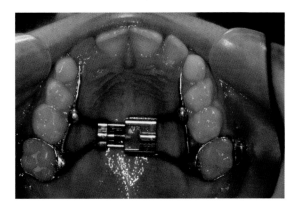

Figure 6.14. Modified rapid maxillary expander (RME) was used in this mixed-dentition patient to correct a posterior cross bite.

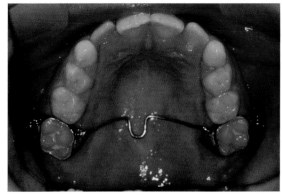

Figure 6.15. At removal of the RME, a soldered transpalatal arch was inserted as a retainer. Note the irritation of the palatal mucosa caused by the lateral arms of the expander.

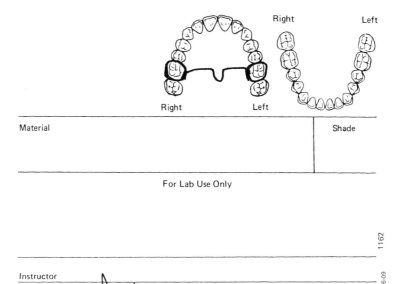

College of Dentistry
The University of Iowa
Department of Orthodontics

Doctor	A. Able	No. 712	Date 9-22-04
Patient	Billy Word		No. 101
Date Needed	9-29-04	Time	1:30 PM

R

Please fabricate a soldered
Transpalatal Arch Wire (TPA)
with .036 rd wire soldered
to 1st molar bands.

Right   Left

Right   Left

Material   Shade

For Lab Use Only

Instructor

Signature

1162
76010/6-09

Figure 6.16. Laboratory prescription for a trans-palatal arch.

Insertion of a Passive Lingual or Palatal Arch

A passive arch must not rotate or move the molars in either a lingual or buccal direction. A passive arch must not move the incisors labially or the molars distally. A passive lower arch also cannot be too short; otherwise, it will lose, rather than maintain, arch length. The passive arch should not interfere with the occlusion or with the eruption of teeth. A passive arch should not irritate soft tissues.

Before cementation of the lower lingual arch, see that it fits passively around the molars and that the wire rests on the lingual surfaces of the lower incisors midway between their incisal edges and gingival margins. Placing loops in the arch wire allow the clinician to adapt the wire to the lingual surfaces of the lower incisors before cementing the bands. When cementing a lower lingual arch, settle the bands onto the molars and bring the wire into contact with the lingual surfaces of the incisors by pushing down on the mesial margins of the bands. Pushing too much on the distal margins of the bands during cementation will lift the wire up and out of contact with the lingual surfaces of the incisors.

When inserting the Nance holding arch, check its fit on the molars and be careful that the acrylic pad touches gently on the palatal soft tissues. The acrylic pad should rest on a large area of the palate to provide adequate anchorage to keep the upper first molars from tipping forward. Polishing the acrylic button on the surface that contacts the palatal tissues will reduce the possibility of irritation to palatal soft tissues. Impaction of food beneath the acrylic pad can cause soft tissue irritation. Dental floss can be used to clean debris between the acrylic pad and the palatal mucosa when the appliance is cemented on the teeth. If palatal soft tissues beneath the acrylic button become markedly irritated, then the appliance must be removed.

When a passive lingual or palatal arch is removed prematurely due to some problem, it should be replaced as soon as possible to avoid loss of arch length.

Fixed-Removable Lingual and Palatal Arches

A fixed-removable lingual arch consists of bands on the first molars that have attachments on their lingual surfaces for the insertion and removal of a lingual or palatal wire. These arches are used to move teeth. Adjustments in the shape of the wire can lengthen the arch by moving incisors forward and molars backward. Widening of the wire can move the molars and other posterior teeth buccally, thus increasing arch width and arch length. Constriction of the wire can move the molars lingually when this would improve a posterior crossbite problem. The appliance can also rotate upper or lower molars. The Wilson 3D Lingual Arch is shown in Figures 6.17 and 6.18. A close-up view of the lower left molar band shows the two vertical tubes into which the removable arch wire fits (Fig. 6.18). An optional spring is shown on the left side that can be used to tip backward the lower second molar.

The construction, insertion, and adjustment of fixed-removable lingual arches require great skill, so that the appliance does not move the teeth in an undesirable manner. The appliances can tip the teeth not banded as well as tip and torque the banded molars. The rule at the beginning of the insertion is that the appliance is first fitted passively in the tubes on the lingual surfaces of the molar bands. After the wire fits passively, then it is adjusted to deliver the tooth moving force. When fitted passively in the molar band tubes, these appliances can be used for space and arch dimension maintenance.

Figures 6.19 through 6.22 show how a removable lower lingual arch moved tooth #23 into proper alignment. The mixed-dentition analysis predicted a −0.6 mm TSALD. Tooth #23 erupted lingually to the line of arch (Fig. 6.19). The lower removable lingual arch that moved tooth #23 labially is shown in Figure 6.20. The removable arch was inserted into horizontal tubes welded on the lingual surfaces of each molar (Fig. 6.21). Loops in the wire mesial to the molar bands were opened gradually to move forward both lower lateral incisors. Shaving the mesial surfaces of the primary canines, or extracting them, as was done for this patient, would create arch length for aligning the incisors. Positioning the anterior wire on the cingula of the lower incisors applies the force closer to the centers of resistance of the lower incisors for optimum movement of the teeth. The aligned incisors are shown after treatment ended when a soldered lingual arch had replaced the removable lingual arch (Fig. 6.22).

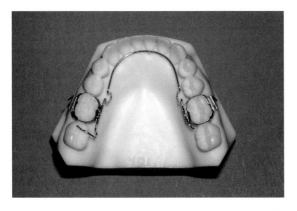

Figure 6.17. Wilson 3D Lingual Arch is a fixed-removable lingual arch shown with an optional spring to upright a lower second molar (Rocky Mountain Orthodontics).

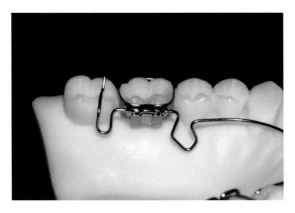

Figure 6.18. Removable Wilson Arch wire fits into two vertical tubes welded on the lingual surface of the molar band.

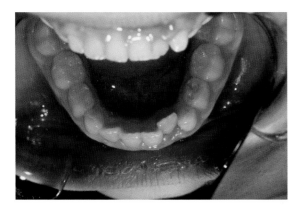

Figure 6.19. This patient had a lingually displaced lower left lateral incisor and a rotated right lateral incisor.

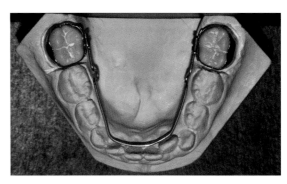

Figure 6.20. Fixed-removable lower lingual arch was made to move the lateral incisors into the arch. The lower primary canines were extracted.

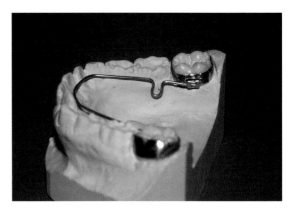

Figure 6.21. Removable lingual wire fit into a horizontal tube welded on the lingual surface of the molar band.

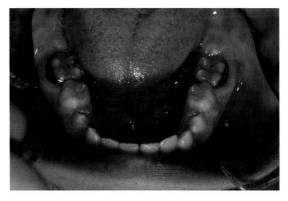

Figure 6.22. Removable lingual arch was replaced by a fixed lingual arch, seen here after the eruption of canines and first premolars.

Undesirable Side Effects of Passive and Active Lingual and Palatal Arches

Banded molars can be rotated, moved buccally and lingually, extruded on one side, and intruded on the other side in ways that are not desired. Passive arches will actually be quite active, if the bands were dislodged when the working cast was poured. Bending of the lingual arch wire prior to its cementation can move teeth in ways that are not intended. Lower incisors can be moved forward and intruded when appropriate adjustments are not made to the wire prior to cementation or during the cementation of a passive arch. Periodic observation of patients is essential whenever a lingual arch is placed in their mouth. If undesirable tooth movements are detected at recall visits, the problem can be corrected by adjusting or remaking the lingual arch appliance.

The lower lingual arch shown in Figure 6.23 unintentionally rotated the patient's lower first molars. A patient whose lower lingual arch was interfering with the eruption of her lower right canine is shown in Figures 6.24 through 6.26. The soldered lower lingual arch shown in Figure 6.24 is deflecting the eruption of the lower right canine. A new fixed-removable lower lingual arch was placed in the mouth with 18-mil-diameter finger springs soldered to the wire to move the erupting canines buccally (Fig. 6.25). The lower arch is shown after the alignment of the canines in Figure 6.26.

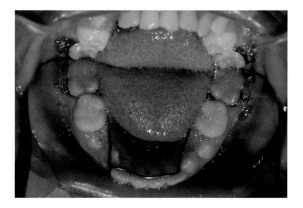

Figure 6.24. This lower lingual arch is deflecting the erupting right canine in a lingual direction.

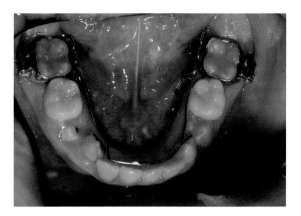

Figure 6.25. Fixed-removable lower lingual arch was made with two 18 mil finger springs soldered to the 36 mil lingual wire in order to push the erupting canines buccally.

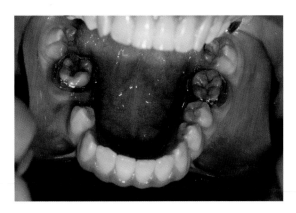

Figure 6.23. This lingual arch inadvertently rotated the lower right first molar.

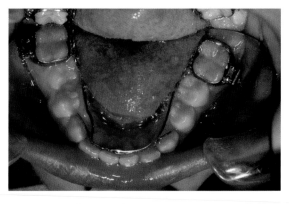

Figure 6.26. After several adjustments of the finger springs, each adjustment requiring removal of the lingual arch, the canines moved buccally.

Laboratory Prescription and Construction of a Lower Loop Lingual Arch

A laboratory prescription form is shown with instructions to the technician in Figure 6.27. A written description of the appliance includes wire type and size. The lingual arch is drawn on the form. The lingual arch wire is stainless steel (ss) in a diameter of 36-thousandths of an inch (0.036) or 36 mil.

Figures 6.28 through 6.51 illustrate the laboratory construction of a lower loop lingual arch.

College of Dentistry
The University of Iowa
Department of Orthodontics

Doctor A. Able   No. 712   Date 10-20-04

Patient Annie Body   No. 1834

Date Needed 10-27-04 Time 4:30 PM

℞

Please fabricate a soldered lower lingual holding arch (LLHA) using .036 rd ss wire with adjustment loops mesial to permanent 1st molars

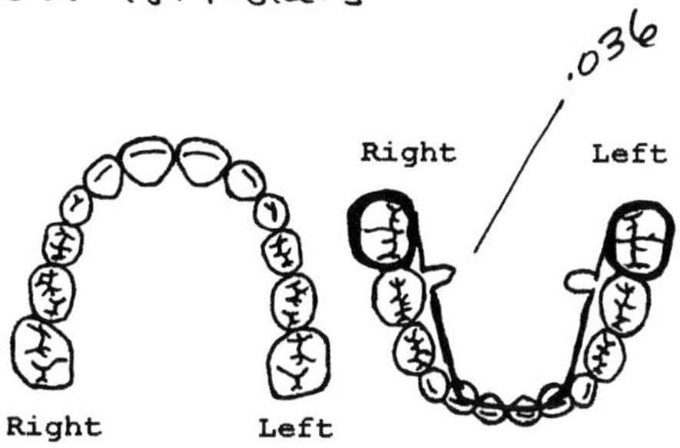

.036

Right / Left

Right   Left

Material	Shade

For Lab Use Only

Instructor

Signature

76010/6-09

Figure 6.27. Laboratory prescription form for a lower lingual arch with adjustment loops.

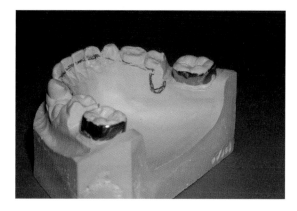

Figure 6.28. Pencil outline of lingual wire drawn on cast.

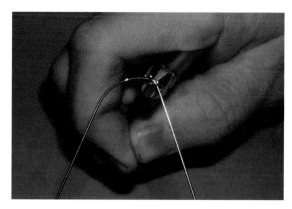

Figure 6.31. Bend the wire with a three-prong pliers.

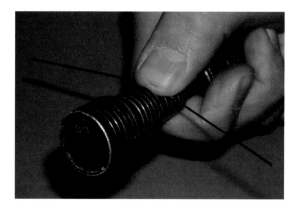

Figure 6.29. Place a parabolic bend in the 36-mil wire with a wire-bending turret or any suitable cylinder.

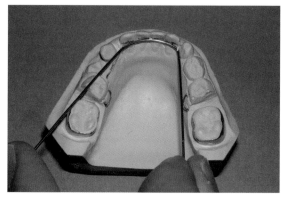

Figure 6.32. Fit the wire on the cast and mark it to bend the left side of the wire.

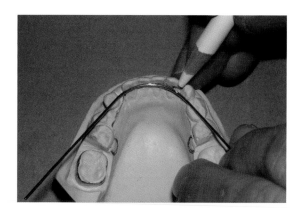

Figure 6.30. Mark wire at midline and 2 to 3 mm back from the distal contact of the lateral incisor.

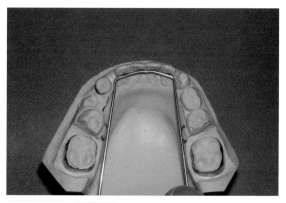

Figure 6.33. Mark the wire to bend it to better fit the lingual surface of the lateral incisors.

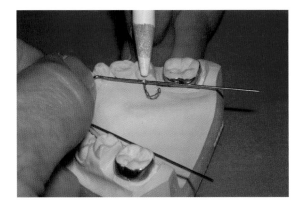

Figure 6.34. Mark the wire to bend the loop.

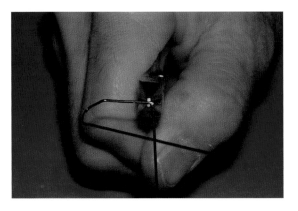

Figure 6.35. Bend the loop with bird beak (No. 139) pliers, keeping the wire slightly away from the lingual soft tissues.

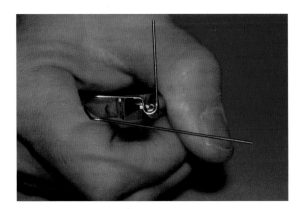

Figure 6.36. Finish the loop with the No. 139 pliers.

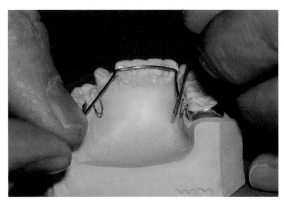

Figure 6.37. Loop is angled slightly away from the lingual tissues.

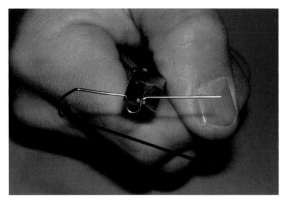

Figure 6.38. Bend the wire toward the band with the No. 139 pliers.

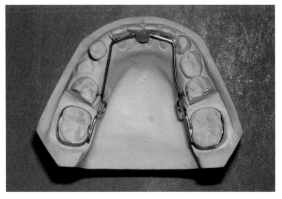

Figure 6.39. Fabricated arch wire is held in position with a small bead of wax.

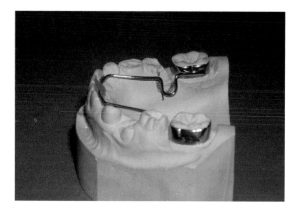

Figure 6.40. Ends of the arch wire are centered on the lingual surfaces of the bands.

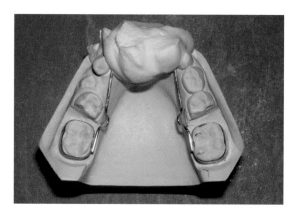

Figure 6.41. Plaster is placed on the anterior portion of the wire to stabilize it during soldering.

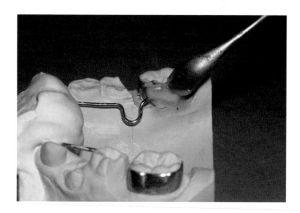

Figure 6.42. Wire and band are coated with flux.

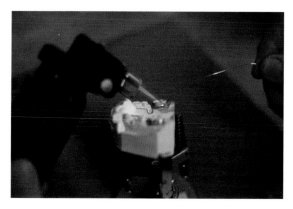

Figure 6.43. Solder is melted over the wire and band with a butane torch.

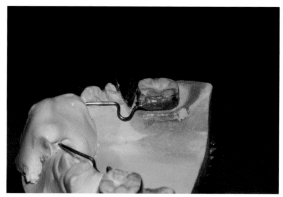

Figure 6.44. Finished solder joint covers the wire but does not flow onto the mesial or distal band surfaces. A knife is used to remove the appliance from the cast.

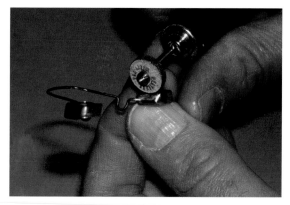

Figure 6.45. Begin finishing with a rough stone to remove excess solder.

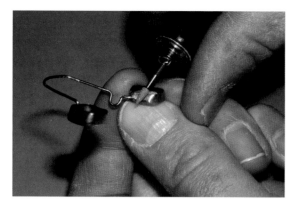

Figure 6.46. Use a small green stone to smooth solder joints.

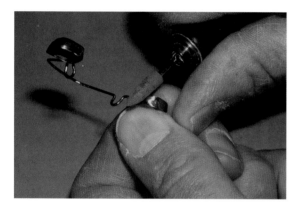

Figure 6.47. Use a rubber point to remove heavy scratches left by the green stone.

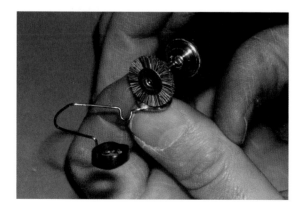

Figure 6.48. Use a brush with Tripoli to reduce rubber point scratches.

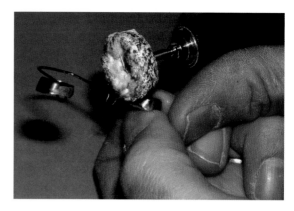

Figure 6.49. Finish with a rag wheel and rouge for high polish.

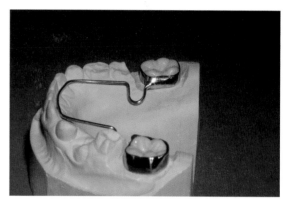

Figure 6.50. Side view of the completed lingual arch: solder covers the wire and is polished, and loop has proper width and height.

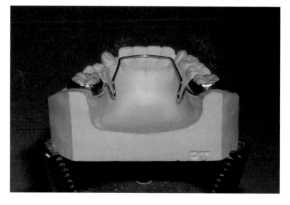

Figure 6.51. Posterior view of the completed lingual arch: the wire is above the cingula of the incisors, and loops are angled away from the tissues.

Failure of a Lower Lingual Arch

The wire may break because of repeated bending of the wire due to mastication or manipulation by the tongue. Some patients push the anterior wire upward with the tongue, effectively ending its usefulness. When chewing forces act over a long time, the wire usually breaks near the solder joint holding the wire on the molar bands. During soldering, the heat anneals the wire near the solder joint, creating a weakness in the wire. Two patients with broken wires are shown in Figures 6.52 through 6.55. In Figure 6.52, the broken lingual arch is shown from the front. The lingual arch appears to be intact and in contact with the lower incisors. In Figure 6.53, a break in the lingual arch is observed on the left side just mesial to the solder joint. Another patient is shown from the front in Figure 6.54. In this patient, the break at the right solder joint allowed the anterior wire to disengage from the lower incisors (Fig. 6.54). A photograph of the broken lingual arch is shown after its removal from the mouth in Figure 6.55.

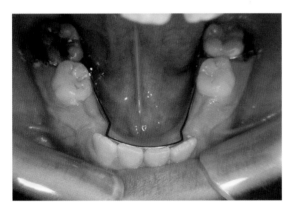

Figure 6.52. Occlusal view of a patient with a broken lingual arch.

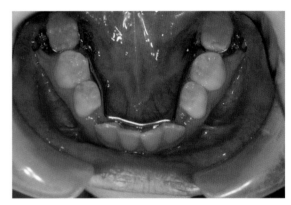

Figure 6.54. Occlusal view of a patient with a broken lingual arch.

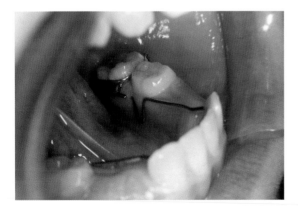

Figure 6.53. Lingual view of wire broken mesial to the left molar band.

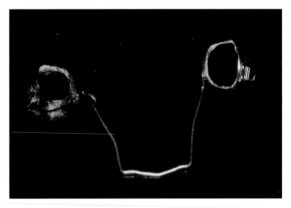

Figure 6.55. View of the removed lingual arch showing the wire broken at a failed solder joint on the right molar.

REFERENCES

Brennan, M. M., and Gianelly, A. A. 2000. The use of the lingual arch in the mixed dentition to resolve incisor crowding. Am. J. Orthod. Dentofac. Orthop. 117:81–85.

Brunelle, J. A., Bhat, M., and Lipton, J. A. 1996. Prevalence and distribution of selected occlusal characteristics in the U.S. population, 1988–1991. J. Dent. Res. 75(Spec. Issus):706–713.

Dugoni, S., Lee, J. S., Valera, J., and Dugoni, A. 1995. Early mixed dentition treatment: post-retention evaluation of stability and relapse. Angle Orthod. 65:311–319.

Little, R. M. 1975. The Irregularity Index: a quantitative score of mandibular anterior alignment. Am. J. Orthod. 68:554–563.

Moorrees, C. F. A., and Chadha, J. M. 1965. Available space for the incisors during dental development. Angle Orthod. 35:12–22.

Northway, W. M. 2000. The not so harmless maxillary primary first molar extraction. J. Am. Dent. Assoc. 131:1711–1720.

Ronnerman, A., and Thilander, B. 1978. Facial and dental arch morphology in children with and without early loss of deciduous molars. Am. J. Orthod. 73:47–58.

Management of Anterior Crossbites

7

Prevalence of Anterior Crossbite Malocclusions

The U.S. Public Health Service surveyed the incidence of anterior crossbites in a large sample of whites, blacks, and Mexican Americans from 1988 to 1991 (Brunelle, Bhat, and Lipton 1996).

The subjects examined ranged from 8 to 50 years old. Subjects with zero overjet totaled 4.4% of the sample. Subjects having from –1 to –4 mm of anterior crossbite totaled 0.8% of the sample. The percentage of potential patients who need treatment for this malocclusion problem is about 5% (Table 7.1).

Table 7.1. Distribution of Overjet among Americans Ages 8 to 50 Years, 1988–1991*

	Overjet (mm)	Percent of Persons	Cumulative Percent
Mandibular incisors	–4	0.3	0.3
	–3	0.1	0.4
	–2	0.1	0.5
	–1	0.3	0.8
Maxillary incisors	0	4.4	5.2
	1	14.0	19.2
	2	25.9	45.1
	3	23.7	68.8
	4	15.2	84.0
	5	7.7	91.7
	6+	8.3	100.0

*From Brunelle, Bhat, and Lipton (1996).

Essentials of Orthodontics: Diagnosis and Treatment
by Robert N. Staley and Neil T. Reske
© 2011 Blackwell Publishing Ltd.

Angle Classification

Observe the Angle Classification of the molars and canines. The best candidates for minor orthodontic treatment are those with a Class I molar and canine occlusion or a super Class I occlusion in centric occlusion in association with a forward anteroposterior shift from centric relation to centric occlusion.

Centric Relation to Centric Occlusion Functional Shift on Closure

Examine the patient who has an anterior crossbite for any evidence of a forward anteroposterior shift during closure of the mandible. Ask the patient if he can touch the incisal edges of his upper and lower incisor teeth together, in order to determine whether a forward shift is taking place. If the patient's mandible shifts forward during closure from centric relation to centric occlusion, correction of the anterior crossbite will result in a posterior displacement of the mandible. If the patient with a forward shift has Class I molars in centric occlusion, correction of the anterior crossbite will eliminate the forward shift and tend to make the molar occlusion end-to-end. If the patient with a forward shift has a Class II molar relationship in centric occlusion, treatment of the crossbite will eliminate the shift and tend to make the molar occlusion more severely Class II. If the patient with a forward shift has a Class III molar relationship in centric occlusion, treatment of the crossbite will eliminate the forward shift and tend to make the molar relation less severely Class III. For patients who have an anterior crossbite associated with a forward anteroposterior shift, a slightly super Class I molar occlusion in centric occlusion before treatment is most desirable, because correction of the anterior crossbite would eliminate the shift and tend to alter the molar occlusion to Class I.

If no forward anteroposterior shift is present, the molar relationship will not change as a result of the crossbite treatment, making the diagnosis and treatment more straightforward.

Overbite

Moderate to deep overbite of the incisors is a favorable condition for successful treatment of an anterior crossbite, because the deeper overlap of the incisors will help retain the incisors brought out of crossbite. A removable appliance with a posterior acrylic bite block is needed in deep overbite patients to allow an appliance to move the upper incisors forward out of crossbite. Normal to deep overbite patients can be treated with both removable and fixed appliances. Because removable appliances have less control of the teeth than fixed appliances, removable appliances are best suited for patients whose teeth need to move short distances and are not rotated.

When a patient has little overbite or an anterior openbite, correction of the crossbite will require extrusion of the upper and perhaps lower incisors after the crossbite is corrected, in order to establish normal overbite. Without any overbite at the end of treatment, the upper incisor(s) can easily relapse into a crossbite. A maxillary Hawley retainer is needed to keep the tooth from relapsing back into crossbite. As an upper incisor is tipped forward with either a removable or a edgewise fixed appliance, its change in labial-lingual inclination tends to move the incisal edge upward (vertically), which in turn opens the bite. The finger spring of a removable appliance will often intrude the upper incisor as it pushes the crown forward, an action that also opens the bite. For these reasons, an edgewise fixed appliance is the best appliance for treating patients who have minimal overbite or frank anterior openbite. An edgewise appliance can move an incisor forward and also extrude it as needed to create overbite. Even then, the retention of the crossbite is a long-term concern. Patients with a frank anterior openbite should be referred to a specialist.

Adequate Arch Length

A tooth in crossbite cannot be moved out of crossbite, if the existing space in the arch cannot accommodate the tooth. If arch length is insufficient, the first priority in treatment is to create sufficient arch length. In minimal arch length deficiencies, shaving off a little enamel from the tooth itself and its surrounding teeth may be adequate. No more than 0.2 or 0.3 mm should be removed from a permanent tooth. Larger amounts of interproximal enamel can be removed from primary teeth that will eventually exfoliate. If spaces exist between other anterior teeth, these spaces should be closed to create adequate arch length and accommodate the tooth in crossbite. As arch length deficiency increases, it is more likely that a fixed orthodontic appliance will be needed to accomplish the treatment.

Spaces can be opened between teeth with finger springs mounted in a Hawley appliance and with compressed coil springs in the edgewise fixed appliance.

Inclination of Maxillary Incisor Roots

If the tooth in crossbite is positioned lingual to the line of arch (the line along the crest of an alveolar ridge that represents where the anatomic contact points of the teeth should be located ideally on that alveolar ridge) in the anterior palate, it will have to move a long distance to get it out of crossbite. The resulting increase of the labial-lingual inclination of the tooth will create a functional and aesthetic problem and increase the probability that the tooth will relapse back into crossbite. In order to correct the increased inclination problem, an edgewise fixed orthodontic appliance with a large rectangular arch wire must be used to torque the tooth and move its root labially into normal inclination. The farther a tooth in crossbite is positioned away from the line of arch, the more likely it is that the labial-lingual inclination of the tooth must be corrected with an edgewise fixed orthodontic appliance. The most appropriate teeth for minor treatment with a removable appliance are located a short distance from the line of arch.

Teeth most easily moved out of crossbite are those that are inclined lingually toward the palate. The orthodontic movement of these teeth during the correction of the crossbite should bring them into more normal inclination. Teeth that are inclined lingually are the best teeth to treat with a removable appliance.

Rotation of Tooth in Crossbite

If the tooth in crossbite is rotated on its long axis, a fixed orthodontic appliance is the most appropriate choice for treatment of the crossbite. Removable appliances cannot easily rotate teeth. A rotated tooth has a high potential for relapse following its treatment. When possible, a fixed retainer is bonded to the lingual surface of the rotated tooth and its surrounding teeth at the end of treatment in order to prevent the relapse of the rotation. When both central incisors are rotated prior to treatment, it is best to bond a fixed retainer to the lingual surfaces of both teeth to prevent relapse of the rotation after treatment.

Number of Teeth in Crossbite

The difficulty of the treatment increases with the increase in number of teeth in crossbite. When several anterior teeth are in crossbite, an edgewise fixed appliance provides the best treatment.

Alignment of Lower Anterior Teeth

Alignment of the lower anterior teeth, if needed, should be done after the crossbite problem has been corrected. Alignment of lower teeth before the crossbite is corrected will complicate the correction of the crossbite by increasing the distance required to move the upper teeth forward, and will delay the elimination of a functional shift, should one be present.

Treatment of Anterior Crossbites with Removable Appliances

A removable inclined plane (Bruckl appliance) can be used to correct anterior crossbites and

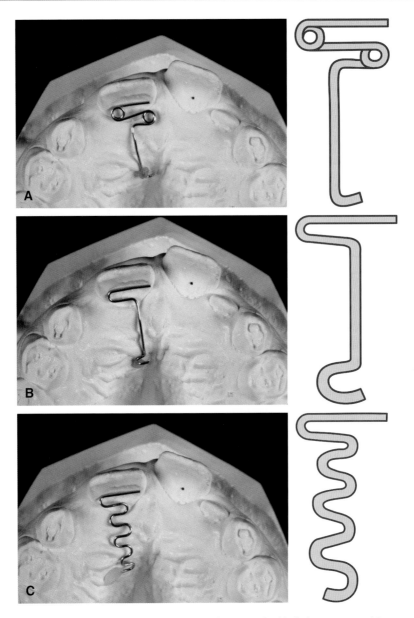

Figure 7.1. Finger springs used in the correction of anterior crossbites: (**A**) double helix or recurved finger spring, (**B**) question mark finger spring, (**C**) Z or S finger spring, (**D**) eyelet arm finger spring, and (**E**) mushroom finger spring.

retain the corrected occlusion (Jirgensone, Liepa, and Abeltins 2008).

A Hawley appliance can be used to correct an anterior crossbite (Hawley 1919). Several types of finger springs are shown in Figure 7.1. The double helical spring has a long range of action with reduced force (Fig. 7.1A). The question mark spring has a short range of action and a strong force (Fig. 7.1B). The Z or S spring has a long range of action and strong force (Fig. 7.1C). The eyelet arm spring is similar to the question mark spring (Fig. 7.1D). The mushroom spring

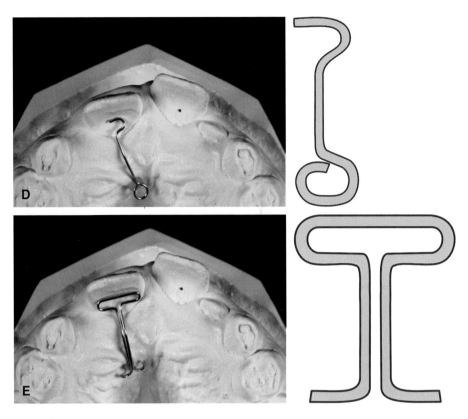

Figure 7.1. *Continued*

is a combination of two question mark springs and has a short range and strong force (Fig. 7.1E). The mushroom spring is often used to move posterior teeth buccally. All the finger springs are fabricated from 18-mil (0.018 inch) stainless steel; have a leg of wire, which is embedded in the acrylic body of the appliance; and are activated by extending the spring toward the incisor in crossbite. The springs are bent in the laboratory to adapt passively against the lingual surface of an incisor with the free end of the spring usually on the mesial side of the lingual surface. From this initial position, adjustments to activate the spring must keep the wire well adapted to the lingual surface of the incisor. To keep the spring against the lingual surface of the incisor, it is usually bent toward the cingulum as well as advanced forward. The force on the cingulum tends to intrude the incisor. The force needed to tip a tooth with a finger spring ranges

from 30 to 50 grams (Crabb and Wilson 1972). Small adjustments to activate the finger springs will produce forces in this range.

For the springs to work effectively, the appliance must have secure clasps, such as the Adams clasp, to keep the appliance anchored on the molars when the spring is activated against the incisor in crossbite (Adams 1984). If the clasps do not securely hold to the anchor teeth, activation of the finger spring will dislodge the appliance from the teeth. The patient must wear the appliance at all the times, except when eating.

The teeth in anterior crossbite usually have some degree of overbite. Posterior bite blocks are added to the Hawley appliance to open the bite enough to easily bring the incisor forward out of crossbite. After the crossbite is corrected, the posterior bite block should be reduced to permit normal occlusion of the upper and lower teeth. A Hawley retainer is then fabricated to hold the

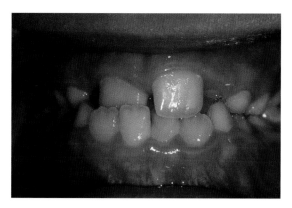

Figure 7.2. In centric occlusion, the patient's upper right central incisor is in crossbite.

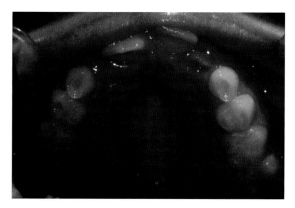

Figure 7.4. Upper right central incisor is inclined lingually, a favorable position.

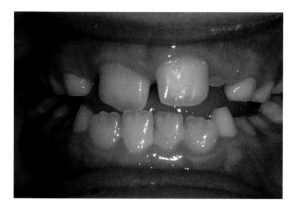

Figure 7.3. Upper and lower right central incisors touch in centric relation, evidence for an anterior functional shift.

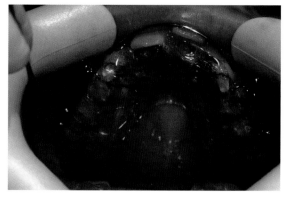

Figure 7.5. Maxillary Hawley appliance is shown with posterior bite blocks to open the bite to facilitate the labial movement of the upper right central incisor.

corrected tooth in its new position for about 1 year. After that, the retainer should be removed in mixed-dentition patients to allow for unimpeded growth of the maxilla. Older patients could continue to wear the retainer at night time, if needed.

A patient with an anterior crossbite is illustrated in Figure 7.2. His upper right central incisor was in lingual crossbite. The patient had super Class I molar relationships and could touch the incisal edges of his upper and lower right central incisors (Fig. 7.3). This upper right central incisor has two favorable conditions: (1) it is lingually inclined and (2) it has adequate room in the arch (Fig. 7.4). The Hawley appliance used

in the patient is shown in Figure 7.5. The posterior acrylic bite plates are visible in Figure 7.5. Double helical finger springs were placed lingual to tooth #8 and tooth #10. The finger spring lingual to #10, which was beginning to erupt, was made as a precaution in case #10 erupted into crossbite. The Hawley appliance is shown from the occlusal view on the working cast on which it was fabricated in Figure 7.6. The two palatal finger springs are clearly seen on the palatal side of the appliance (Fig. 7.7). Adams clasps on the first molars hold the appliance on the anchor teeth. The laboratory prescription for the Hawley appliance is shown in Figure 7.8. The

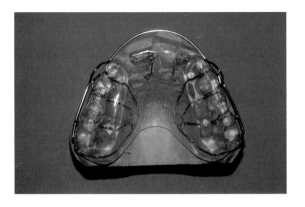 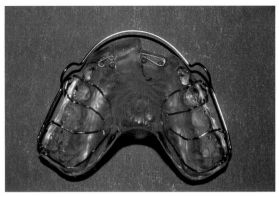

Figure 7.6. Hawley appliance is shown with two finger springs—one to move the right central incisor, the other to move the left lateral incisor if it erupts into crossbite.

Figure 7.7. View of the palatal side of the appliance shows the double helical finger springs and Adams clasps on the first primary and permanent molars.

College of Dentistry
The University of Iowa
Department of Orthodontics

Doctor **K.A. South** No. **81599** Date **10-21-04**

Patient **SISSY WACHTER** No. **91578**

Date Needed **10-28-04** Time **8 AM**

Rx **Please fabricate a Maxillary Modified Hawley with .032 labial bow soldered to .026 Adams Clasps on permanent 1st molars. Also use .026 Adams clasps on primary 1st molars and .018 double helical springs on tooth #8 and #10 to push them anteriorly out of crossbite. Include occlusal coverage on posterior teeth to open bite 3MM.**

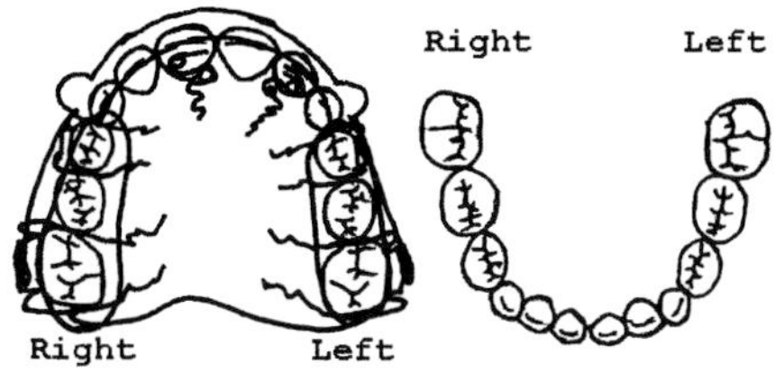

Right   Left

Right   Left

Material   Shade

For Lab Use Only

Instructor

Signature

76010/6-09

Figure 7.8. Laboratory prescription for a maxillary Hawley appliance to correct an anterior crossbite.

patient chose not to wear the appliance and subsequently discontinued treatment.

Treatment of Anterior Crossbites with Fixed Appliances

The correction of an anterior crossbite by opening the bite with glass ionomer cement has been reported (Tzatzakis and Gidarakou 2008). Glass ionomer cement is built up on the occlusal surfaces of the mandibular first molars or primary second molars sufficiently to create a transient anterior openbite. The authors reported that the primary and permanent teeth in crossbite moved quickly into normal position.

The use of a bonded compomer bite plane to correct an anterior crossbite has been reported (Croll and Helpin 2002).

Edgewise fixed appliances using nickel titanium arch wires can rapidly correct an anterior crossbite in conjunction with either a lower posterior acrylic bite plate or glass ionomer cement on the occlusal surfaces of the lower molars to open the bite sufficiently to easily move the upper incisor out of crossbite (Skeggs and Sandler 2002).

A patient with her upper right lateral incisor in crossbite is shown in Figure 7.9. The patient's first molars were in Class I occlusion and no anteroposterior shift was detected. The position of the lateral incisor in crossbite is shown from the occlusal view in Figure 7.10. The incisor is inclined lingually, a favorable finding. However, arch length is inadequate locally by about 0.8 mm. This amount of arch length can be gained by shaving enamel off the mesial surface of the upper right primary canine (Fig. 7.10). A fixed edgewise appliance was placed on the upper permanent first molars and permanent incisors (Fig. 7.11). Before the fixed appliance was placed on the teeth, a posterior acrylic bite plate was fabricated and placed in the lower arch and was equilibrated into even occlusion on both sides of the arches (Fig. 7.11). The lower posterior bite plate facilitated the unimpeded labial movement of tooth #7.

An effective mechanic to move tooth #7 consisted of an 18-mil nickel titanium arch wire tied

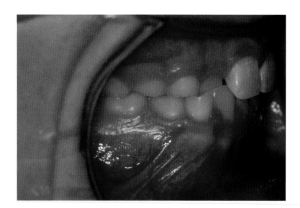

Figure 7.9. This patient's upper right lateral incisor was in crossbite.

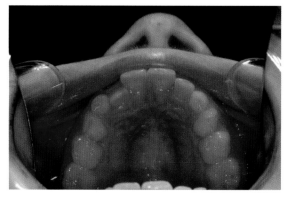

Figure 7.10. Deficiency in arch length for the lateral incisor required removal of enamel from the mesial surface of the right primary canine.

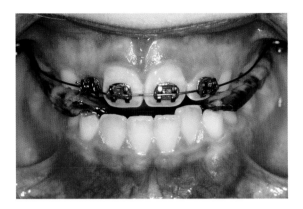

Figure 7.11. Edgewise fixed appliance in conjunction with a removable acrylic lower bite plate were used to correct the crossbite.

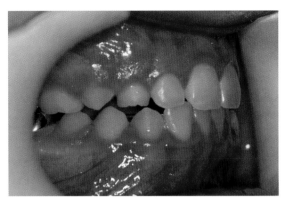

Figure 7.13. Lateral incisor is shown after removal of the fixed appliance.

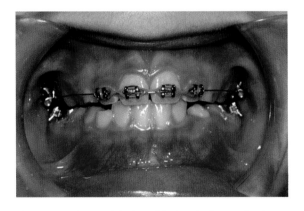

Figure 7.12. Upper right lateral incisor is shown after it was moved out of crossbite.

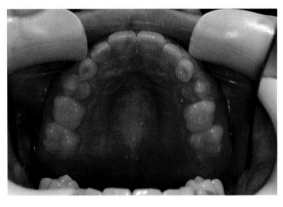

Figure 7.14. Lateral incisor is properly aligned in the upper arch.

into the braces with stainless steel ligatures on teeth #7, #8, #9, and #10. The patient is shown after the correction of the crossbite in Figure 7.12. A lower lingual arch was placed to move the lower left lateral incisor out into the arch from its lingual position (Fig. 7.12, lower bands visible). The occlusion is shown after the appliance was removed in Figure 7.13. After treat-ment, the upper right lateral incisor is nicely positioned along the upper arch (Fig. 7.14). Placement of a Hawley retainer to be worn for about 1 year is an essential part of the treatment. A guide for retainer wear is full-time for 6 months and nighttime wear thereafter. A laboratory pre-scription for the fabrication of the lower acrylic bite plate is shown in Figure 7.15.

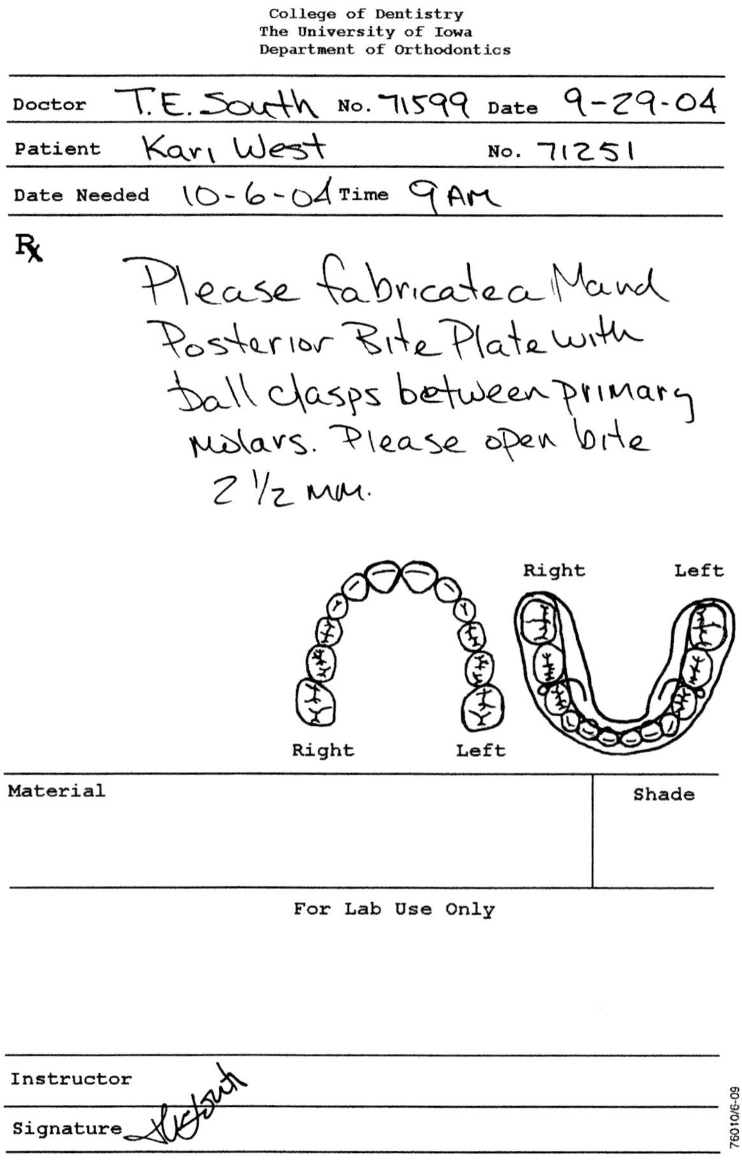

College of Dentistry
The University of Iowa
Department of Orthodontics

Doctor   T.E. South   No. 71599   Date   9-29-04

Patient   Kari West   No. 71251

Date Needed   10-6-04   Time   9 AM

℞

Please fabricate a Mand
Posterior Bite Plate with
ball clasps between primary
molars. Please open bite
2 ½ mm.

Right   Left

Right   Left

Material | Shade

For Lab Use Only

Instructor

Signature

76010/6-09

Figure 7.15. Laboratory prescription for a lower acrylic posterior bite plate.

Construction of a Removable Maxillary Appliance to Close a Diastema and Correct a Lateral Incisor in Crossbite

The construction of the appliance is illustrated in Figures 7.16 through 7.27. A double helical coil spring will move the upper left lateral incisor out of crossbite. Steps in the bending of the helical spring are illustrated in Figures 7.28 through 7.43. The first helix is bent counterclockwise upward from the cast surface, and the second helix is bent clockwise downward to the cast surface (Fig. 7.38). Closure of the diastema between the central incisors by moving tooth #9

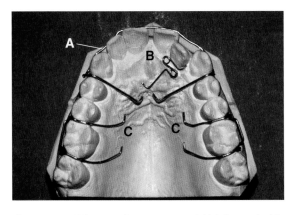

Figure 7.16. Wires on the cast are a labial bow, double helical finger spring, and Adams clasps on the first molars.

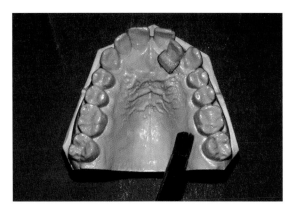

Figure 7.19. Separating medium is applied to the cast.

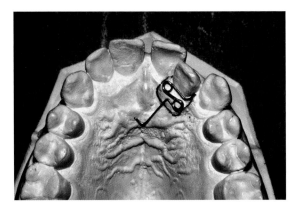

Figure 7.17. Double helical coil spring touches the cingulum of the incisor.

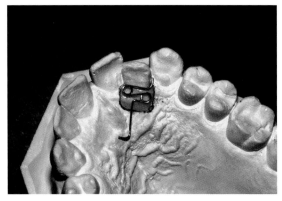

Figure 7.20. Helical coil spring is positioned on wax.

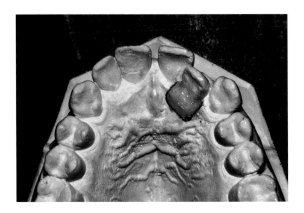

Figure 7.18. Layer of wax 0.5 mm thick is placed on the cast beneath the helical coil spring.

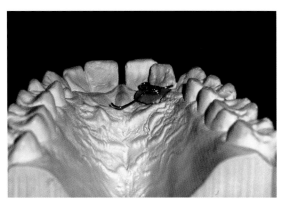

Figure 7.21. Helical coil spring is positioned away from the palatal surface 0.5 mm.

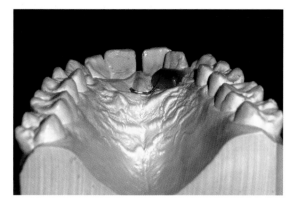

Figure 7.22. Coil spring is covered by 0.5 mm of wax, except for its retention that will be embedded in acrylic.

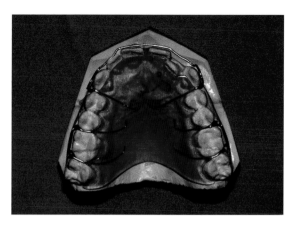

Figure 7.25. Acrylic body is polished on its tongue side, not on the side facing the palatal mucosa.

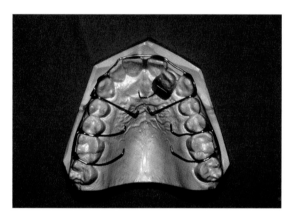

Figure 7.23. Labial bow and Adams clasps are held in position by wax.

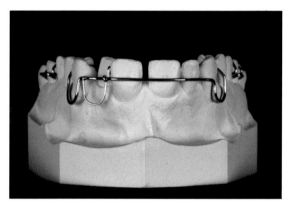

Figure 7.26. Loop spring is soldered on the labial bow to close the diastema between the central incisors.

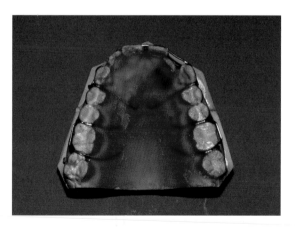

Figure 7.24. Acrylic resin is sprinkled on the cast to form the body of the appliance.

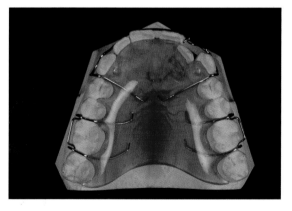

Figure 7.27. Completed appliance is shown.

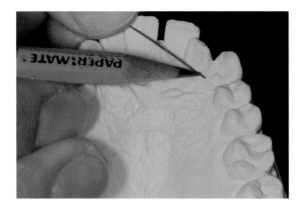

Figure 7.28. An 18-mil stainless steel wire is marked for the first bend of a double helical finger spring.

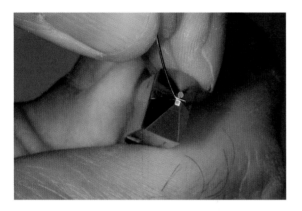

Figure 7.29. First bend is made around the rounded beak of No. 139 pliers.

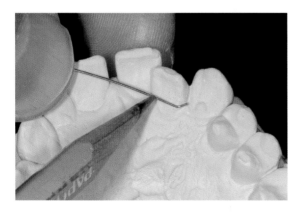

Figure 7.30. Wire is marked for bending the first helical coil spring.

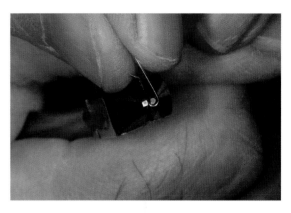

Figure 7.31. Begin the first coil of the first helix by bending the wire around the round beak of the pliers and above the wire that engages the tooth surface.

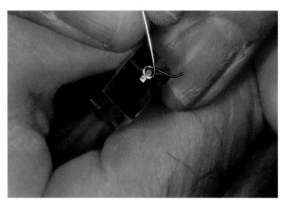

Figure 7.32. Reposition the pliers to continue forming the first coil of the first helix. Keep the helical coil parallel with the wire arm that engages the tooth surface.

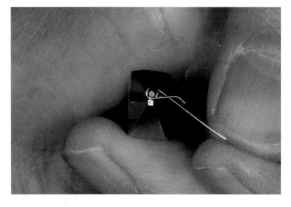

Figure 7.33. Complete the second coil of the first helical spring.

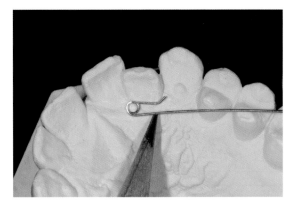

Figure 7.34. Wire is marked for bending the second helical coil spring.

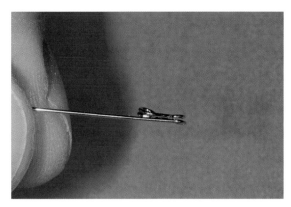

Figure 7.37. Wires forming the two helices are parallel and compact in the vertical plane.

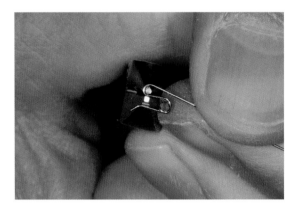

Figure 7.35. First coil of the second helix is bent around the rounded pliers' beak and below the wire arm that engages the tooth surface.

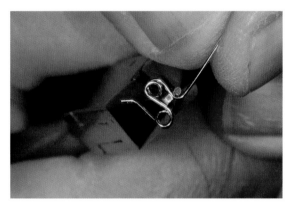

Figure 7.38. Bend the wire to form the retention arm.

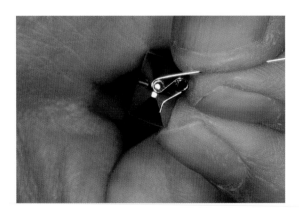

Figure 7.36. Second coil of the second helix is formed.

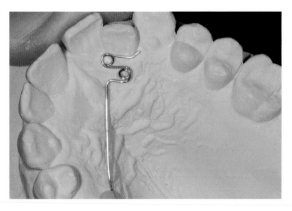

Figure 7.39. Mark the wire for the loop at the end of the retention arm.

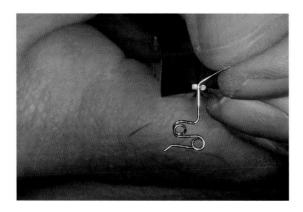

Figure 7.40. Bend the loop in the retention arm.

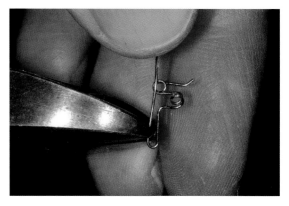

Figure 7.42. Cut the excess wire from the retention arm.

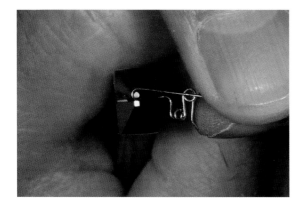

Figure 7.41. Finish bending the loop in the retention arm.

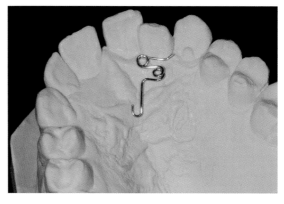

Figure 7.43. Completed double helical coil spring adapted to the cast.

into contact with tooth #8 will create the arch length needed to move the upper left lateral incisor into the arch. The double helical spring is activated by inserting the round beak of a No. 139 pliers in the helix nearest the incisor and unwinding the helix. To keep the part of the spring lying against the lingual surface of the incisor in full contact with the tooth, the second coil spring is also unwound sufficiently to ensure the spring arm will exert its force in the appropriate direction against the lingual surface of the lateral incisor. Incremental adjustments are small so that the force from the spring does not over-power the ability of the Adams clasps to hold the appliance on the teeth.

A loop or arc spring formed from 18-mil stainless steel wire is soldered onto the labial bow to move the left central incisor into contact with the right central incisor (Fig. 7.26). Steps in the construction of the loop spring are shown in Figure 7.44. Bending of the spring is illustrated in Figure 7.44A–C. Electrosoldering is illustrated in Figure 7.44E. The loop is activated by opening it with the flat beak of the No. 139 pliers in small incremental adjustments. A laboratory prescription for this appliance is shown in Figure 7.45.

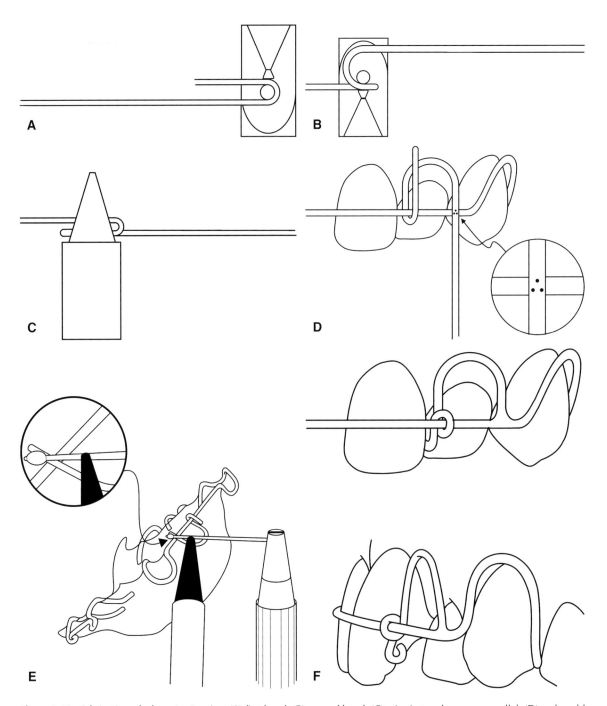

Figure 7.44. Fabrication of a loop (arc) spring: (**A**) first bend, (**B**) second bend, (**C**) wire in two loops are parallel, (**D**) tack weld the loops to the labial bow wire, (**E**) the looped wire is soldered to the labial bow, (**F**) front and side views of the finished spring (Loop design and construction steps courtesy of James P. Vance, C.D.T.).

College of Dentistry
The University of Iowa
Department of Orthodontics

Doctor A. Able No. 712 Date 10-20-04

Patient Annie Bodie No. 83

Date Needed 10-27-04 Time 4:30 P.M.

℞

Please fabricate a Max Hawley with .030 labial bow canine to canine. Use .026 rd SS wire for Adams Clasps on 1st Molars, a .018 double helix spring on tooth #10 to push facially and a .018 arch spring soldered to labial bow to close diastema between #8 + #9

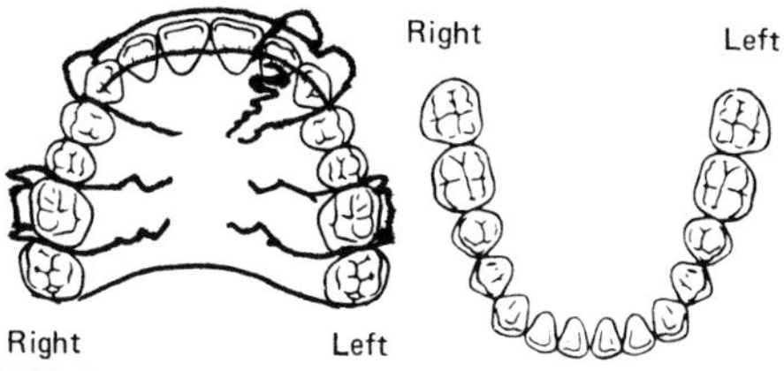
Right
Left
Right
Left

Material

Shade

For Lab Use Only

1162

Instructor

Signature

76010/6-09

Figure 7.45. Laboratory prescription for the Hawley appliance with finger and loop springs.

REFERENCES

Adams, C. P. 1984. The design, construction & use of removable orthodontic appliances. Bristol: John Wright & Sons Ltd.

Brunelle, J. A., Bhat, M., and Lipton, J. A. 1996. Prevalence and distribution of selected occlusal characteristics in the U.S. population, 1988–1991. J. Dent. Res. 75(Spec. Issue):706–713.

Crabb, J. J., and Wilson, H. J. 1972. The relation between orthodontic spring force and space closure. Dent. Pract. 22:233–240.

Croll, T. P., and Helpin, M. L. 2002. Simplified anterior cross bite correction using a bonded compomer bite plane. J. Clin. Orthod. 36:356–358.

Jirgensone, I., Liepa, A., and Abeltins, A. 2008. Anterior cross bite correction in primary and mixed dentition with removable inclined plane (Bruckl appliance). Stomatologija 10:140–144.

Hawley, C. A. 1919. A removable retainer. Int. J. Orthod. Oral Surg. 2:291–298.

Skeggs, R. M., and Sandler, P. J. 2002. Rapid correction of anterior cross bite using a fixed appliance: a case report. Dent. Update 29:299–302.

Tzatzakis, V., and Gidarakou, I. K. 2008. A new clinical approach for the treatment of anterior cross bites. World J. Orthod. 9:355–365.

Management of Posterior Crossbites

8

Definition of Posterior Crossbite

In normal occlusion, the buccal surfaces of the upper posterior teeth project farther buccally than the buccal surfaces of the lower posterior teeth. This projection is termed **buccal overjet**. In posterior crossbite malocclusions, the buccal surfaces of lower teeth project farther buccally than the buccal surfaces of the upper posterior teeth. Posterior crossbites have six possible explanations: (1) The upper arch is too narrow, (2) the lower arch is too wide, (3) a lateral functional shift occurs during closure of the mandible, (4) one or more teeth are displaced toward the palate in the maxillary alveolar ridge, (5) one or more teeth are displaced toward the buccal side of the mandibular alveolar ridge, and (6) combinations of the above explanations.

Essentials of Orthodontics: Diagnosis and Treatment by Robert N. Staley and Neil T. Reske © 2011 Blackwell Publishing Ltd.

The number of teeth in crossbite can vary from one upper tooth and one lower tooth to all the posterior teeth on one or both sides of the arch. The number of teeth involved in crossbite is a guide to the severity of the problem: the more teeth involved, the more difficult is the treatment.

Prevalence of Posterior Crossbite Malocclusions

The U.S. Public Health Service surveyed the incidence of posterior crossbites in a large sample of whites, blacks, and Mexican Americans from 1988 to 1991 (Table 8.1) (Brunelle, Bhat, and Lipton 1996). The prevalence of posterior crossbites for all persons was 9.4%. No significant differences were observed between the races and genders. A positive association was observed between increased prevalence of posterior crossbites and increased incisor irregularity.

Table 8.1. Prevalence of Posterior Crossbite by Age, Gender, and Race of Americans Ages 8 to 50 Years, 1988–1991

	Age Groups (Percent of Persons [SE])			
	All Ages	8–11 Years	12–17 Years	18–50 Years
All persons	9.4 (0.8)	8.5 (1.2)	7.9 (1.5)	9.9 (1.0)
Males	9.1 (1.2)	7.2 (2.6)	6.0 (1.5)	10.2 (1.3)
Females	9.6 (0.8)	9.9 (2.0)	9.7 (2.1)	9.5 (1.0)
Race/ethnicity				
Whites	9.6 (1.0)	8.8 (1.4)	7.6 (2.1)	10.2 (1.3)
Blacks	9.2 (1.1)	6.6 (1.1)	7.7 (2.2)	10.4 (1.2)
Mexican Americans	8.5 (0.9)	6.9 (1.7)	8.4 (1.2)	8.9 (0.9)

From Brunelle, Bhat, and Lipton (1996).

Angle Classification

Patients having Class I occlusions without crowding are the best candidates for limited treatment of posterior crossbites. Patients who have Class II and Class III malocclusions with posterior crossbites are best treated by a specialist, because their treatment is complex and lengthy.

Intermolar Width Measurements

In unilateral and bilateral posterior crossbite malocclusions, measurement of the upper and lower intermolar widths and comparison of these widths to the widths of males and females who have normal occlusion will help determine whether the upper arch, lower arch, or both are part of the etiology of the crossbite (adult arch width norms are given in Figure 3.5, chapter 3).

The difference between the upper and lower intermolar widths will provide an estimate for the amount of expansion needed to correct the crossbite. Approximately 1.5 mm in males and 1.2 mm in females should be added (absolute sum) to the intermolar width difference to expand the arch enough to ensure normal buccal overjet. The intermolar width difference is also a guide to select patients for limited treatment. Intermolar width differences between 1 mm and 6 mm are recommended for limited treatment. Patients with differences greater than 6 mm are best treated by specialists.

The intermolar width difference is also a guide for selecting appliances to correct the crossbite. Removable appliances are adequate for correcting crossbites requiring 1 mm to 5 mm of intermolar expansion. Corrections requiring 5 mm or more of intermolar expansion are best treated by fixed appliances, such as the quad helix and fixed W spring appliances. Crossbites requiring 6 mm or more of correction are best treated with rapid maxillary expansion (RME) appliances. Rapid expanders separate the maxillary suture, thereby treating the underlying etiology of skeletal narrowness and moving the teeth more bodily, which increases the probability of obtaining a more stable treatment of the posterior crossbite.

Age of Patient

Posterior crossbites are best treated in children and adolescents. Adults have maxillary sutures that are hard to open and many need surgically assisted RME (SARME) to effectively correct a posterior crossbite.

Buccolingual Inclination of the Posterior Teeth

If an upper molar in crossbite is inclined lingually, the inclination is favorable, because correcting the crossbite will improve its inclination by tipping the tooth to a more normal inclination. If an upper molar in crossbite is inclined buccally, the inclination is unfavorable, because correcting the crossbite will increase the buccal inclination to an even greater abnormal buccal inclination. Excessive buccal inclination of upper molars may be the result of a skeletal narrowness of the upper arch that caused a dental compensation (excessive buccal inclination) of the upper molars to accommodate for the skeletal discrepancy between the maxilla and mandible. In such cases, fixed RME appliances are recommended for treatment, because they will expand the suture and help control the inclination of the buccally inclined molars.

Abnormal buccal inclination of a lower molar in crossbite is favorable, because moving the molar to a more normal inclination will help to correct the crossbite. A lingually inclined lower molar in posterior crossbite is unfavorable. Excessive lingual inclination of the lower posterior teeth must be reckoned with in calculating the need for maxillary expansion. Buccal movement of lingually inclined lower posterior teeth to more normal inclination increases the goal for maxillary expansion. In patients with lingually inclined lower posterior teeth, the lower arch is expanded along with the upper arch.

Etiology of Bilateral and Unilateral Posterior Crossbites

In centric occlusion, two basic types of posterior crossbites are observed: bilateral and unilateral.

Bilateral posterior crossbites have a close correspondence between centric occlusion and centric relation in Class I and Class II malocclusions. In Class III malocclusions, an anterior crossbite is often associated with a bilateral posterior crossbite, thereby introducing the possibility of an anteroposterior functional shift. Bilateral posterior crossbites have two basic etiologies: (1) the upper arch has narrower than normal width and the lower arch has normal or larger than normal arch width and (2) the upper arch has normal width and the lower arch has larger than normal width. Bilateral crossbites with both of

these etiologies are therefore treated with appliances that move teeth on both sides of the upper arch in a buccal direction. Measuring the upper and lower arch widths will help the clinician understand the etiology of the crossbite and decide how much expansion is needed to correct the posterior crossbite.

Unilateral posterior crossbites have five etiologies:

(1) The upper arch has narrower than normal width and the lower arch has normal or larger than normal width, (2) the upper arch has normal width and the lower arch has larger than normal width, (3) premature tooth contacts deflect the mandible laterally during closure and the upper and lower arch widths are normal, (4) etiology #1 in combination with premature tooth contacts, and (5) etiology #2 in combination with premature tooth contacts. Effective treatment of unilateral posterior crossbites requires a diagnosis based on careful clinical observation for premature tooth contacts and measuring the upper and lower arch widths and comparing them to a norm.

Most patients who have a **unilateral posterior crossbite** shift their mandibles toward the side of the crossbite when closing into centric occlusion. This **lateral functional shift** may be caused only by a premature contact (etiology No. 3) or by discrepancies in the upper and lower arch widths (Thilander and Lennartsson 2002). When a unilateral posterior crossbite is associated with a lateral functional shift and a discrepancy in arch widths, it is in reality a bilateral posterior crossbite treatable with appliances that move both sides of the upper arch in a buccal direction. Correction of the crossbite in these patients should eliminate the lateral functional shift. Studies have suggested that the relation between condyle and fossa in persons with unilateral posterior crossbites may become asymmetric (Miyawaki et al. 2004; Nerder, Bakke, and Solow 1999), possibly inducing asymmetric growth of the mandible (Lam, Sadowsky, and Omerza 1999; Pinto et al. 2001). It is further thought that the prolonged asymmetric closure of the mandible in patients with a unilateral crossbite may predispose them to disc displacement and temporomandicular joint (TMJ) clicking (Egermark, Magnusson, and Carlsson 2003; Pullinger, Seligman, and Gornbein 1993). Positive associations between unilateral posterior crossbite and TMJ clicking were reported in several studies (Egermark, Magnusson, and Carlsson 2003; Kritsineli and Shim 1992; Pullinger, Seligman, and Gornbein 1993; Thilander et al. 2002). A recent study of 1291 school-age children, 10 to 16 years old, found no association between posterior unilateral crossbite and TMJ clicking (Farella et al. 2007). Additional well-designed studies are needed to clarify the truth about these associations.

When a lateral shift cannot be readily observed in a patient with a unilateral posterior crossbite, ask the patient to open widely, to determine whether the upper and lower dental midlines are coincident in the open position. If the midlines are coincident when open and deviated when closed, this is evidence that a lateral shift is operating during closure of the mandible. A diagnostic splint can also be used to demonstrate the presence of absence of a lateral shift.

If no lateral shift can be detected, the patient may have a **true unilateral posterior crossbite**. Most appliances expand bilaterally. In patients with true unilateral posterior crossbites, an expander operating bilaterally will cause the non-crossbite side to move into buccal crossbite as the crossbite side is corrected. Unilateral mechanics such as cross arch elastics are used with a bilateral expander to treat the buccal crossbite side in true unilateral crossbites. In complex true unilateral posterior crossbite patients, surgically assisted RME may be an effective treatment. Patients with true unilateral crossbites should be referred to a specialist.

Vertical Dimension

Overbite is another predictor of difficulty in the treatment of posterior crossbites. Normal overbite is a favorable finding. During the treatment of most posterior crossbites, the bite is opened at least temporarily. If a patient has an anterior openbite or a very deep overbite associated with a posterior crossbite, he should be referred to a specialist.

Treatment of Posterior Crossbites

A systematic review of literature found five randomized clinical trials and eight controlled clinical trials that studied orthodontic treatment of posterior crossbites (Harrison and Ashby 2001). The review authors concluded that evidence reported by Lindner (1989) and Thilander et al. (1984) suggests that the removal of premature contacts of primary teeth is effective in preventing a posterior crossbite from being perpetuated to the mixed dentition and adult teeth. When grinding alone is not effective, using an upper removable expansion plate to expand the upper teeth will decrease the risk of a posterior crossbite from being perpetuated to the permanent dentition. We conclude that bilateral and unilateral posterior crossbites with a lateral functional shift should be corrected in the primary, mixed, or early permanent dentitions with an emphasis on early detection and treatment with the hope of not perpetuating the crossbite and functional shift to the adult dentition.

Correction of Posterior Crossbites with Removable Appliances

For best results, the upper molars of patients receiving expander treatment by a removable appliance should be upright or inclined lingually. Molars that are buccally inclined are not suitable for these appliances that primarily tip molars in a buccal direction. Retention for about 1 year with a Hawley retainer or a trans-palatal arch following active treatment is recommended.

The **removable W spring expander** is useful in mixed dentition patients who need less than 5 mm of maxillary arch expansion. The treatment of a 9-year 2-month-old mixed-dentition patient with a Class I molar relation and a unilateral posterior crossbite on her right side is shown in Figures 8.1 through 8.6. She had a

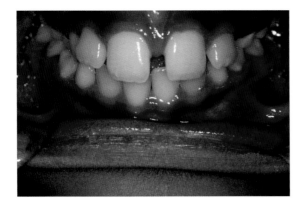

Figure 8.1. Patient with a unilateral posterior crossbite and lateral functional shift to the right side. (Courtesy of Dr. John Casko.)

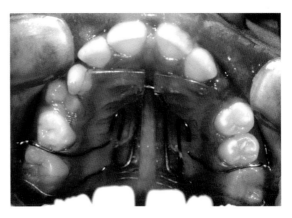

Figure 8.4. View of the removable W spring expander in the mouth. (Courtesy of Dr. John Casko.)

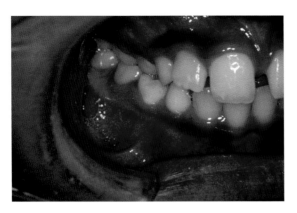

Figure 8.2. View of teeth in crossbite. (Courtesy of Dr. John Casko.)

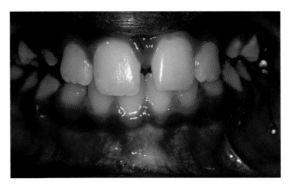

Figure 8.5. After correction of the crossbite, the functional shift was eliminated and the dental midlines were together. (Courtesy of Dr. John Casko.)

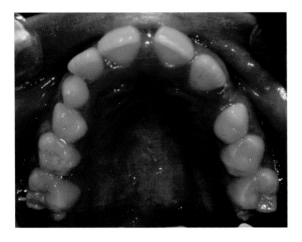

Figure 8.3. Occlusal view of the narrow upper arch. (Courtesy of Dr. John Casko.)

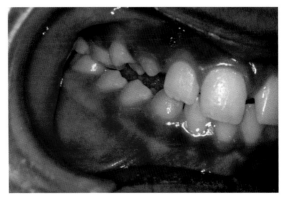

Figure 8.6. Teeth were no longer in crossbite on the right side. (Courtesy of Dr. John Casko.)

College of Dentistry
The University of Iowa
Department of Orthodontics

Doctor D. Varga   No. 854 Date 6-18-04

Patient Fritz Voosh   No. 62988

Date Needed 6-25-04 Time 4:30 PM

℞

Please fabricate a Maxillary
Removable W-spring expansion
appliance with a .036 rd wire
and .026 rd Adams Clasps on
1st molars

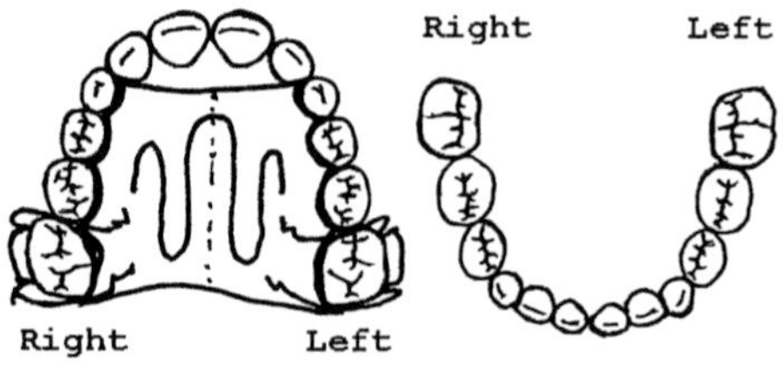

Right   Left

Right   Left

Material   Shade

For Lab Use Only

Instructor

Signature

76010/6-09

Figure 8.7. Laboratory prescription for a removable W spring expansion appliance.

lateral functional shift of her mandible toward the crossbite side that resulted in a deviation of her lower dental midline to the right side (Fig. 8.1). The crossbite involved the permanent and primary molars (Fig. 8.2). Her upper arch intermolar width was 2 standard deviations narrower than the mixed-dentition norm (Table 8.2) (Fig. 8.3). Her lower arch intermolar width was within normal limits. Her intermolar width difference was –1.2 mm. To create adequate buccal overjet, she needed an additional 1.2 mm expansion for a total of about 2.4 mm. A removable W spring

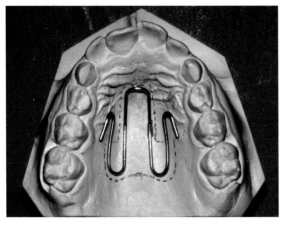

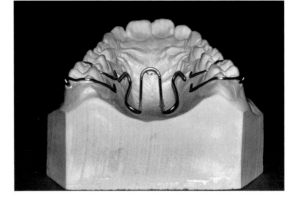

Figure 8.9. Posterior view of the W spring and Adams clasps.

Figure 8.8. W spring wire shown on the palate of a cast.

Table 8.2. Arch Widths at Permanent First Molars in Mixed-Dentition White Subjects with Normal Occlusion at Age 8 Years

		Maxilla				Mandible			
Gender	N	Mean	SD	Min	Max	Mean	SD	Min	Max
Male	18	51.3	2.8	45.1	59.0	50.4	1.7	46.7	52.1
Female	17	47.8	1.8	43.7	50.7	47.0	2.0	44.5	51.7

From Grabouski, J., Staley, R., Kummet, C., unpublished data.

expander is shown in the patient's mouth (Fig. 8.4). Correction of the crossbite eliminated the functional shift, and the lower dental midline became coincident with the upper dental midline (Fig. 8.5). This correction was the result of a cooperative patient and excellent care by the orthodontist. The permanent and primary molars remained out of crossbite, and the permanent canine and first premolar were erupting 1 year 4 months after the start of treatment (Fig. 8.6).

A laboratory prescription for a removable W spring expander is shown in Figure 8.7. Construction of the removable W spring expander appliance is illustrated in Figures 8.8 through 8.15. The W spring wire is bent from a 36-mil stainless steel wire. The two Adams clasps are bent from 26-mil stainless steel wire (Adams 1984). The W spring is shaped to fit the palatal contours (Figs. 8.8 to 8.10). The wire is separated from the palatal surface with a 1-mm layer of wax. The outline for the layer of wax is illus-

trated in Figure 8.11. The waxed spring has retention arms that are free to be embedded into the acrylic body of the appliance (Fig. 8.12). A view from the posterior shows the adaptation to the palate of the retention arms of the W spring and Adams clasps (Fig. 8.13). The acrylic body is shown in Figure 8.14, which was made by applying acrylic liquid and powder resins to the cast. The acrylic body was polished and cut carefully down its middle to create the finished appliance, as seen in Figure 8.15.

Activation of the removable W spring appliance requires a very tight fit of the Adams clasps to the molars. The arrowheads of the clasp can be bent toward the molar crown with No. 139 pliers to increase the grasp of the clasp. The interproximal wires can also be bent with a three-prong pliers to engage the arrowheads more tightly to the molar crown. Finally, the removable W spring should be activated with small increments so that the expansion force

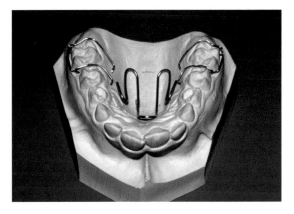

Figure 8.10. Anterior view of the W spring and Adams clasps.

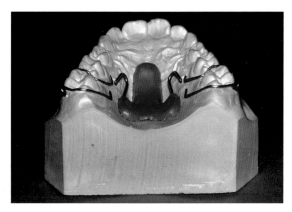

Figure 8.13. Posterior view of waxed W spring and Adams clasps.

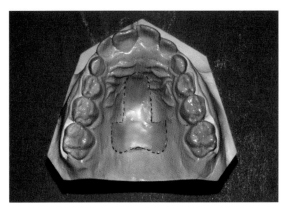

Figure 8.11. View of the wax-out area on the palate with a coating of separating medium on the cast.

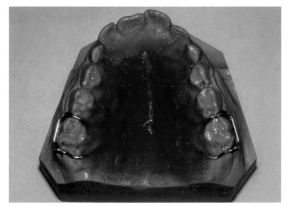

Figure 8.14. Acrylic resin applied to the cast.

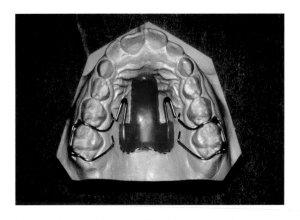

Figure 8.12. W spring waxed in place on the palate. Adams clasps waxed into position.

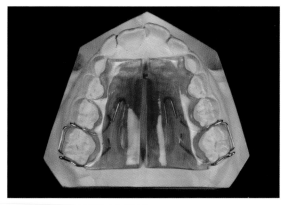

Figure 8.15. The finished and polished W spring appliance.

College of Dentistry
The University of Iowa
Department of Orthodontics

Doctor A. Able No. 712 Date 6-18-04

Patient Joe Campanelli No. 125

Date Needed 6-25-04 Time 10 AM

℞

Please fabricate a Maxillary
split acrylic expander with
.032 ball clasps between canines
and 1st premolars and .026 Adams
clasps on 1st Molars. use a
6mm universal expansion screw.

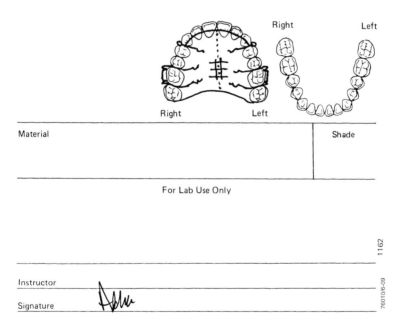

Material   Shade

For Lab Use Only

Instructor

Signature

1162

76010/6-09

Figure 8.16. Laboratory prescription for a maxillary split acrylic expander.

from the spring does not overpower the Adams clasps. The spring is activated by expanding the loops with the squared beak of No. 139 pliers, while keeping the two halves of the appliance parallel (Tenti 1986).

The removable **split acrylic expander** with a jackscrew is another removable appliance that can be used to widen maxillary intermolar width. A laboratory prescription for the construction of a removable split acrylic expander is shown in Figure 8.16. Figure 8.17 illustrates this appliance on the cast of a patient in the permanent dentition. Adams clasps provide the best anchorage for the appliance. Jackscrews are made with and

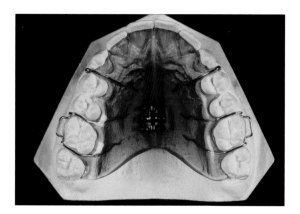

Figure 8.17. Split acrylic appliance on a cast.

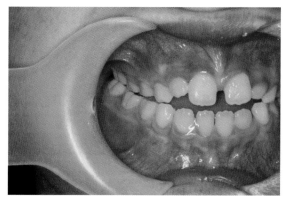

Figure 8.19. Before treatment view of the right sides of the arches. (Courtesy of Dr. Karin Southard.)

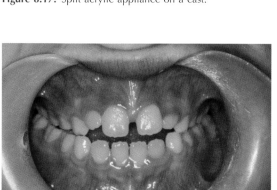

Figure 8.18. Patient with a bilateral posterior crossbite and anterior openbite. (Courtesy of Dr. Karin Southard.)

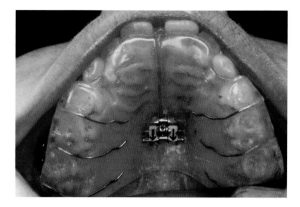

Figure 8.20. Occlusal view of the split acrylic expander in the mouth. (Courtesy of Dr. Karin Southard.)

without a spring. Standard jackscrews without the internal spring work best. Each turn of the standard screw widens the appliance by about 0.25 mm. The activation schedule should be slow to avoid overpowering the Adams clasps. If undercuts are not available on the molar crowns, composite resin can be added to the crown to create undercut areas that the Adams clasps can engage.

A 9-year 9-month-old patient with a bilateral posterior crossbite in the early mixed dentition was treated with a split acrylic expander. The crossbite and its treatment are illustrated in Figures 8.18 through 8.23. The crossbite involved the permanent first molars and primary molars

(Figs. 8.18 and 8.19). Her upper intermolar arch width was 1 standard deviation wider than the mixed-dentition norm. The crossbite was the result of her lower intermolar width that was 3 standard deviations wider than the mixed-dentition norm. The intermolar width difference was −3.8 mm. After adding 1.2 mm for adequate buccal overjet, an increase during treatment of about 5 mm in her upper intermolar width was required. When considering possible future growth of the mandibular arch and the anterior open-bite, this is a difficult treatment. The appliance used to correct the crossbite is shown in Figure 8.20. The occlusion after treatment is shown in Figures 8.21, 8.22, and 8.23. This com-

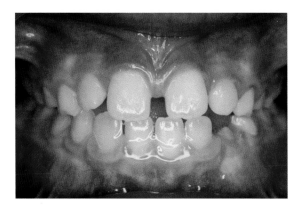

Figure 8.21. Front view of the teeth after treatment. (Courtesy of Dr. Karin Southard.)

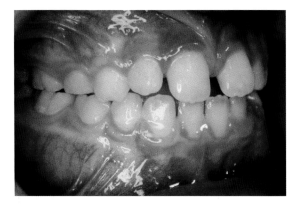

Figure 8.22. View of the teeth on the right side after treatment. (Courtesy of Dr. Karin Southard.)

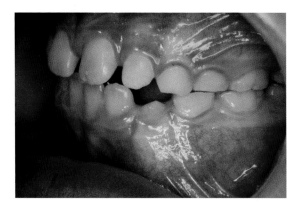

Figure 8.23. View of the teeth on the left side after treatment. (Courtesy of Dr. Karin Southard.)

pliant patient and excellent provider care resulted in correction of the crossbite and the openbite.

Correction of Posterior Crossbites with Fixed Expander Appliances

An advantage of the fixed expanders over the removable expanders is greater control of treatment by eliminating the patient's ability to remove the appliance. The fixed expander moves the molar teeth more bodily, rather than primarily tipping them. Also, the fixed expander can be activated without concern that the expansion forces will dislodge the appliance from the teeth. The expanded arch is retained for 1 year with a soldered trans-palatal arch.

The fixed W spring appliance is particularly useful in the expansion of patients who have unilateral cleft lip and palate in which the ability of the W spring appliance to expand the maxillary segments asymmetrically best meets the needs for expanding the asymmetric maxilla of the patient. A fixed retainer for these patients is often a soldered trans-palatal arch between the first molars, which has bilateral wire arms going forward to the canines supporting the lingual surfaces of the upper posterior teeth.

The **fixed W spring appliance** is similar to the previously described removable W spring expander. A fixed W spring appliance was used to correct a unilateral posterior crossbite in the primary dentition of a 4-year 10-month-old girl (Figs. 8.24 to 8.29). The patient's upper intermolar arch width (42.7 mm) was within normal limits of the mean width of 5-year-old girls with normal occlusion (Table 8.3), and her lower intermolar width (45.6 mm) was 3 standard deviations wider than the female norm (Table 8.3). This posterior crossbite is a result of her abnormally wide lower arch. The intermolar width difference was –2.9 mm, so the addition of 2.0 mm for adequate buccal overjet brought the total needed expansion to 4.9 mm. The lower dental midline was deviated toward the right, the side in crossbite (Fig. 8.24). This deviation was

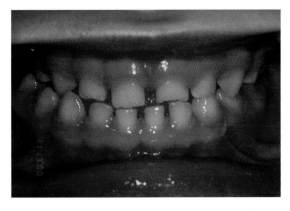

Figure 8.24. Patient with a unilateral posterior crossbite on the right side and functional shift in the primary dentition.

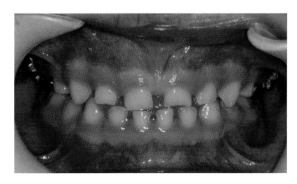

Figure 8.27. After the crossbite was corrected, the dental midlines were closer together.

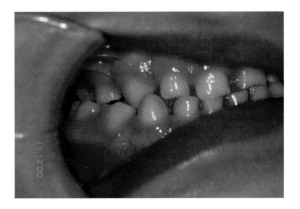

Figure 8.25. View of the right side before treatment.

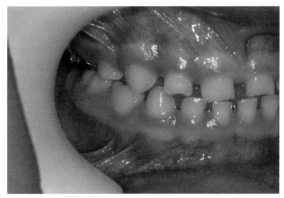

Figure 8.28. View of the right side after treatment.

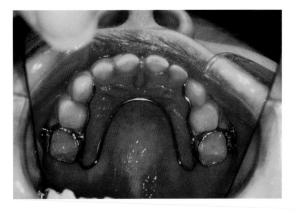

Figure 8.26. Occlusal view of the fixed W spring expander before expansion.

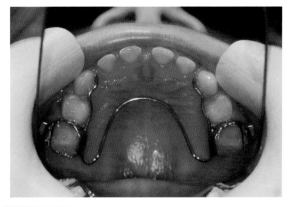

Figure 8.29. Occlusal view of the fixed W spring expander after correction of the crossbite.

Table 8.3. Arch Widths at Primary Second Molars in 5-Year-Old White Subjects with Normal Occlusion (mm)

| Gender | N | Maxilla | | | | | Mandible | | | | |
		Mean	SD	Min	Max	Mean	SD	Min	Max	A – J
Males	16	43.4	2.4	37.3	48.1	40.7	1.9	36.5	44.4	2.7
Females	14	41.6	1.6	39.6	44.3	39.5	1.6	38.1	43.1	2.1

From R. N. Staley, 2009, unpublished data.

associated with a lateral functional shift during closure of the mandible. The fixed W spring appliance was made with a 36-mil wire (Fig. 8.26). The loops are activated as described for the removable W spring. Comparing the expanded appliance to the original cast as a reference helps to keep the appliance properly shaped to the arch. Drawing an outline of the bands and arms of the appliance on paper before and after activation also helps to maintain the shape of the expanded appliance. Typically, the W spring expander is activated from 3 to 5 mm at each visit, depending on the needs of the patient. After the first expansion of the appliance, subsequent expansions require removal of the appliance, activation, and re-cementation of the appliance. The corrected occlusion is shown in Figures 8.27 and 8.28. The lower dental midline moved closer to the upper midline as the functional shift was eliminated. The expanded arch is viewed from the occlusal in Figure 8.29. A laboratory prescription for the fixed W spring appliance is shown in Figure 8.30.

The **quad helix** is another fixed expander that is frequently used by clinicians. The treatment of a patient 10 years 7 months old with the quad helix is illustrated in Figures 8.31 through 8.36. The patient had a Class II subdivision right malocclusion [E, E, I, I] (Fig. 8.32). The patient's upper intermolar width was 2 standard deviations narrower than the adult norm (see Chapter 3). Her lower intermolar width was 1 standard deviation wider than the adult norm. The intermolar difference was −4.45 mm. With the addition of 1.2 mm for adequate buccal overjet, the patient needed 5.65 mm of upper molar width increase. She had a minimal lateral functional shift toward the right side. The quad helix used

in treatment is shown in Figure 8.23. This appliance is a variation of the W spring appliance. It is important that the four helices are bent in a plane parallel to the occlusal plane, and not parallel to the palatal surface. The opening of the helices during activation should produce a horizontal vector of force against upper posterior teeth. The indications for the use and activation of the quad helix are essentially the same as for the fixed W spring. The expander is constructed from 30-mil stainless steel wire soldered to molar bands. A front view of the dentition after treatment is shown in Figure 8.34. The corrected right side is still in a mild Class II occlusion (Fig. 8.25). A removable trans-palatal arch was used to retain the expansion for 1 year. A laboratory prescription for a quad helix appliance is shown in Figure 8.37.

The **modified rapid maxillary expander (modified RME)** effectively corrects crossbites requiring more than 5 mm of expansion. The appliance consists of two molar bands, a standard jack screw, and wire arms that extend from the molar to the primary canines and molars (Fig. 6.14). The appliance is designed for use in the mixed dentition.

The forces applied to the dental arch by the appliance are strong enough to open the midpalatal suture. Opening of the suture is desirable, because, if retained properly, this widening of the maxilla helps to retain the correction of the crossbite. The opening of the maxillary suture is an example of **distraction osteogenesis**. A schedule for activation of the rapid expander based on clinical research provides guidelines for younger and older patients (Zimring and Issacson 1965). The jackscrew opens approximately 0.25 mm with each turn of the screw. The **turn schedule**

College of Dentistry
The University of Iowa
Department of Orthodontics

Doctor   A. Able   No. 712   Date 6-11-04

Patient   Tyrone Trzos   No.

Date Needed 6-18-04 Time 9 AM

℞

Please fabricate a fixed
w-spring appliance with a
.036 rd wire soldered to
bands on primary 2nd Molars.

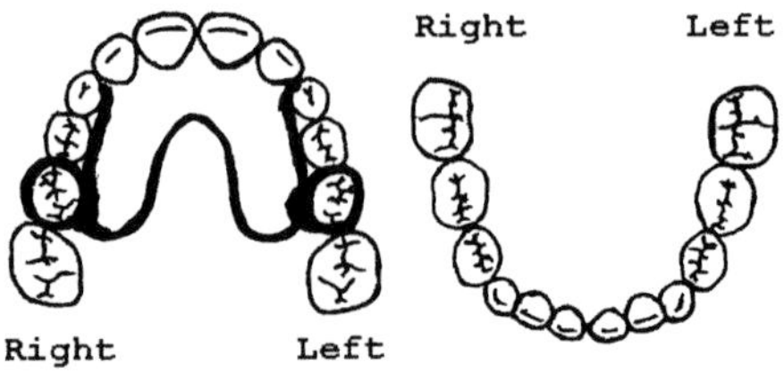

Right   Left

Right   Left

Material   Shade

For Lab Use Only

Instructor

Signature   *A. Able*

Figure 8.30. Laboratory prescription for a fixed W spring appliance in a primary dentition.

for young growing patients is two turns each day for the first 4 or 5 days, and one turn each day for the remainder of the expander treatment. The activation schedule can be slowed down if the patient experiences significant discomfort. A slower turn schedule is recommended for the rapid expander made with acrylic adjacent to the palatal mucosa. The turn schedule recommended for adult patients, who should be treated by a specialist, is much slower.

If the expander becomes loose and must be removed during active expansion, the patient may experience dizziness and perhaps pain. Keep the patient seated in the dental chair until the

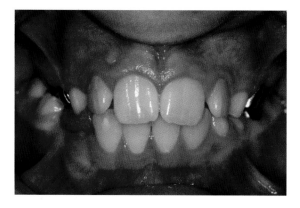

Figure 8.31. Front view of patient with a unilateral posterior crossbite on the right and lower midline deviated right.

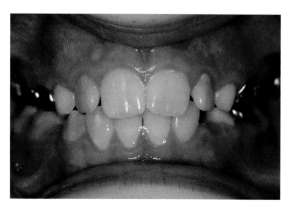

Figure 8.34. Front view after treatment. Note improvement of lower dental midline.

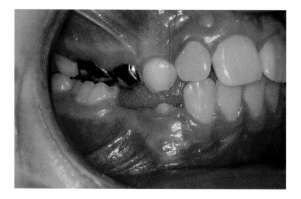

Figure 8.32. View of the teeth on the right side before treatment.

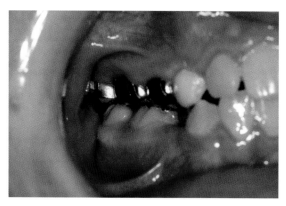

Figure 8.35. View of the right side after correction of the crossbite.

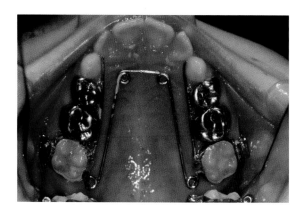

Figure 8.33. View of the quad helix appliance at beginning of treatment.

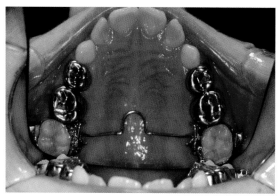

Figure 8.36. Occlusal view of the removable trans-palatal arch used as a retainer for 1 year.

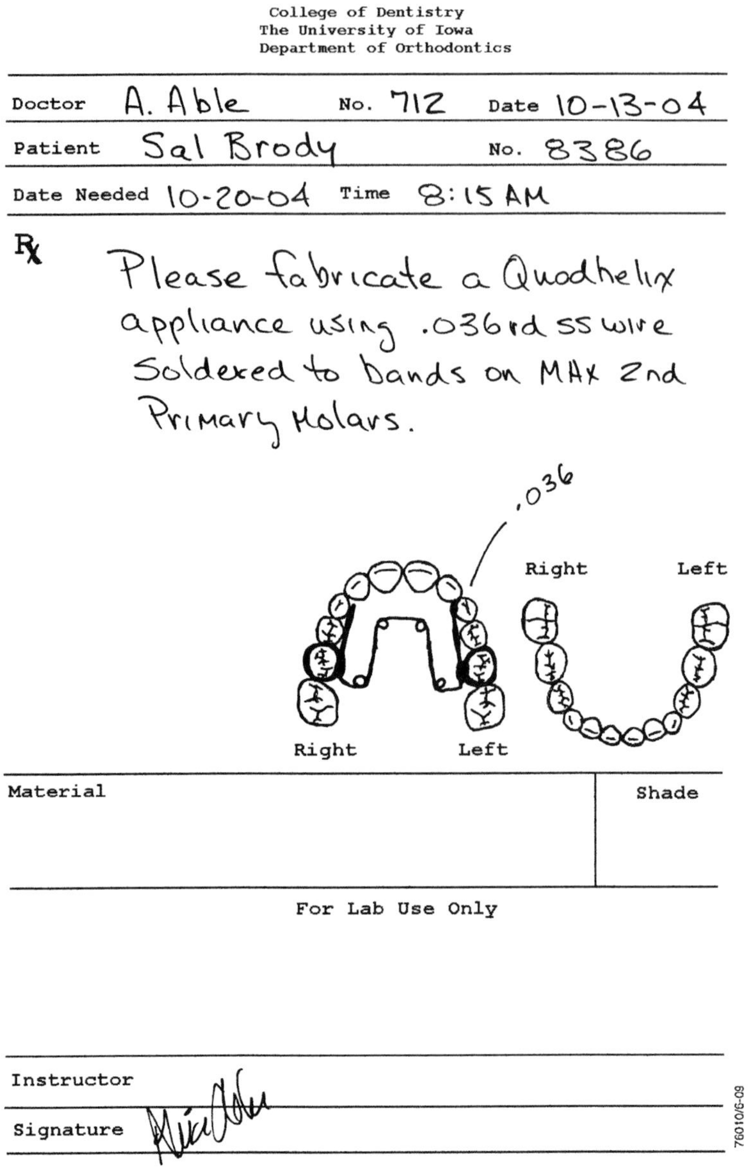

College of Dentistry
The University of Iowa
Department of Orthodontics

Doctor   A. Able   No. 712   Date 10-13-04

Patient   Sal Brody   No. 8386

Date Needed 10-20-04   Time 8:15 AM

℞   Please fabricate a Quadhelix
appliance using .036 rd ss wire
Soldered to bands on MAX 2nd
Primary Molars.

.036

Right   Left

Right   Left

Material   Shade

For Lab Use Only

Instructor

Signature

Figure 8.37. Laboratory prescription for a quad helix expander.

expander is re-cemented. Following expansion, the appliance is left in the mouth for 3 months. When the expander is removed, the best retainer is a soldered trans-palatal arch that is left in the mouth for 1 year. After 3 months, when the expander is removed from the teeth, new bands are fitted for the soldered trans-palatal arch, and

the expander is re-cemented into the upper arch until the trans-palatal arch is fabricated and cemented in the arch.

A patient treated with a modified RME is shown in Figures 8.38 to 8.43. This 7-year 7-month-old boy had a unilateral posterior cross-bite on the right side with an associated func-

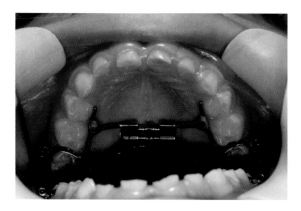

Figure 8.38. Modified rapid maxillary expander cemented in the upper arch.

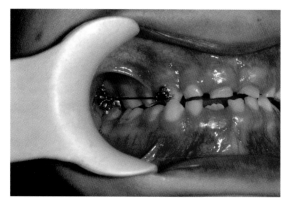

Figure 8.40. After the expansion was completed, the primary canines remained in crossbite.

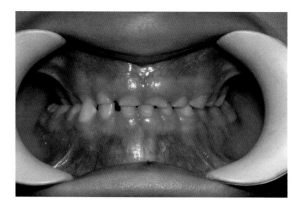

Figure 8.39. Patient with a unilateral posterior crossbite on the right side and functional shift. View from front.

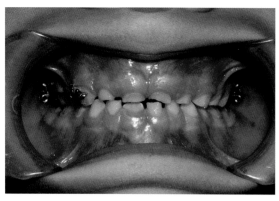

Figure 8.41. Lever arm corrected the canine crossbite. The dental midlines are closer together.

tional shift toward the side of the crossbite (Fig. 8.38). The patient's upper intermolar width was 1 standard deviation narrower than the mixed-dentition norm (Table 8.2). His lower intermolar width was within normal limits of the mixed-dentition norm. His intermolar width difference measured −5.5 mm. When another 1.5 mm for adequate buccal overjet is added to the intermolar difference, the expansion needed is 7 mm. The lower dental midline is to the right of the upper dental midline as the result of a lateral functional shift (Fig. 8.38). The modified RME used in the treatment of this patient is shown (Fig. 8.39). After the expander corrected the posterior cross-

bite, the patient's right primary canines were still in crossbite (Fig. 8.40). Part of the etiology of this patient was a premature contact between the right primary canines. The primary canines could have been reduced in size with a diamond dental burr or one of them extracted to eliminate the premature contact. In this patient, a rectangular segmental arch wire, 18 × 22 mil, was placed in the right molar band to act as a lever arm to move the bracketed maxillary primary canine out of crossbite (Figs. 8.40 and 8.41). The lower dental midline was closer to the upper dental midline after correction of the crossbite (Fig. 8.41). After 3 months of retention, the modified

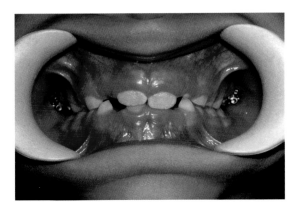

Figure 8.42. Front view after the expander was removed and a trans-palatal arch was cemented.

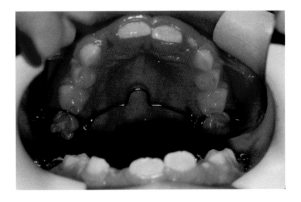

Figure 8.43. Occlusal view of the transpalatal arch retainer.

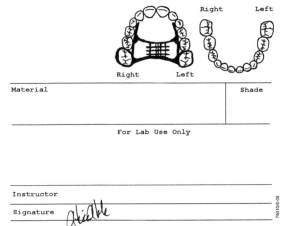

College of Dentistry
The University of Iowa
Department of Orthodontics

Doctor A. Able   No. 712   Date 9-15-04
Patient Peggy Fine   No. 62081
Date Needed 9-22-04 Time 8 AM

℞ Please fabricate a Modified RME
8 mm of expansion is desired.
Please use a 12 mm Palex II screw.
Extend .045 rd ss arms from bands
on 1st Molars to Mesial of canines.

Right   Left

Right   Left

Material   Shade

For Lab Use Only

Instructor

Signature

Figure 8.44. Laboratory prescription for a modified rapid palatal expander.

RME appliance was removed and replaced by a removable trans-palatal arch (Figs. 8.42 and 8.43). A laboratory prescription for a modified RME is shown in Figure 8.44.

The construction of a Hyrax RME is shown in Figures 8.45 to 8.52. The fabrication of a modified RME is very similar to the steps described here. First, bands are fitted on the upper first premolars and first molars (Fig. 8.45). An alginate impression is taken of the upper arch with the bands properly fitted. The bands are then removed from the teeth and placed into the impression (Fig. 8.46). A stone working cast is poured, and 45-mil wires are placed along the lingual surfaces of the posterior teeth (Fig. 8.47).

The wires attached to the jackscrew are bent to fit the appliance into the palate (Fig. 8.48). The jackscrew is placed up into the palate to give the patient's tongue room, but not so far up that the expanding screw can irritate and damage palatal tissues. The metal parts are stabilized with plaster (Fig. 8.49). The wire joints to be soldered are covered with flux and soldered together (Fig. 8.50). The soldered appliance must be removed from the cast and be finished and polished (Figs. 8.51 and 8.52).

An **edgewise fixed appliance** and elastic modules can be used to correct simple crossbites. An 11-year-old patient had a simple crossbite of an upper left first premolar (Figures 8.53 to 8.56).

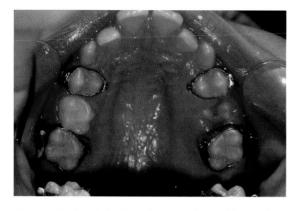

Figure 8.45. Bands fitted on first premolars and first molars.

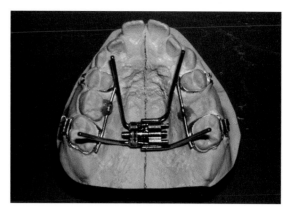

Figure 8.48. Hyrax jackscrew and wire arms fitted into the palate.

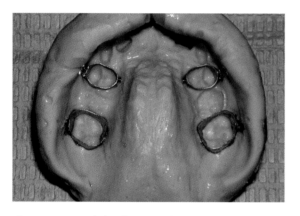

Figure 8.46. Bands fitted into an alginate impression.

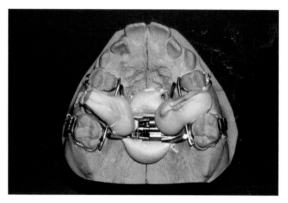

Figure 8.49. Jackscrew and wires stabilized with plaster.

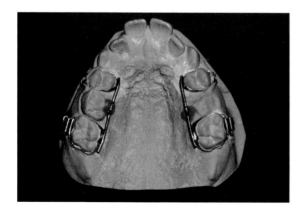

Figure 8.47. Stone cast with bands and 45 mil wires.

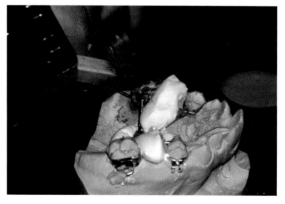

Figure 8.50. Joints between the bands and wires are fluxed and soldered.

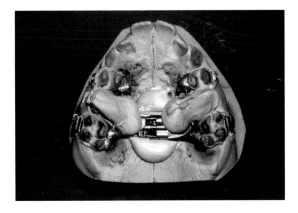

Figure 8.51. Soldered appliance on the working cast.

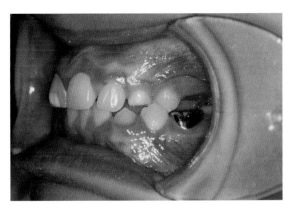

Figure 8.54. Upper left first premolar is in lingual crossbite.

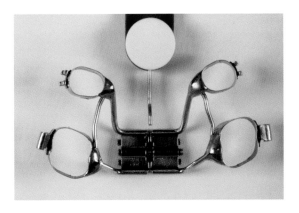

Figure 8.52. Hyrax expander has been polished. A blue and white safety key turns the jackscrew.

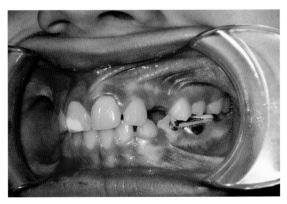

Figure 8.55. Premolar has been moved out of crossbite.

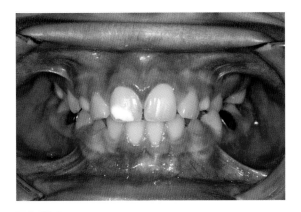

Figure 8.53. Patient in the late mixed dentition with the crossbite of an upper premolar.

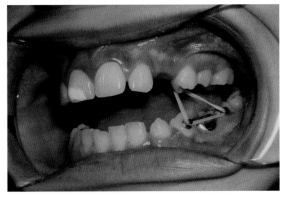

Figure 8.56. Elastic used to correct the crossbite and the bonded button and hook on the lower premolar and molar are shown.

The crossbite is shown in Figures 8.53 and 8.54. The tooth is shown after it had been moved out of crossbite using a fixed appliance and elastic module (Fig. 8.55). Lingual buttons were placed on the lingual surface of the upper first premolar and the buccal surface of the lower first premolar. A hook was bonded to the buccal surface of the lower first molar (Figs. 8.55 and 8.56). The patient was asked to wear, except at mealtimes, an elastic module (rubber band) $^3/_{16}$ inches in diameter with 6 ounces of force to correct the crossbite (Fig. 8.56).

REFERENCES

Adams, C. P. 1984. The design, construction & use of removable orthodontic appliances. Bristol: John Wright & Sons Ltd.

Brunelle, J. A., Bhat, M., and Lipton, J. A. 1996. Prevalence and distribution of selected occlusal characteristics in the U.S. population, 1988–1991. J. Dent. Res. 75(Spec. Issue):706–713.

Egermark, I., Magnusson, T., and Carlsson, G. E. 2003. A 20-year follow-up of signs and symptoms of temporomandibular disorders and malocclusions in participants with and without orthodontic treatment in childhood. Angle Orthod. 73:109–115.

Farella, M., Michelotti, A., Iodice, G., Milani, S., and Martina, R. 2007. Unilateral posterior crossbite is not associated with TMJ clicking in young adolescents. J. Dent. Res. 86:137–141.

Harrison, J. E., and Ashby, D. 2001. Orthodontic treatment for posterior crossbites. Cochrane Database Syst. Rev. (1):CD000979.

Kritsineli, M., and Shim, Y. S. 1992. Malocclusion, body posture, and temporomandibular disorder in children with primary and mixed dentition. J. Clin. Pediatr. Dent. 16:86–93.

Lam, P. H., Sadowsky, C., and Omerza, F. 1999. Mandibular asymmetry and condylar position in children with unilateral posterior crossbite. Am. J. Orthod. Dentofac. Orthop. 115:569–575.

Lindner, A. 1989. Longitudinal study on the effect of early interceptive treatment in 4-year-old children with unilateral crossbite. Scand. J. Dent. Res. 97:432–438.

Miyawaki, S., Tanimoto, Y., Araki, Y., Katayama, A., Kuboki, T., and Takano-Yamamoto, T. 2004. Movement of the lateral and medial poles of the working condyle during mastication in patients with unilateral posterior crossbite. Am. J. Orthod. Dentofac. Orthop. 126:549.

Nerder, P. H., Bakke, M., and Solow, B. 1999. The functional shift of the mandible in unilateral posterior crossbite and the adaptation of the temporomandibular joints: a pilot study. Eur. J. Orthod. 21:155–166.

Pinto, A. S., Buschang, P. H., Throckmorton, G. S., and Chen, P. 2001. Morphological and positional asymmetries of young children with functional unilateral posterior crossbite. Am. J. Orthod. Dentofac. Orthop. 120:513–520.

Pullinger, A. G., Seligman, D. A., and Gornbein, J. A. 1993. A multiple logistic regression analysis of the risk and relative odds of temporomandibular disorders as a function of common occlusal features. J. Dent. Res. 72:968–979.

Tenti, F. V. 1986. Orthodontic appliances fixed and removable. Genova, Italy: Caravel.

Thilander, B., and Lennartsson, B. 2002. A study of children with unilateral posterior crossbite, treated and untreated in the deciduous dentition—occlusal and skeletal characteristics of significance in predicting the long-term outcome. J. Orofac. Orthop. 63:371–383.

Thilander, B., Rubio, G., Pena, L., and de Mayorga, C. 2002. Prevalence of temporomandibular dysfunction and its association with malocclusion in children and adolescents: an epidemiological study related to specified stages of dental development. Angle Orthod. 72:146–154.

Thilander, B., Wahlund, S., and Lennartson, B. 1984. The effect of early interceptive treatment in children with posterior cross-bite. Eur. J. Orthod. 6:25–34.

Zimring, J. F., and Issacson, R. J. 1965. Forces produced by rapid maxillary expansion. (III) Forces present during retention. Angle Orthod. 35:178–186.

Management of Incisor Diastemas

9

Prevalence of Maxillary Diastemas

The prevalence of a diastema between the maxillary central incisors of 2-mm or greater width in the U.S. population is shown in Table 9.1 (Brunelle, Bhat, and Lipton 1996). When all race groups are pooled, males had a diastema significantly more frequently than females. The prevalence of diastemas in blacks (16.2%) was significantly higher than the prevalence in whites (4.9%) and in Mexican Americans (6.6%), who had statistically similar frequencies of occurrence. Eight- to 11-year-old children in all groups had a higher prevalence of maxillary diastemas than did 12- to 17-year-old adolescents and 18- to 50-year-old adults, primarily because the younger subjects did not have a full complement of erupted permanent teeth.

Etiologic Factors to Consider

Many opinions about the cause and relapse of the median diastema between the upper central incisors have appeared in the periodical literature

Essentials of Orthodontics: Diagnosis and Treatment by Robert N. Staley and Neil T. Reske © 2011 Blackwell Publishing Ltd.

(Shashua and Årtun 1999). A follow-up study of 97 consecutively treated patients 4 to 9 years after orthodontic correction gives reliable evidence about the diagnosis and treatment of median distemas (Shashua and Årtun 1999). The relapse incidence was 49%. Logistic regression analysis showed only two significant associations between pretreatment factors and high risk for relapse: (1) diastemas wider than 2 mm and (2) having a family member with a similar diastema. Pretreatment spacing of the upper anterior teeth approached significance. At follow-up, fremitus (mobility of a maxillary incisor when sensed by a forefinger placed on the labial surface while the patient clenched his teeth) was the only parameter at follow-up that was significantly associated with the reopening of space. The following factors were not significantly associated with relapse of diastema closure: (1) abnormal frenum, (2) midline interosseous cleft, and (3) deep overbite. The authors stated that a frenectomy should not be performed to enhance the stability of treatment closing a diastema (Shashua and Årtun 1999). In a longitudinal study of a group of 9-year-old subjects with abnormal frenum, no difference was found in spontaneous closure of the diastema between subgroups that had and did not have a frenectomy (Bergström, Jensen, and Mortensson 1973).

Table 9.1. Prevalence of Maxillary Diastema ≥2 mm by Age, Gender, and Race in Americans 1988–1991

	All Ages Percent of (SE)	8–11 Years Percent of (SE)	12–17 Years Percent of (SE)	18–50 Years Percent of (SE)
All persons	6.5 (0.6)	19.3 (2.4)	6.0 (0.7)	4.8 (0.6)
Males	7.7 (0.9)*	20.0 (3.7)	7.2 (1.5)	6.2 (0.9)
Females	5.3 (0.5)	18.7 (2.2)	4.8 (1.1)	3.5 (0.5)
Whites	4.9 (0.6)	17.7 (2.7)	5.5 (0.9)	3.2 (0.6)
Males	6.2 (1.0)	18.5 (4.7)	7.1 (2.2)	4.6 (1.0)
Females	3.8 (0.5)	17.0 (2.6)	3.9 (1.4)	1.9 (0.4)
Blacks	16.2 (0.9)†	29.4 (3.0)	12.5 (2.5)	14.7 (0.8)
Males	16.8 (1.3)	27.4 (3.0)	12.4 (4.0)	16.0 (1.4)
Females	15.6 (1.4)	31.5 (4.2)	12.6 (2.0)	13.7 (1.3)
Mexican Americans	6.6 (0.8)	18.2 (3.4)	4.1 (1.8)	5.0 (0.6)
Males	7.6 (1.1)	19.3 (4.0)	5.0 (2.2)	6.1 (0.9)
Females	5.4 (0.8)	17.0 (3.2)	3.2 (1.5)	3.6 (0.5)

*Males are different from females, $p < 0.01$.
†Blacks are different from whites and Mexican Americans, $p < 0.001$.
From Brunelle, Bhat, and Lipton (1996).

When taking pretreatment records, it is important to ask whether another family member has a diastema similar to the patient. Familial associations indicate that an important genetic component is involved in the development of a median diastema (Shashua and Årtun 1999). In these patients, long-term retention should be mentioned before starting the treatment.

From these findings, clinicians must be prepared to retain indefinitely the closure of large median diastemas. Another approach is to use aesthetic dentistry to enlarge the widths of upper anterior teeth that are smaller than normal. Long-term retention must be the goal for adolescent and adult patients. Children in the mixed dentition who have diastema issues cannot be fully treated until all the upper teeth mesial to the first molars are erupted.

Size of Teeth and Bolton Analysis

On the basis of these findings, the size and spacing of upper incisors should be evaluated when planning treatment. Does the Bolton anterior analysis predict a mandibular excess? If so, closure of the upper diastema should be accompanied with esthetic dentistry to enlarge the upper incisors to correct the Bolton discrepancy. Does the lower arch have spaces that, in effect, create a Bolton mandibular excess? If so, the lower arch spaces must be closed along with the upper anterior diastema. If the lower spaces are not closed, aesthetic dentistry must unduly enlarge the mesiodistal size of the upper anterior teeth to achieve appropriate overbite and overjet.

Upper central incisors are usually stable with regard to size and shape, whereas the upper lateral incisors are prone to greater variation in size and shape (Dahlberg 1953). In most patients whose tooth size plays a role, the upper lateral incisors are too small. All four of the upper incisors may be too small in some patients with a diastema problem. Measurements can be taken of the mesiodistal widths of the incisors to determine the role of tooth size in the diastema problem of a particular patient. The widths of the anterior teeth in American whites with normal occlusion are given in Table 9.2.

When a small Bolton mandibular excess occurs in a Class I patient with normal-sized upper incisors and small spaces between them, the upper spaces could be reduced in size by removal of some interproximal enamel from several lower

Table 9.2. Mesiodistal Widths of Anterior Teeth in White Americans with Normal Occlusion (mm)

	Central Incisor			Lateral Incisor			Canine		
	Mean ± SD	Min	Max	Mean ± SD	Min	Max	Mean ± SD	Min	Max
Maxilla									
Males N = 19	8.8 ± 0.6	7.9	9.8	6.9 ± 0.5	6.2	8.2	8.0 ± 0.4	7.4	8.7
Females N = 19	8.6 ± 0.7	7.6	10.5	6.6 ± 0.6	5.3	7.7	7.8 ± 0.4	7.2	8.4
Mandible									
Males N = 19	5.6 ± 0.6	4.8	7.2	6.0 ± 0.4	5.3	6.9	6.9 ± 0.3	6.3	7.6
Females N = 19	5.4 ± 0.4	4.6	6.2	5.9 ± 0.4	5.3	6.9	6.7 ± 0.4	6.3	7.5

From R. N. Staley, T. L. Juhlin, and C. Kummet, 2009, unpublished data.

teeth, such as premolars and canines, accompanied by retraction of the lower teeth (Bolton 1958). This treatment requires a full arch fixed appliance in the lower arch. Removal of enamel from lower teeth is best limited to a small amount, such as 1 or 2 mm for the entire arch. The space created by enamel removal in the lower arch must be closed before upper arch spaces can be closed or reduced in size.

Some patients with a small median diastema between the two upper central incisors associated with well-aligned upper and lower arches can be treated with composite resin build-ups without orthodontic treatment. This treatment is excellent from the viewpoint of tooth stability following closure of the diastema. Whenever orthodontic appliances move teeth, the potential for postorthodontic tooth movement must be recognized and controlled with a retainer.

Arch Size

If arch size is suspected as an etiologic factor, measuring the widths of the patient's arches and comparing them with those in males and females who have normal occlusion will reveal the presence of this factor. Arch width norms for American whites are given in Figure 3.5, Chapter 3.

Patients who have large upper and lower arches associated with generalized spaces may have a large tongue or generalized small teeth, which are etiologic factors associated with some diastemas. Referral to a specialist is the best management decision for these patients.

Maxillary Labial Frenum

A median diastema between the upper central incisors may be associated with an abnormal maxillary labial frenum. Characteristics to be observed include (1) the frenum attaches into the soft tissues between the incisors or even into the palatal tissues lingual to the incisors, (2) the frenum that attaches to the soft tissues between the incisors is wider than normal, and (3) the soft tissues between the central incisors move and are blanched when the upper lip is pulled to stretch the frenum.

A frenectomy, the surgical removal and repositioning of a frenum, is not recommended based on the evidence given earlier. A 20-year-old female patient with an abnormal maxillary frenum is shown in Figure 9.1. A periapical radiograph of the central incisors shows a midline interosseous cleft (Fig. 9.2). This 20-year-old patient had a frenectomy after closure of the

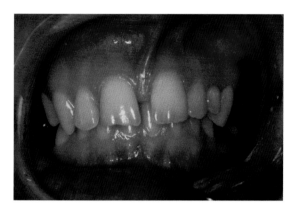

Figure 9.1. Patient with an abnormal maxillary frenum.

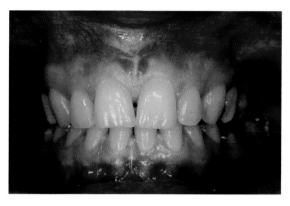

Figure 9.3. Patient's teeth after a frenectomy was performed.

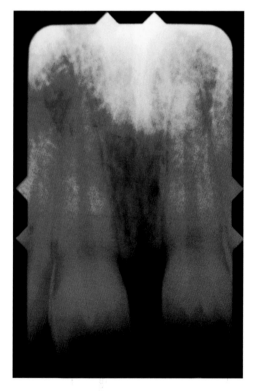

Figure 9.2. Periapical radiograph of the patient with an abnormal frenum.

diastema (Fig. 9.3). One potential negative outcome of a frenectomy is the development of an open gingival embrasure, or black triangle, as observed in this patient (Fig. 9.3) (Kurth and Kokich 2001).

Rotated Incisors

When an incisor is severely rotated, a diastema may appear. Rotation of the tooth to its proper position with a fixed edgewise appliance will reduce or eliminate the diastema problem. Retention of the tooth after treatment to prevent relapse of the rotation is very important. Supracrestal fiberotomy and bonded fixed retainers are used to reduce relapse and retain rotated teeth (Edwards 1988).

Thumb-Sucking Habit

Patients who have a thumb-sucking habit may present with diastemas between the upper incisors. If the patient has a Class I occlusion, interceptive limited treatment involves first stopping the habit and then retracting the incisors. After the habit is stopped, the upper incisors usually return to a more normal position without active orthodontic treatment. Limited orthodontic treatment may be needed to properly position the teeth after the habit has ceased. The use of an appliance in conjunction with psychological support of the patient by the clinician has been shown to be an effective means to help a young patient break the habit (Bourne 2005; Haryett, Hansen, and Davidson 1970).

Angle Classification

Patients with Class I molar and canine occlusion are the most appropriate candidates for limited orthodontic treatment. Patients with Class II and Class III occlusions are best managed by referral to a specialist.

Management with Appliances

Removable appliances are useful when one or two teeth need to be moved, when the diastema is no larger than 2 mm, and when tipping movements from the appliance will not adversely affect the angulation of the tooth. Finger springs originating in the palatal or lingual acrylic are used when diastemas are small and the teeth are located on the crest of the alveolus. Loop springs, also known as arc springs, can be soldered on the labial bow of a Hawley appliance to close a diastema. The spring on a removable appliance should push against the tooth crown at the level of the gingiva to ensure the most favorable movement of the tooth. The anterior palatal acrylic of the removable appliance is given a parabolic shape to guide the tooth or teeth being moved and keep them in the central part of the alveolar ridge. The labial bow on a Hawley appliance can be used to retract all four of the incisors.

When more than one or two teeth must be moved, when rotated teeth must be corrected, and when centering a tooth in a space is required, a fixed edgewise appliance best accomplishes the treatment goals.

Treatment of a Diastema with a Removable Loop Spring Appliance

A 17-year-old patient with a Class I occlusion had a diastema between her maxillary central incisors (Figs. 9.4 to 9.7). In Figure 9.4, the removable appliance to correct the diastema contained two loop springs soldered to the labial bow of a Hawley appliance. Figure 9.5 shows the loop spring on the left side. The appliance is shown from an occlusal view in Figure 9.6. The

appliance is retained in the arch with two ball clasps (Fig. 9.6). The activations of the loop springs using the squared beak of No. 139 bird beak pliers to open the springs are small so as to not overpower the ball clasps. The patient chose not to wear the removable appliance and a fixed appliance achieved the result shown in Figure 9.7. After the diastema was closed, the maxillary central incisors were held together with a metal retainer bonded on the lingual surfaces of the central incisors. The patient was advised to have composite resin aesthetic dentistry treatment to normalize the size and shape of her maxillary lateral incisors. A laboratory prescription for the removable appliance is shown in Figure 9.8.

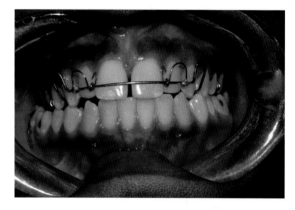

Figure 9.4. Patient with a median diastema and removable appliance to close the diastema.

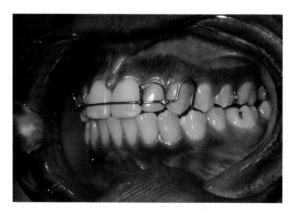

Figure 9.5. View of the teeth and appliance from the left side.

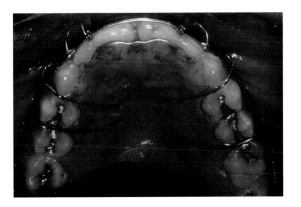

Figure 9.6. Occlusal view of the appliance.

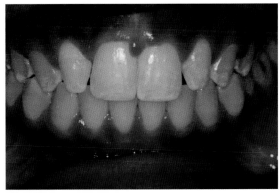

Figure 9.7. Front view of the teeth after closure of the diastema with a fixed appliance.

College of Dentistry
The University of Iowa
Department of Orthodontics

Doctor	A. Able	No. 712	Date 7-12-01
Patient	DAN VARGA		No. 14
Date Needed	7-19-01	Time 8 AM	

℞ Please fabricate a Maxillary Hawley Retainer with .030 labial bow and two .018 rd arch loop springs to close diastema between the Centrals. Place .032 ball clasps between 2nd Premolars and 1st molars. Use Clear acrylic please.

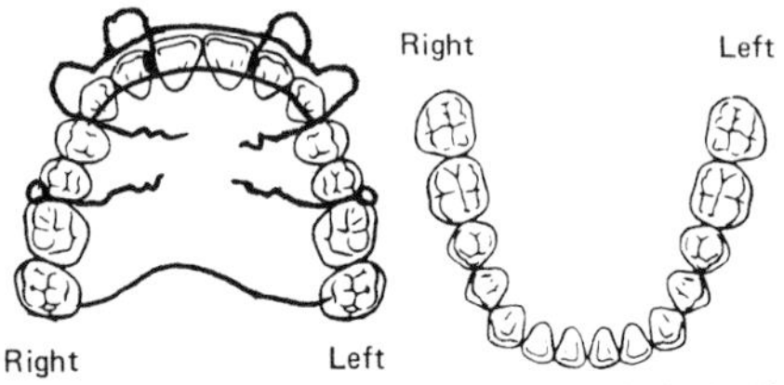

Right   Left

Right   Left

Material	Shade

For Lab Use Only

Instructor

Signature

1162

76010/6-09

Figure 9.8. Laboratory prescription for a removable appliance with two loop springs, labial bow, and ball clasps to close a maxillary diastema.

Treatment of a Diastema with a Finger Spring Removable Appliance

An 8-year 5-month-old girl and parent were concerned about the large median diastema in her upper arch (Figs. 9.9 to 9.14). She also had a small anterior openbite. Her molar occlusion was Class I in the early mixed dentition (Fig. 9.10). A removable appliance to bring the two central incisors together with finger springs is viewed from the front (Fig. 9.12). Also seen are loops embedded in the anterior of the appliance to control tongue position. The appliance is seen from the occlusal in Figure 9.13. After treatment, the diastema between the central incisors was closed and the upper right lateral incisor was almost fully erupted (Fig. 9.14). The upper and lower dental midlines were not coincident, partly due to the diastema closure and partly due to the rightward drifting of the lower incisors. A laboratory prescription for this type of finger spring appliance is shown in Figure 9.15.

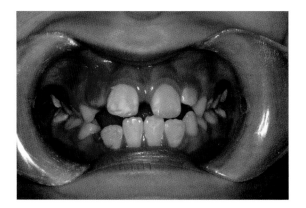

Figure 9.9. Front view of a patient with a median diastema.

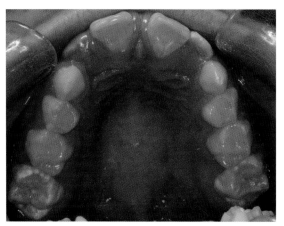

Figure 9.11. Occlusal view of the teeth and diastema.

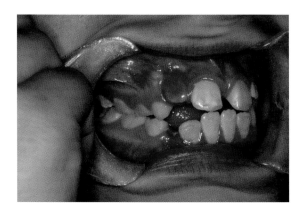

Figure 9.10. View of the right side of the dentition.

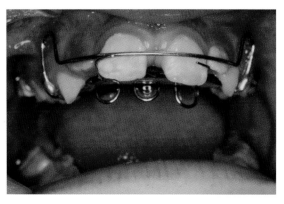

Figure 9.12. Front view of the appliance in the mouth.

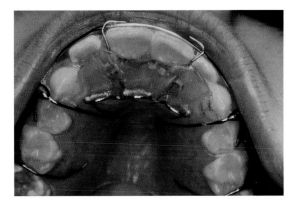

Figure 9.13. Occlusal view of the appliance after closure of the diastema.

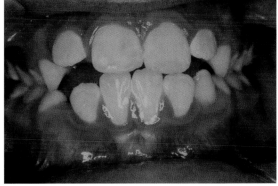

Figure 9.14. Front view after closure of the diastema.

College of Dentistry
The University of Iowa
Department of Orthodontics

Doctor	A. Able	No. 712	Date	8-3-04
Patient	John Morgani		No.	99
Date Needed	8-11-04	Time	3PM	

R̽

Please fabricate a Maxillary Hawley Retainer with .018 rd finger springs with a helix to mesially move centrals to close the diastema.

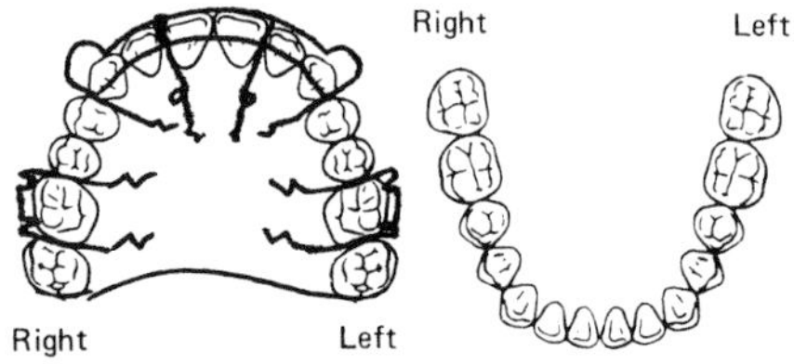

Right   Left

Right   Left

Material   Shade

For Lab Use Only

1162

760100/6-09

Instructor

Signature

Figure 9.15. Laboratory prescription for a removable appliance with two finger springs to close a maxillary diastema.

Treatment of a Diastema Caused by a Thumb Habit

A young patient in the mixed dentition had a thumb sucking habit and end-to-end molar relationships (Figs. 9.16 to 9.20). The habit had opened her bite and opened a diastema between her maxillary central incisors (Fig. 9.16). The patient often held her tongue in the position shown in Figure 9.17. Her tongue was held forward to close the anterior openbite created by the habit. Closure of the anterior opening with the tongue was essential to achieve an anterior seal while swallowing. This tongue behavior is often a byproduct of a thumb sucking habit, even after the habit has stopped. An appliance was constructed to remind the patient not to suck her thumb (Fig. 9.18). The appliance was soldered to bands fitted and cemented to the upper first molars (Fig. 9.18). After discussing the need for stopping the habit, the patient was told that the appliance was a reminder to her not to put her thumb into her mouth. She stopped the habit entirely in about 2 months. The teeth moved into relatively normal positions within 8 weeks after the habit was stopped, as shown in Figure 9.19. The diastema was closed, and the openbite was eliminated. An occlusal view at the same visit

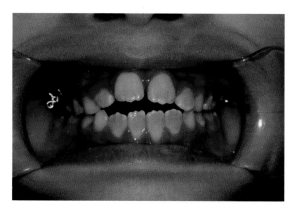

Figure 9.16. Front view of the diastema and anterior bite when the habit appliance was inserted in the mouth.

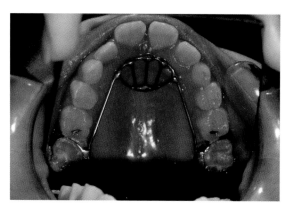

Figure 9.18. Occlusal view of the habit appliance. A soldered crib lies close to the anterior palatal tissues.

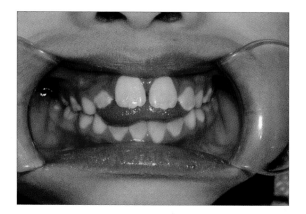

Figure 9.17. View of the patient's tongue filling the anterior openbite.

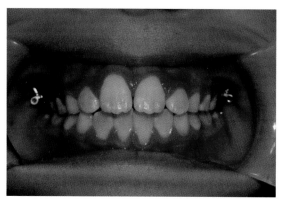

Figure 9.19. Front view 4 months after placement of the habit appliance.

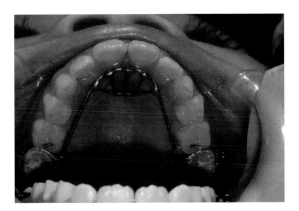

Figure 9.20. Occlusal view 4 months after placement of the habit appliance.

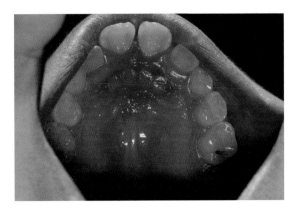

Figure 9.21. Occlusal view of irritated palatal tissues after removal of the habit appliance.

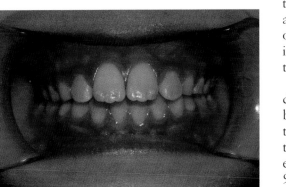

Figure 9.22. Front view of the teeth 1 year after removal of the habit appliance.

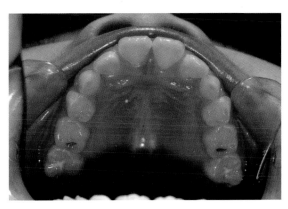

Figure 9.23. Occlusal view of the teeth 1 year after removal of the habit appliance.

shows the improved alignment of the upper incisors after the habit stopped and the teeth had moved physiologically into normal positions (Fig. 9.20). The palate was slightly irritated by the appliance as shown in Figure 9.21. The patient's teeth are shown 1 year after the habit was stopped (Figures 9.22 and 9.23).

Treatment of a Diastema with the Edgewise Fixed Appliance

When the edgewise appliance is used to correct an upper median diastema, the clinician must carefully bond the brackets to the upper anterior teeth to finish the treatment with normal tooth angulations (Mulligan 2003). Proper angulation of the cental incisors will establish a healthy interaction between the incisors and the functional forces produced during mastication.

A 9-year 5-month-old patient in the late mixed dentition was concerned about the diastema between her maxillary central incisors (Figs. 9.24 to 9.27). A simple fixed appliance was placed on the central incisors consisting of a porcelain twin edgewise bracket bonded to each tooth (Fig. 9.25). A segmental arch wire of 20-mil-diameter stainless steel wire was placed in the bracket slots and bent upward at the distal ends of the brackets. A two-link plastic module was stretched

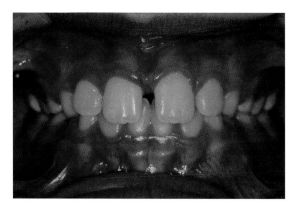

Figure 9.24. Front view of the maxillary diastema.

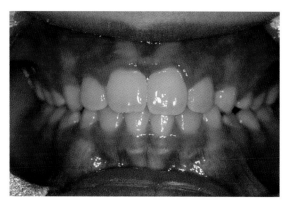

Figure 9.27. In retention, the diastema remained closed.

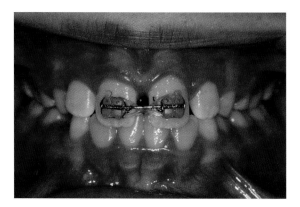

Figure 9.25. Simple edgewise fixed appliance with brackets and plastic module was placed on the central incisors.

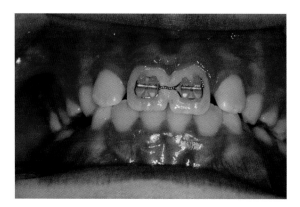

Figure 9.26. After closure of the diastema, the brackets were ligated together with wire.

between the brackets to close the diastema (Fig. 9.25). Stretching the module between the mesial ears of the brackets and using wire ligatures to secure the arch wire keep the module from rotating the incisors as the diastema closes. The diastema closed in a few weeks, opening spaces between the central and lateral incisors on both sides of the arch (Fig. 9.26). The central incisors were held together with ligature wire (Fig. 9.26). Three months later, the patient was seen in retention (Fig. 9.27). A fixed bonded metal lingual retainer (not visible) was attached to the lingual surfaces of the maxillary central incisors before removing the edgewise brackets to keep the diastema closed. The maxillary lateral incisors drifted mesially to close the spaces distal to the central incisors (Fig. 9.27).

A 9-year 6-month-old patient with a Class I molar relation in the early mixed dentition had a diastema between his central incisors that was caused by the rotation of the upper right central incisor by a mesiodens between the central incisors (Figs. 9.28 to 9.31). The mesiodens was surgically removed before these photographs were taken. An occlusal view showed that adequate arch length existed to rotate the central incisor into a more normal position in the arch (Fig. 9.29). A simple fixed appliance consisting of bands on the upper first molars and edgewise brackets on the two upper central incisors, called

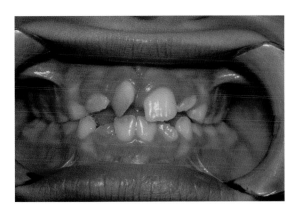

Figure 9.28. Diastema viewed from the front.

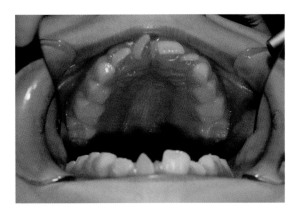

Figure 9.29. Occlusal view illustrates the rotated tooth and arch length available.

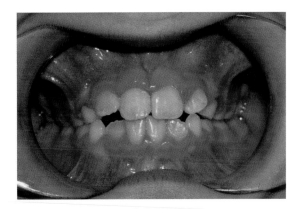

Figure 9.30. After the right central incisor was rotated, the diastema was closed.

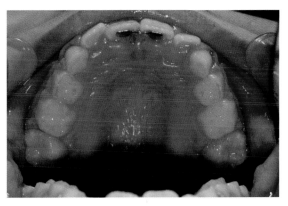

Figure 9.31. Fixed bonded lingual retainer held the teeth together.

a 2 × 2 appliance, was placed to correct the rotation and diastema. A series of nickel titanium archwires from small diameter to larger diameter were used to accomplish the rotation of the upper right central incisor. The patient is shown in Figure 9.30 after the interceptive orthodontic rotation and closure of space. A fixed bonded lingual retainer held the central incisors together and prevented relapse of the rotated central incisor (Fig. 9.31).

An older adolescent patient with a Class I occlusion is shown with diastemas between his incisors that were caused by the small size of his lateral incisors (Figs. 9.32 and 9.33). The Bolton mandibular excess in tooth size is easily recognized. The patient was treated with full upper and lower edgewise fixed appliances to correct his deep bite, align the incisors, and center each upper lateral incisor between the central incisor and canine for composite resin aesthetic dentistry. The teeth are shown after orthodontic and esthetic treatments in Figure 9.33.

A 9-year 6-month-old girl had diastemas between her upper incisors (Figs. 9.34 through 9.39). She had a Class II subdivision malocclusion (E, II, I, I) in the early mixed dentition and was directed to comprehensive treatment. She had a very deep overbite. Overjet was not easily measured to her rotated upper incisors. The left

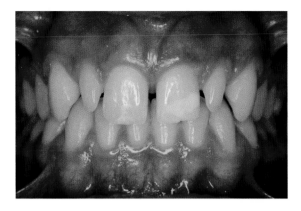

Figure 9.32. Front view before treatment. (Courtesy of Dr. Thomas Southard.)

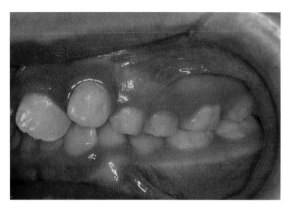

Figure 9.35. View of the left side teeth.

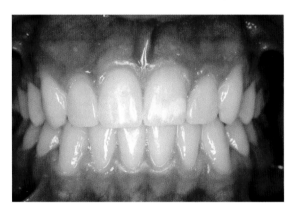

Figure 9.33. Front view after orthodontic treatment with a full edgewise fixed appliance and esthetic build-up of the lateral incisors. (Courtesy of Dr. Thomas Southard.)

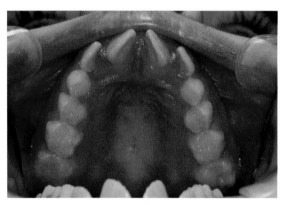

Figure 9.36. Occlusal view of the rotated incisors.

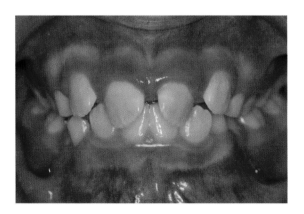

Figure 9.34. Front view of diastemas associated with rotated maxillary central incisors.

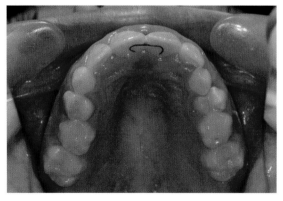

Figure 9.37. Occlusal view after rotation of incisors and closure of the diastemas. A fixed bonded wire retained the teeth.

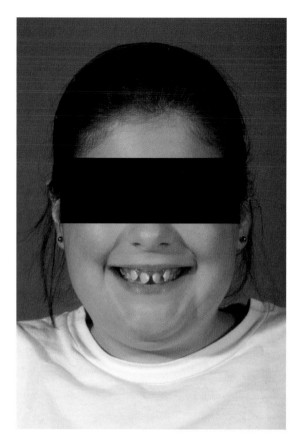

Figure 9.38. Smiling patient before treatment.

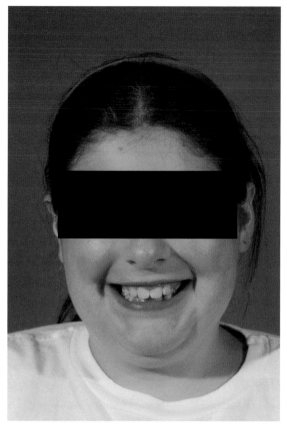

Figure 9.39. Smiling patient after treatment.

side teeth were Class I (Fig. 9.35). An occlusal view shows the rotations of the upper incisors (Fig. 9.36). A full edgewise appliance with nickel titanium wires corrected the rotations of her incisors in a stage 1 treatment. The upper arch is seen after alignment of the incisors (Fig. 9.37). A fixed bonded wire retained the positions of the central incisors (Fig. 9.37). Facial photographs of the patient before treatment (Fig. 9.38) and after treatment (Fig. 9.39) show the improvement in the facial appearance of this patient.

A 7-year 4-month-old girl and her mother were concerned about the size of the median diastema between her upper central incisors (Figs. 9.40 through 9.45). She had a deep overbite of 71% and overjet of 2.8 mm. Her first

molars had Class I relationships. The treatment was not necessary for developmental or occlusal reasons but was done to satisfy the aesthetic concerns of the parent. The occlusal view shows the teeth and spaces in the anterior arch (Fig. 9.41). A simple fixed appliance was used to close the diastema (Fig. 9.42). The closed diastema is viewed from the occlusal (Fig. 9.43). After the appliance was removed, the upper and lower dental midlines were coincident (Fig. 9.44). The retainer used to hold the diastema is shown in Figure 9.45. A fixed bonded retainer could not be used in this patient, because of her deep overbite. Fixed upper lingual retainers in deep bite patients are likely to be dislodged when exposed to heavy forces from mastication.

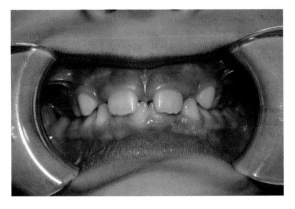

Figure 9.40. Front view of a diastema in a 7-year 4-month-old girl.

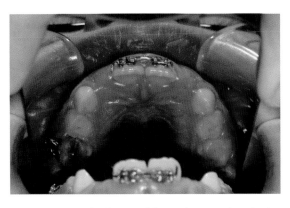

Figure 9.43. Occlusal view of the appliance and teeth after closure of the diastema.

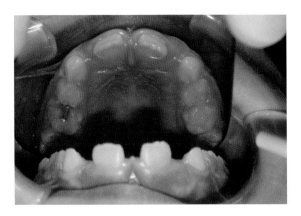

Figure 9.41. Occlusal view of the teeth and diastema.

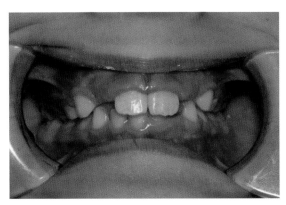

Figure 9.44. Front view after the appliance was removed.

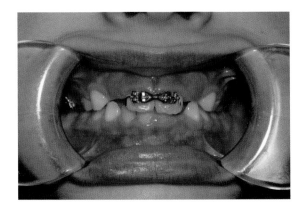

Figure 9.42. Front view of the appliance after closure of the diastema.

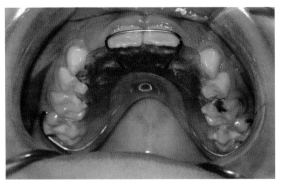

Figure 9.45. Occlusal view of the Hawley retainer in the upper arch.

REFERENCES

Bergström, K., Jensen, R., and Mortensson, B. 1973. The effect of superior labial frenectomy in cases with midline diastema. Am. J. Orthod. 63:633–638.

Bolton, W. A. 1958. Disharmony in tooth size and its relation to the analysis and treatment of malocclusion. Angle Orthod. 28:113–130.

Bourne, C. O. 2005. The comparative effectiveness of two digit-sucking deterrent methods. West Indian Med. J. 54:257–260.

Brunelle, J. A., Bhat, M., and Lipton, J. A. 1996. Prevalence and distribution of selected occlusal characteristics in the U.S. population, 1988-1991. J. Dent. Res. 75(Spec. Issue):706–713.

Dahlberg, A. A. 1953. Concepts of occlusion in physical anthropology and comparative anatomy. J. Am. Dent. Assoc. 46:530–535.

Edwards, J. G. 1988. A long-term prospective evaluation of the circumferential supracrestal fiberotomy in alleviating orthodontic relapse. Am. J. Orthod. 93:380–387.

Haryett, R. D., Hansen, F. C., and Davidson, P. O. 1970. Chronic thumbsucking. Am. J. Orthod. 57:164–178.

Kurth, J. R., and Kokich V. G. 2001. Open gingival embrasures after orthodontic treatment in adults: prevalence and etiology. Am J. Orthod. Dentofac. Orthop. 120:116–123.

Mulligan, T. F. 2003. Diastema closure and long-term stability. J. Clin. Orthod. 37:560–574.

Shashua, D., and Årtun, J. 1999. Relapse after orthodontic correction of maxillary median diastema: a follow-up evaluation of consecutive cases. Angle Orthod. 69:257–263.

Molar Uprighting and Space Regaining

10

Introduction

The dentist who removes either a primary or a permanent tooth or observes a patient shortly after the loss of a tooth has an obligation to inform the patient or parent of the likelihood that teeth adjacent to an extraction site will move in an unfavorable manner. Most of the unfavorable tooth movement occurs in the arch from which the tooth is removed; however, teeth in the opposing arch can also overerupt into the extraction site. In many patients who lose primary molars or permanent teeth, the unfavorable movement of teeth adjacent to the extraction site will require orthodontic treatment to restore good occlusion and prepare the patient for prosthesis. After the adjacent teeth have moved in an undesirable manner, the orthodontic recapture of lost arch length may not fully restore the original arch length. In summary, the time and expense of orthodontic treatment will far exceed the time and expense to prevent undesirable tooth movement adjacent to an extraction site. Space maintenance appliances include the lingual holding arch, a palatal holding arch, and the Hawley retainer.

Essentials of Orthodontics: Diagnosis and Treatment by Robert N. Staley and Neil T. Reske
© 2011 Blackwell Publishing Ltd.

Ectopic Eruption of Permanent First Molars

In 3% to 4% of the American population, permanent first molars erupt ectopically (Kimmel, Gellin, Bohannan, and Kaplan 1982). Ectopic eruption has a familial tendency, occurring more frequently (19%) in siblings (Kurol and Bjerklin 1982). The phenomenon occurs more frequently (25%) in children with cleft lip and palate (Carr and Mink 1965). Maxillary molars are more frequently affected by ectopic eruption than are mandibular molars (Young 1957). In a study of 315 children, the frequency of ectopic eruption was 8% of the sample for maxillary molars and less than 1% for mandibular molars (O'Meara 1962) One-half of the patients present with unilateral ectopic eruption, and one-half, bilaterally (Young 1957). Ectopic eruption of first molars does not differ by gender or race (Kimmel et al. 1982).

Ectopically erupting molars fall into two types: reversible (self correcting) and irreversible. The frequency of the reversible type was reported as 66% in an American sample of 1,619 children (Young 1957) and as 59% in a sample of 2,903 Swedish children (Kurol and Bjerklin 1986). Only a few of the ectopic permanent first molars seen at age 7 and older became reversible (Bjerklin

151

and Kurol 1981). Based on this evidence, we conclude that after the age of 7, the vast majority of patients will experience irreversible ectopic eruption and treatment can proceed to correct the problem. Self-correction and eruption are considerably less frequent in cleft lip and palate patients (Carr and Mink 1965). Non–cleft children under the age of 7 with ectopic molars should be observed to allow time for the molar to self-correct.

Two studies found that patients with ectopically erupting maxillary molars often lack adequate arch length and have a retropositioned and smaller-than-normal maxilla (Canut and Raga 1983; Pulver 1968). One study found that three factors differentiated the irreversible ectopic eruption patients from those with normal eruption: the ectopic group had (1) a steeper angle of eruption, (2) a larger permanent first molar width, and (3) a tendency for a shorter maxilla (Bjerklin and Kurol 1983). Two early review articles summarize ectopic eruption and discuss

clinical management of the problem (Kennedy and Turley 1987; Kurol and Bjerklin 1986).

The distal surface of the primary molar may be resorbed in varying degrees by the ectopically erupting permanent molar crown. In some instances, the ectopic permanent first molar resorbs most of the primary molar's roots, causing premature exfoliation of the primary second molar and eruption of the first molar into the arch space needed by the second premolar. Barberia-Leache, Suarez-Clua, and Saavedra-Ontiveros (2005) described four grades of magnitude for lesions in maxillary primary second molars caused by an ectopically erupting permanent first molar: (1) **Grade I** [mild] involved limited resorption of cementum and dentin; (2) **Grade II** [moderate] involved resorption of the dentin without pulp exposure; (3) **Grade III** [severe] involved resorption of the distal root leading to pulp exposure; Grade IV [very severe] involved resorption that affects the mesial root of the primary second molar. The grades are illustrated in Figure 10.1.

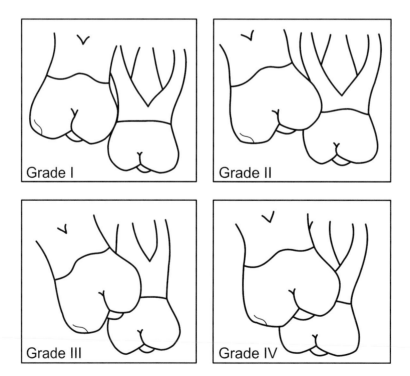

Figure 10.1. Grades for the magnitude of lesions in maxillary primary second molars caused by ectopically erupting first molars.

Barberia-Leache et al. (2005) reported that 4.3% of 509 consecutive Spanish patients between 6 and 9 years old experienced ectopic eruption of maxillary first molars. No gender difference was found. Ectopic eruption occurred unilaterally in 36.4% and bilaterally in 63.6% of the patients, which are not significantly different occurrences. In the unilateral occurrence patients, significantly more ectopic molars were found on the right side than on the left side. Of the 36 ectopic molars in 22 children, 69% were reversible and 31% were irreversible. The majority of Grade I and II molars were reversible and the majority of Grade III and IV molars were irreversible. Some Grade III molars were reversible and some Grade I molars were irreversible.

Early detection of the ectopic eruption of a maxillary permanent first molar and radiographic examination of the problem will help determine the best approach to the problem. Periodic observation is appropriate in younger patients, while patients older than 7 years require treatment.

Uprighting Molars in the Mixed Dentition

The premature loss of a primary second molar because of ectopic eruption of the permanent first molar or because of caries is usually accompanied by the mesial tipping of the adjacent permanent first molar. The erupted first molar then impacts the adjacent nonerupted second premolar. When the problem occurs with an upper permanent first molar, the molar occlusion becomes Class II, and when the problem occurs with a lower first molar, the molar occlusion becomes Class III. In both cases, an asymmetric malocclusion develops unless the problem occurs bilaterally. If these problems are not treated in the mixed dentition, they will probably require orthodontic treatment in the permanent dentition. A panoramic radiograph of a 10-year 4-month-old male patient is shown in Chapter 5, Figure 5.6; in which a lower right permanent first molar is tipped forward over an ankylosed primary second molar that in turn has prevented the eruption of a developing second premolar. In Chapter 5, Figure 5.9, the loss of a primary second molar in an 8-year-old girl has allowed the upper first molar to move forward and impact her upper right second premolar. In Chapter 5, Figure 5.10, a 9-year 7-month-old girl has prematurely lost a lower left primary second molar that allowed the first molar to move forward and impact the lower left second premolar.

Ectopic Eruption of Upper First Molars

A boy aged 9 years 2 months presented with the premature loss of his upper right primary second molar (Figs. 10.2 and 10.3). He had a Class II subdivision right malocclusion with his upper right permanent first molar in a Class II relationship with his lower right permanent first molar. The mesial shifting of his upper first molar impacted his nonerupted upper right second premolar (Figs. 10.3 and 10.4). After the eruption of his upper right first premolar, a removable appliance was constructed with a helical finger spring to move the upper molar distally into a Class I relationship (Fig. 10.5). The patient lost his removable appliance after wearing it for

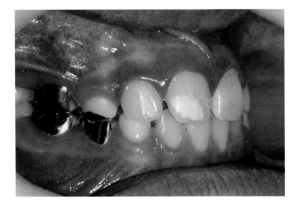

Figure 10.2. Patient with premature loss of his upper right primary second molar.

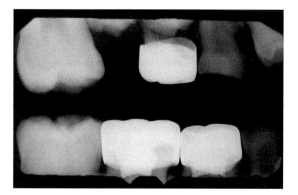

Figure 10.3. Bite wing radiograph showing the impacted upper right second premolar.

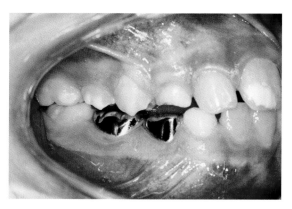

Figure 10.6. The occlusion on the right side is shown after the eruption of the upper right second premolar.

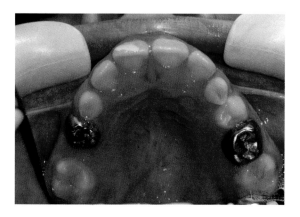

Figure 10.4. Occlusal view of the upper arch with the mesially displaced right permanent first molar.

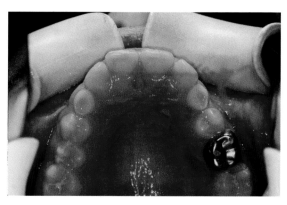

Figure 10.7. Occlusal view of the erupted upper right second premolar is shown.

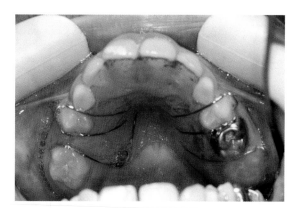

Figure 10.5. Shamy removable appliance was made to move the right first molar distally.

2 months. An edgewise fixed appliance was made to complete the distal movement of the first molar. After receiving the fixed appliance, the patient said that he wished he had not lost his removable appliance! A Nance palatal holding arch retained the regained arch length. At age 10 years 2 months his occlusion is seen after the eruption of his upper second premolar (Figs. 10.6 and 10.7).

The prescription for making the removable appliance is shown in Figure 10.8. The helical coil finger spring for this patient was made from 21 × 28 mil rectangular wire after the design of Shamy (1972). The helix of the spring has a diameter of 2 to 3 mm, is located 8 mm above the

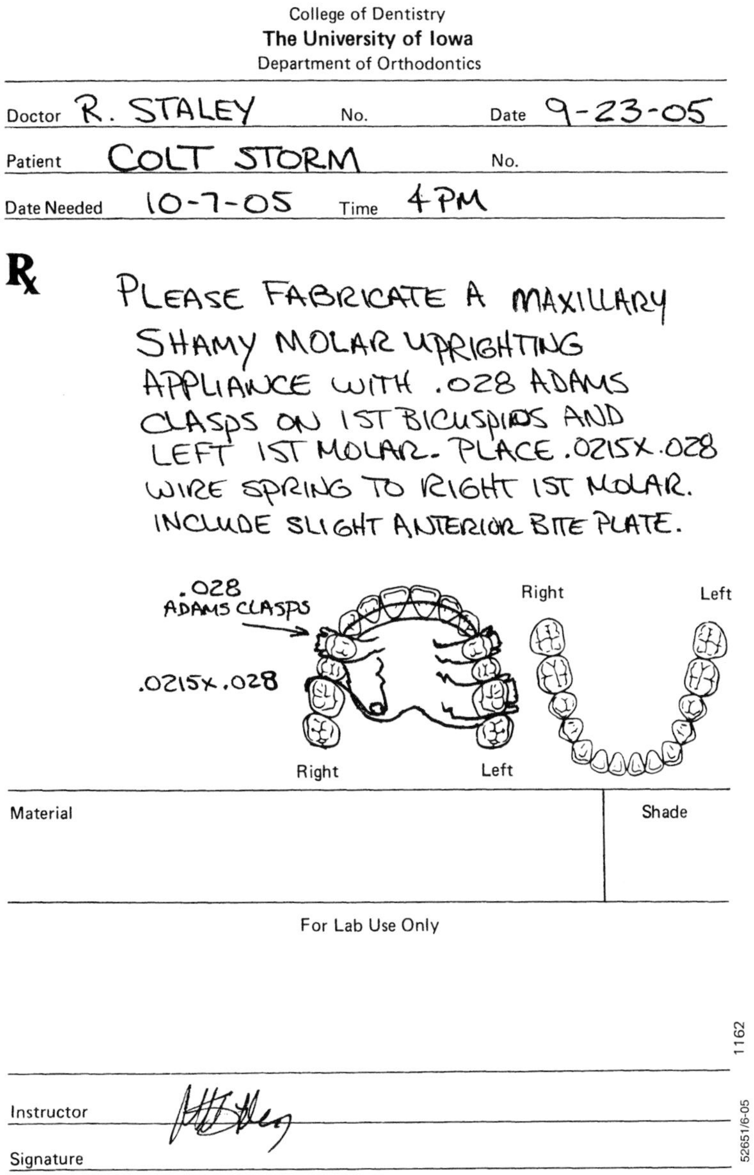

College of Dentistry
The University of Iowa
Department of Orthodontics

Doctor R. STALEY   No.   Date 9-23-05

Patient COLT STORM   No.

Date Needed 10-7-05   Time 4 PM

℞   PLEASE FABRICATE A MAXILLARY
SHAMY MOLAR UPRIGHTING
APPLIANCE WITH .028 ADAMS
CLASPS ON 1ST BICUSPIDS AND
LEFT 1ST MOLAR. PLACE .0215X.028
WIRE SPRING TO RIGHT 1ST MOLAR.
INCLUDE SLIGHT ANTERIOR BITE PLATE.

Material   Shade

For Lab Use Only

Instructor   _____

Signature   _____

1162
52651/6-05

Figure 10.8. Laboratory prescription for an upper Shamy molar uprighting appliance.

lingual gingival margin, and is centered above the middle of the molar crown (Fig. 10.9A). The Shamy appliance was stabilized with Adams clasps on the upper first premolars and the upper left first molar (Adams 1984). The arrowheads of the clasps are adjusted to grip the anchor teeth very tightly, to hold the anchor teeth together and resist the force exerted by the finger spring. An anterior bite plate on the appliance opens the bite 1 to 2 mm to facilitate the movement of the upper molar. The spring is activated by opening the helix with No. 139 bird beak pliers. The arm of the finger spring is activated distally to about the middle of the occlusal surface of the first

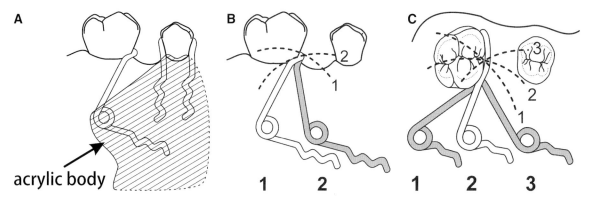

Figure 10.9. Shamy molar distalizing spring: palatal view (**A**), effect of anteroposterior position of the helix on vertical movement of the spring (**B**), and effect of the anteroposterior position of the helix on buccolingual movement of the spring (**C**).

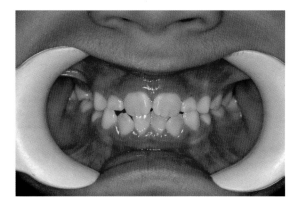

Figure 10.10. Front view of the occlusion.

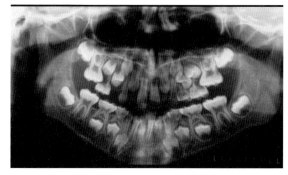

Figure 10.11. Pretreatment panoramic radiograph showing the ectopic eruption of the upper permanent first molars.

molar. The arm of the spring is kept as close as possible to the gingival tissues adjacent to the mesial surface of the tooth so the force exerted by the spring is near the center of resistance of the first molar. During activation, the correctly positioned spring arm (Fig. 10.9B, 1) moves occlusally along an arc determined by the helical coil spring (Fig. 10.9B). This movement requires periodic adjustment of the clasp arm to keep it in contact with the gingival part of the crown. The spring must engage the mesiolingual surface of the molar to guide the tooth distally and buccally along the arch without moving it lingually into crossbite (Fig. 10.9C). The correct position

of the uprighting spring is illustrated in Figure 10.9C, 2. Treatment time to move a molar distally 4 mm is about 4 months, assuming 1 mm per month of tooth movement (Iwasaki, Crouch, Reinhardt, and Nickel 2004).

Another boy aged 5 years 10 months presented with both upper permanent first molars erupting ectopically (Figs. 10.10 through 10.15). A panoramic radiograph (Fig. 10.11) shows his right molar is a Grade IV impaction and his left molar (Fig. 10.13) is a Grade III impaction (Barberia-Leache et al. 2005). The upper primary second molars were extracted to allow eruption of the permanent first molars after considering the great

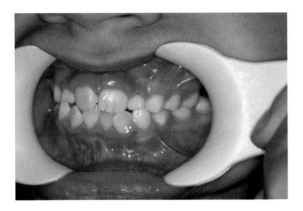

Figure 10.12. View of the teeth on the right side.

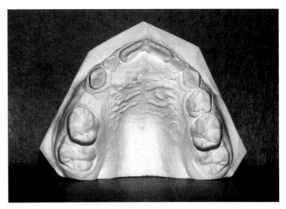

Figure 10.15. Occlusal view of the patient's upper cast illustrates the impaction of both permanent first molars.

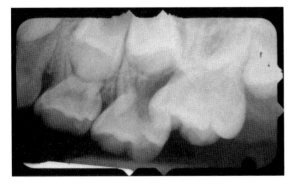

Figure 10.13. Grade III impaction of the upper permanent first molar is shown in this radiograph.

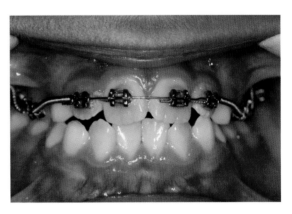

Figure 10.16. Front view of the fixed appliance used to move the upper first molars distally.

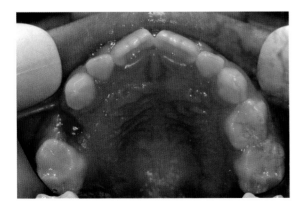

Figure 10.14. Occlusal view of the teeth in this patient.

degree of resorption of the roots of the upper primary second molars. After the permanent first molars were sufficiently erupted, a fixed appliance was placed on the upper teeth to move the first molars distally with trapped coil springs delivering moderate forces (Figs. 10.16 and 10.17). After the upper molars were moved to a Class I occlusion, the molars were retained with a Nance palatal holding arch (Figs. 10.18 and 10.19). The patient is shown at 10 years of age after his second premolars had erupted (Figs. 10.20 and 10.21).

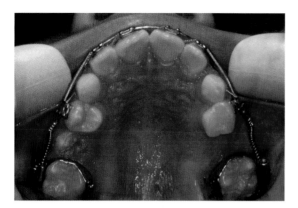

Figure 10.17. Occlusal view of the fixed appliance showing the coil springs that pushed the first molars distally.

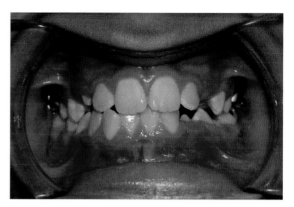

Figure 10.20. Front view of the teeth after the premolars were erupted.

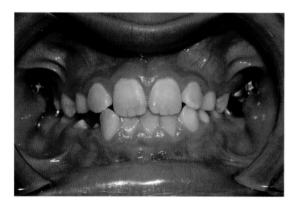

Figure 10.18. Front view of the teeth after the fixed appliance was removed.

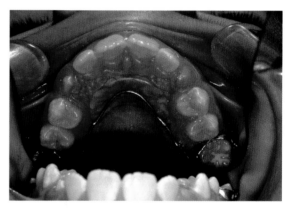

Figure 10.21. Occlusal view of the upper arch showing the erupted premolars and palatal holding arch.

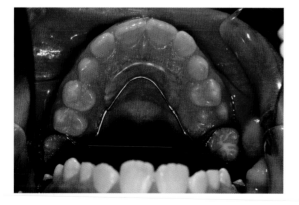

Figure 10.19. Occlusal view showing the palatal holding arch retainer.

Ectopic Eruption and Tipping of Lower First Molars

An 8-year 6-month-old girl lost her lower primary second molars, and presented soon after the loss of her lower left primary second molar. The left permanent first molar was in good position; however, the lower right first molar had drifted forward (Fig. 10.22). A mandibular removable Shamy (1972) appliance was given to the patient (Fig. 10.23). The mandibular spring was made from 21 × 28 mil rectangular wire. The spring is

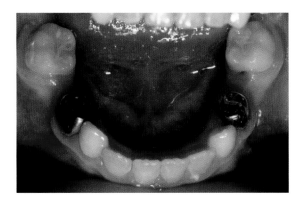

Figure 10.22. The lower arch of a patient with a mesially displaced lower right permanent first molar.

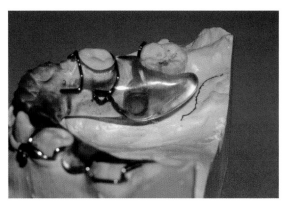

Figure 10.24. Adams clasps and helical finger spring of the appliance are shown.

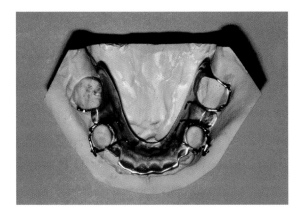

Figure 10.23. Removable Shamy appliance was made to regain arch length.

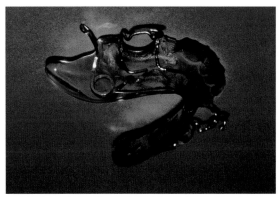

Figure 10.25. Helical spring is shown from the lingual side of the appliance.

shown in Figures 10.24 and 10.25. The spring would operate as described earlier for the maxillary Shamy appliance. A laboratory prescription for the appliance is shown in Figure 10.26. The patient would not wear the appliance and stopped coming for orthodontic appointments. Had this appliance regained arch length, it would have been replaced with a lower lingual holding arch to maintain arch length for the eruption of the premolars and canines.

A 9-year 11-month-old girl presented with the early loss of a lower left primary second molar resulting in the impaction of her lower left second premolar and a Class III subdivision left malocclusion (Figs. 10.27 through 10.30). In Figure 10.27, the deviation of the lower dental midline to the left side can be seen. The periapical film in Figure 10.30 shows the impaction of the lower left second premolar and a favorable space between the lower left first and second molars

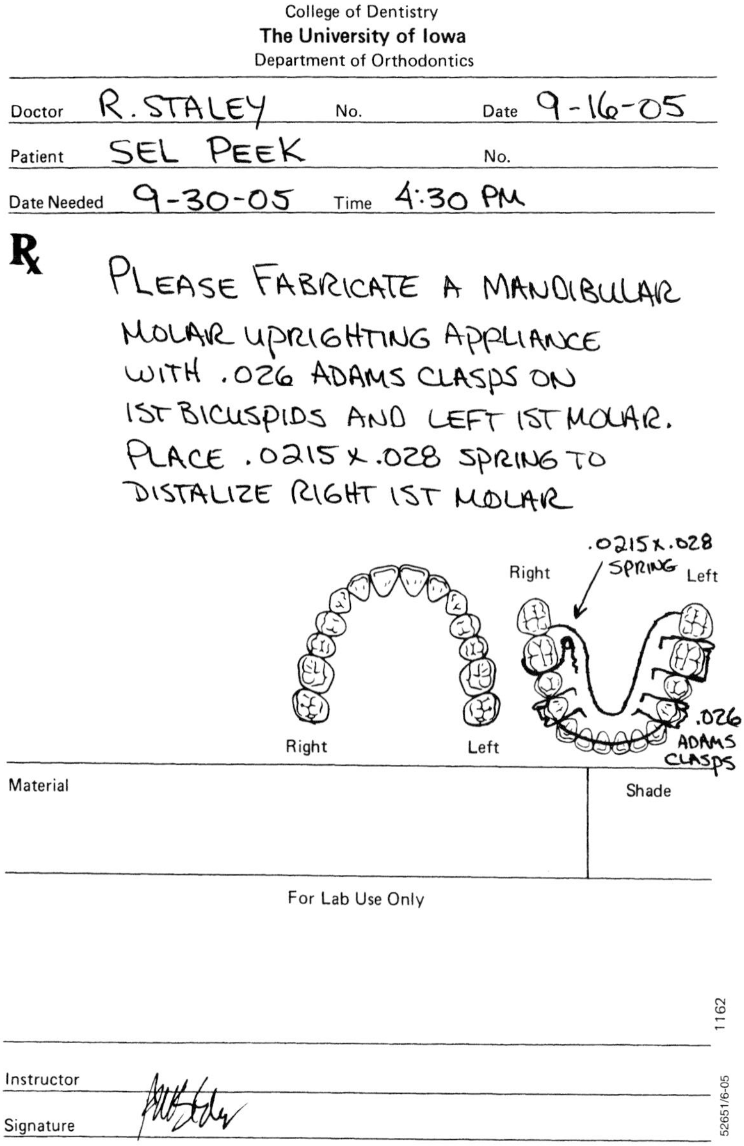

College of Dentistry
The University of Iowa
Department of Orthodontics

Doctor	R. STALEY	No.	Date 9-16-05
Patient	SEL PEEK		No.
Date Needed	9-30-05	Time 4:30 PM	

℞

PLEASE FABRICATE A MANDIBULAR
MOLAR UPRIGHTING APPLIANCE
WITH .026 ADAMS CLASPS ON
1ST BICUSPIDS AND LEFT 1ST MOLAR.
PLACE .0215 x .028 SPRING TO
DISTALIZE RIGHT 1ST MOLAR

.0215 x .028
SPRING
Right   Left

Right   Left

.026
ADAMS
CLASPS

Material _____ Shade _____

For Lab Use Only

Instructor _____
Signature _____

1162

5265 1/6-05

Figure 10.26. Laboratory prescription for a lower Shamy molar uprighting appliance.

that can be used to move the lower first molar distally. The patient's pretreatment panoramic radiograph is shown in Chapter 5, Figure 5.10. A fixed edgewise appliance was used to move the lower left first molar distally (Figs. 10.31 through 10.34). The appliance used a trapped coil spring to move the lower left first premolar mesially and the lower left first molar distally (Figs. 10.32 through 10.34). At the removal of the appliance, the lower midline had moved to the right toward the upper midline (Fig. 10.35) and the lower left second premolar had fully erupted (Fig. 10.36).

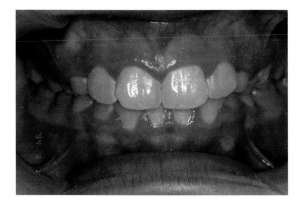

Figure 10.27. Front view of the teeth of a patient who prematurely lost her lower left primary second molar. Notice the shift of the lower dental midline to the left.

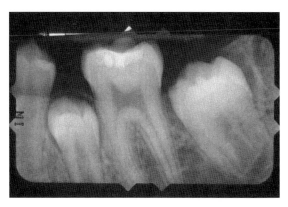

Figure 10.30. Periapical radiograph showing the impaction of the lower left second premolar and the tipped permanent first molar.

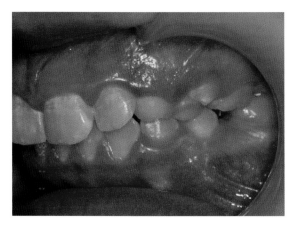

Figure 10.28. View of the left side showing the mesially displaced lower left permanent first molar.

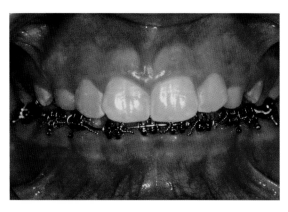

Figure 10.31. Front view of the edgewise fixed appliance used to move the lower left permanent first molar distally.

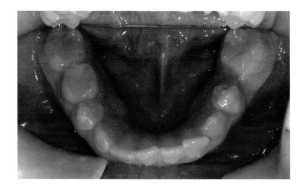

Figure 10.29. Occlusal view of the lower arch showing the loss of arch length in the lower left quadrant.

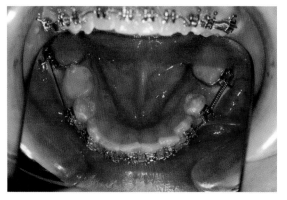

Figure 10.32. Occlusal view of the space regaining fixed appliance.

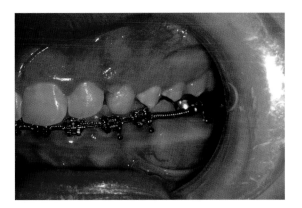

Figure 10.33. View showing the eruption of the lower left second premolar.

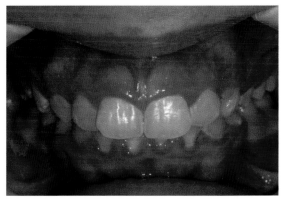

Figure 10.35. Front view after the fixed appliance was removed. Notice the improvement of the lower dental midline.

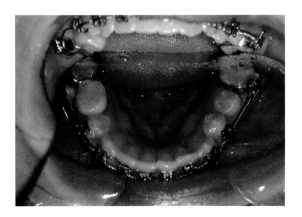

Figure 10.34. Occlusal view of the erupted second premolar.

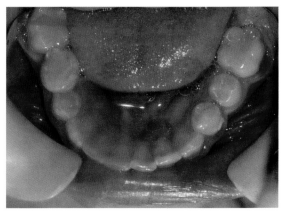

Figure 10.36. Occlusal view after the fixed appliance was removed.

Mesial Tipping of Permanent Molars after Loss of a First Molar

In the permanent dentition, the loss of a **first molar** by extraction can be followed by the mesial drifting and tipping of the second molar and distal drifting of premolars into the extraction site (Fig. 10.37A). In Figure 10.37, tracings from several panoramic radiographs show the undesirable movements of lower second and third molars following the loss of a first molar. If a mixed-dentition patient loses a first molar while the second molar is not yet erupted, the second molar may erupt forward in the arch and finally take the position of the first molar, or be nearly in contact with the second premolar. If the second molar erupts over a long period of time, the first molar in the opposing arch may over-erupt and keep the second molar from fully erupting. If the first molar is lost after the second molar is fully erupted, the second molar will usually tip forward into the extraction site of the first molar (Fig. 10.37A). A third molar usually tips forward with the second molar after the loss of a first molar in the adult dentition (Fig. 10.37, C and D). Sometimes when a first molar is lost, the second molar remains in its original position, because the good occlusion of the opposing upper teeth keeps it from moving mesially.

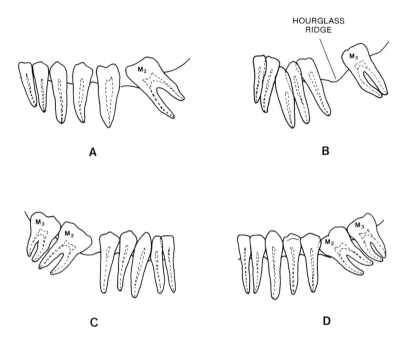

Figure 10.37. Tracings from panoramic radiographs of four patients with mandibular molars tipped into molar extraction sites: after loss of the first molar (**A, C, D**); after loss of the first and second molars (**B**).

When older adolescents and adults lose a first molar, the alveolar ridge at the extraction site eventually resorbs. Resorption of alveolar bone at the extraction site is hastened when the buccal and/or lingual alveolar plates are lost during an extraction. The resorbed ridge is narrow and is called an **hour glass ridge** because of its appearance from the occlusal view (Fig. 10.37B). Hour glass resorption is more common in the lower than in the upper arch. Orthodontic movement of a tooth through the resorbed ridge to eliminate the need for prosthesis may be possible but may be very difficult. The mesial root of the molar can be partially resorbed during its movement through a resorbed ridge. The smaller premolars can more easily move through resorbed ridges than molars. If the occlusion has a Class III tendency or if premolar and anterior teeth are crowded, moving the premolars distally can help close a molar extraction site with an orthodontic appliance. Garcia-Fernandez (2000) introduced a distraction osteogenesis procedure to widen an hour glass ridge before attempting to protract a molar through an edentulous alveolar ridge. The objective of molar protraction mechanics is to finish with the upper and lower dental midlines coincident and the canines Class I. In a unilateral space closure, these objectives are difficult to obtain with conventional orthodontic mechanics. Implants and temporary anchorage devices can be used as rigid anchors to move second and third molars forward without having a detrimental effect on the position of the other teeth (Roberts, Marshall, and Mozsary 1990; Roberts, Nelson, and Goodacre 1994).

Rather than closing the extraction site of a first molar, orthodontic appliances are commonly used to upright and move distally the mesially tipped second molar and move the adjacent premolars forward prior to prosthetic replacement of the lost tooth. Uprighting and moving the second and third molar crowns distally will extrude their crowns and open the bite, so the patient must be told that occlusal equilibration will be needed to close the bite during and after this treatment. The orthodontic treatment must be coordinated with the restorative dentist who will construct an appropriate prosthesis.

Prevention of Molar Tipping after the Loss of a First Molar

Dentists can best serve their patients by preventing the tipping of teeth after the extraction of a first molar. The teeth adjacent to the extraction site can be kept from drifting into the site with a Hawley retainer until the patient has received a prosthetic replacement. Before the extraction, the dentist should also inform the patient that a second molar and healthy third molar can be moved forward by an orthodontist to close the extraction site, if orthodontic movement is started within 10 days after the extraction. This applies also to the extraction of a carious second molar behind which is a healthy third molar. Teeth are most optimally moved through **fresh extraction** sites in which the alveolar bone has not yet resorbed. The buccal and lingual alveolar bone plates must be preserved during extraction to ensure that a molar distal to the extraction site can be successfully moved into the extraction site. Dentists should uphold the highest standards of care by informing the patient about these preventive and treatment options and strongly urge the patient to promptly pursue either prosthetic replacement or orthodontic treatment.

Impaction of Second Molars

A lower **second molar** may erupt only partially as it tips mesially and becomes caught under the crown of an erupted first molar. In Figure 10.38,

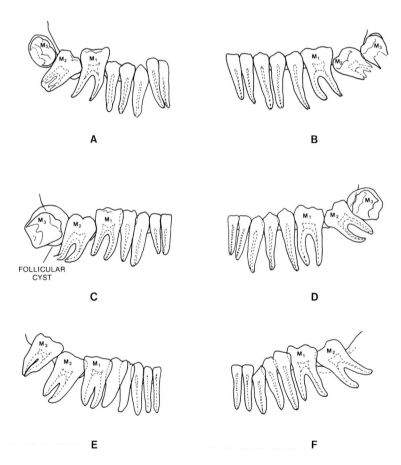

Figure 10.38. Tracings from panoramic radiographs of six patients with impacted mandibular second molars.

tracings of several panoramic radiographs illustrate impacted lower second molars. Impaction of lower second molars is evidence of inadequate mandibular arch length. If an impacted third molar lies distal to the impacted second molar (as illustrated in Figure 10.38, B–E), consider extracting the third molar to create arch length to accommodate uprighting of the second molar. In adolescent patients, the molar in the opposing arch is usually present but not overerupted; however, in adult patients, the opposing molar may be overerupted. When the opposing tooth is overerupted, it will seriously limit how far the tipped molar can extrude while being uprighted. In these cases, removal of enamel from the occlusal surfaces of both molars will be needed to keep from opening the bite of the patient. The overerupted molar can also be intruded with an orthodontic appliance before the tipped molar is uprighted.

Loss of Both First and Second Molars

Sometimes both molars are lost to extraction and a third molar is left malpositioned at the distal end of the ridge. Also, one or two premolars and a first molar may be lost, leaving a lone malpositioned second or third molar at the distal end of the arch. Fixed appliances cannot easily control the movement of a tipped molar so far from the other teeth in the arch. The end of the arch wire becomes an extended cantilever beam that cannot efficiently move the tooth. An implant placed near the malpositioned tooth will allow the tooth to be efficiently moved. A removable appliance can be used to upright a tipped molar in these cases, provided that only a simple tipping movement is required and that at least three posterior anchor teeth are available for Adams clasps, one of which is on the side with the tipped molar. Equilibration of the occlusal surface of the uprighted molar will be required to keep the bite from opening.

T-Loop Uprighting Spring and Edgewise Fixed Appliance

The T-loop spring in an edgewise fixed appliance is effective in uprighting a mesially tipped molar. A segmental T-loop appliance is illustrated in Figure 10.39. The T-loop is bent with either bird beak pliers or loop forming pliers. The first step in treatment after banding the molars and bracketing of other teeth is leveling of the anchor teeth shown in Figure 10.38, A and B. The appliance can be either segmental as shown or include, more ideally, the whole arch. Leveling involves the use of flexible and smaller wires at first followed by larger and larger wires until an 18×25 mil rectangular stainless steel wire can be inserted into the edgewise bracket slots on the anchor teeth. The molar to be uprighted is not included in the leveling wires.

The T-loop spring wire is shown in Figure 10.39C. The loop is bent with the part going into the molar tube at a lower level than the part that inserts into the appliance on the anchor teeth. The distal leg of the wire should be bent downward as shown in Figure 10.40A. The T-loop spring winds up when the wire is inserted into the molar tube and the brackets of the anchor teeth (Fig. 10.39, D and E). The loop unwinds as the wire uprights the tipped molar. The design of the T-loop spring wire helps to control extrusion of the molar (Fig. 10.39F). If distal movement of the tipped molar is desired to open space in the arch for prosthesis, the wire distal to the molar can be cut flush with the distal terminus of the buccal tube. The T-loop can be opened mesiodistally to move the molar farther distally if desired. If distal movement of the molar is not desirable, then the wire distal to the molar is bent down (cinched). Cinching the T-loop spring will rotate the roots of the molar mesially and the crown distally. The wire mesial to the canine in a segmental appliance is bent down or inward toward the embrasure in all circumstances. When the missing molar will be replaced by prosthesis, spaces remaining between the premolars and canines are closed by trapping an open coil spring between the uprighted molar and nearest premolar. To keep

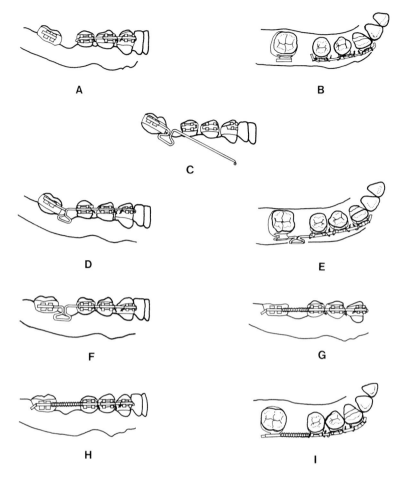

Figure 10.39. T-loop uprighting appliance: segmental arch wire (**A**, **B**), T-loop spring not activated (**C**), T-loop spring activated (**D, E**), after uprighting molar (**F**), and arch wire with coil spring to close spaces between anchor teeth (**G, H, I**).

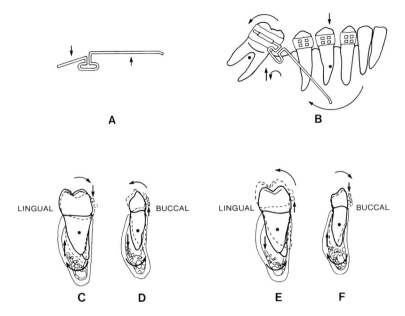

Figure 10.40. Forces generated by the T-loop spring: lateral view of the spring (**A**), rotation of the teeth in the mesiodistal plane (**B**), vertical forces generated by the vertical step in the spring (**C, D**), and vertical forces generated from the clockwise grand rotation (**E, F**).

the action of the coil spring under control, the arch wire must be bent down at the distal of the molar tube and mesial to the canine bracket, or in full arch appliances bent down at the distal end of both molar tubes (Fig. 10.39, G–I).

Forces Generated by the T-loop Uprighting Spring

The forces generated by the T-loop wire are shown in Figure 10.40. For additional information about how teeth move, see Chapter 12. A lateral view of a segmental T-loop spring is shown in Figure 10.39A. Figure 10.39B shows how the segmental wire rotates teeth in the mesiodistal plane. The wire rotates the molar with a counterclockwise couple that acts around the center of the buccal tube. The wire creates a series of couples that act around the centers of the brackets of the premolars and canine. The couple (a pair of forces that are equal in magnitude, opposite in direction, and act in the same plane that rotate a tooth around a point located

in the center of a bracket or tube) on the second premolar is clockwise, the couple on the first premolar in counterclockwise, and the couple on the canine is clockwise, as the couples from molar to canine obey Newton's third law of motion. The molar also rotates around its center of resistance (the black dot between the roots) if the T-loop also pushes the molar distally. When the molar rotates primarily around its center of resistance, its crown will rise vertically much more than when it rotates around the center of the tube. The upward movement of the crown as the molar rotates around its center of resistance causes an opening of the bite, which is usually not desirable. To counter this tendency for molar extrusion during uprighting, use larger stiffer rectangular arch wires, keep the loop as small as practical (reduces flexibility and is kinder to adjacent soft tissues), and bend the distal segment of the wire at a lower level than the wire that engages the anchor teeth.

The premolar-canine segment rotates en masse around some point between the second premolar and canine (black dot in the root of the first premolar) as the mesial leg of the sectional wire rotates down and backward (Fig. 10.39B). The molar also rotates about this point in an upward and forward direction. This grand rotation moves in a clockwise direction. The horizontal step between the mesial and distal legs creates a grand rotation of the teeth that moves them in an opposite counterclockwise direction. As the molar uprights, these forces balance out, leaving the teeth in new positions that conform to the shape of the sectional arch wire. After the molar is uprighted, replace the T-loop spring with a level arch wire to align the teeth and prevent the T-loop spring from moving the teeth eventually into undesirable positions.

A view from the distal surface of the teeth in the buccolingual plane shows the affects of the vertical forces on the teeth (Fig. 10.40, C–F). Because it is important to control vertical changes, a clinician places counteracting force systems to keep vertical changes minimal. The vertical step in the horizontal levels of the mesial and distal legs of the arch wire (Fig. 10.40A) produces a counterclockwise grand rotation with the vertical forces shown in Figure 10.40, C and D. The vertical forces arising from the vertical step in the T-loop arch wire shown in Figure 10.40, C and D, counteract the vertical forces that arise from the activated T-loop spring shown in Figure 10.40, E and F. The clockwise grand rotation arising from activating the T-loop spring moves the premolars downward and moves the molar upward as shown in Figure 10.40, E and F. The downward force translates the premolar downward a short distance and moves its crown buccally as the tooth rotates around its center of resistance. When the arch wire binds in the bracket slot, the premolar will rotate in the buccolingual plane around the center of the rectangular arch wire. The upward force on the molar will roll the crown lingually as the tooth extrudes and rotates about its center of resistance. When the rectangular wire binds in the buccal tube, the molar will rotate around the center of the arch wire (Fig. 10.40, E and F). The movements of the teeth and forces in Figure 10.40, C and D, are the reverse for those described in detail for Figure 10.40, E and F.

Patient Treated with a T-Loop Uprighting Spring

An 11-year 4-month-old girl who had an impacted lower left second molar is shown in Figures 10.41 through 10.46. Her lower left second molar is impacted behind her lower left first molar (Figs. 10.41 and 10.42). A periapical radiograph shows an altered alveolar bone profile between the first and second molars commonly observed mesial to tipped lower molars (Fig. 10.42). A T-loop spring, incorporated into a full lower arch wire was used to upright the impacted second molar (Fig. 10.43). The T-loop spring

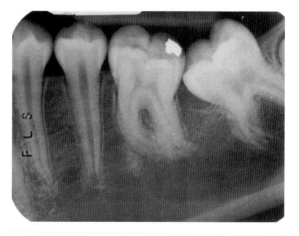

Figure 10.41. Panoramic radiograph shows the impacted lower left permanent second molar.

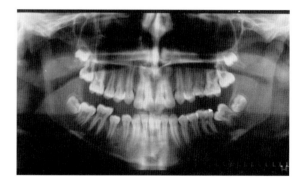

Figure 10.42. Periapical radiograph shows the impacted tooth with an altered interdental alveolar bone profile.

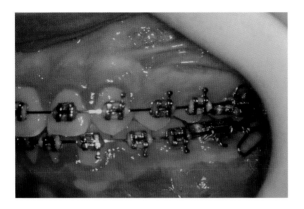

Figure 10.43. View of the edgewise appliance and the T-loop spring on the patient's right side.

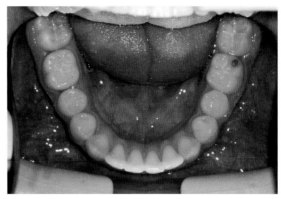

Figure 10.45. View of the lower arch after the removal of the fixed appliance.

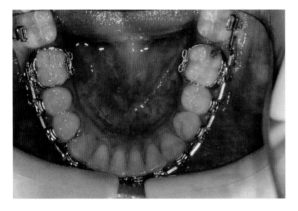

Figure 10.44. View of the molar after it was uprighted by the spring. A new lower arch wire replaced the T-loop wire to protract the uprighted second molar.

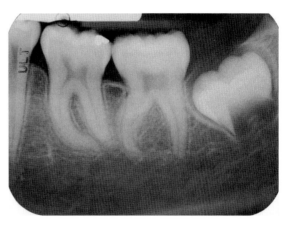

Figure 10.46. Periapical radiograph of the uprighted molar shows a more normal alveolar bone profile between the first and second molars.

moved the second molar distally as it uprighted the tooth (Fig. 10.44). An occlusal view of the lower arch after the appliance was removed is shown in Figure 10.45. A periapical radiograph after treatment shows the atypical form of the mesial root of the second molar that limited the extent to which the molar could be uprighted (Fig. 10.46). The radiograph in Figure 10.46 also shows remodeling of the alveolar bone located mesial to the second molar compared to its configuration before treatment (Fig. 10.42), a beneficial result of the uprighting.

Helical Uprighting Spring

A fixed edgewise appliance with a helical uprighting spring is illustrated in Figure 10.47. Because the helical spring extrudes the molar that it uprights, it should not be used where the molar to be uprighted has no opposing molar. The helical spring is best used in patients who have a fully erupted opposing molar, because the opposing tooth will counteract the extrusion force of the spring during mastication and when the teeth are brought together in occlusion. The anchor

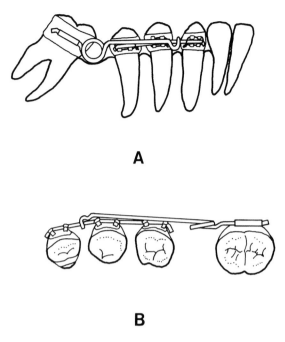

Figure 10.47. Helical uprighting spring: buccal view (**A**), occlusal view (**B**).

teeth are first leveled with a series of leveling arch wires up to a larger wire such as an 18 × 25 mil stainless steel rectangular wire. A full arch wire is preferable to the segmental wire illustrated in Figure 10.47.

Bird beak pliers or loop forming pliers are used to form the helical spring from an 18 × 25 mil stainless steel wire. The wire is kept on the same horizontal level on each side of the helix (Fig. 10.48A). The helix is bent toward the gingiva so that the helix does not interfere with the occluding teeth of the opposite arch (Fig. 10.48A). The diameter of the helix is about 3 to 4 mm and should be small enough to avoid injury of the gingival tissues. Bend the helix so that it winds up when the spring is activated and unwinds when it delivers the uprighting force (Figs. 10.47A and 10.48B). The mesial leg of the helical spring has a hook that activates the spring when it engages the arch wire running through the anchor teeth brackets (Fig. 10.47A). The vertical loop at the mesial end of the spring allows for mesial-distal adjustment of the hook, if needed (Figs.

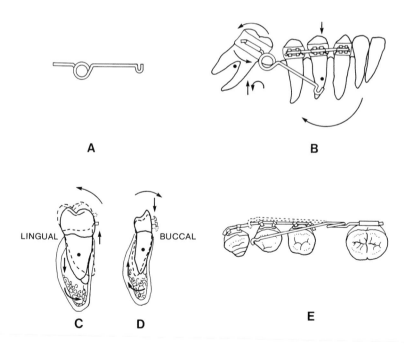

Figure 10.48. Forces generated by a helical uprighting spring: lateral view of spring (**A**), an unactivated spring showing forces generated in the mesiodistal plane (**B**), vertical forces on the molar and second premolar (**C, D**), and occlusal view of unactivated spring (**E**).

10.47A and 10.48B). The spring wire is bent (cinched) distal to the molar tube (Figs. 10.47A and 10.48B). After the molar is uprighted, a new arch wire is inserted to either close space that may be present or further open the space mesial to the uprighted molar for prosthesis (Fig. 10.39, G–I).

Forces Generated by the Helical Uprighting Spring

The forces generated by the helical uprighting spring are illustrated in Figure 10.48, B–D. The forces acting the mesiodistal plane are shown in Figure 10.47B. If the helical spring is activated by hooking its arm over the arch wire between the first premolar and canine, the spring puts a downward force on the arch wire between the canine and first premolar. The downward force rotates the canine-premolar segment en masse in a clockwise grand rotation that moves the canine downward and backward and moves the second premolar upward and forward around some point (black dot) between the canine and second premolar. To minimize this grand rotation, the arm of the helical spring should be located on the arch wire as near as possible to the center of mass of the three anchor teeth in this segmental version of the appliance. A full arch wire would further minimize this grand rotation. If the arm of the helical spring is hooked between the premolars, the downward force would create a counterclockwise grand rotation. The downward force also translates the canine and premolars downward a short distance. A reactive vertical force extrudes the molar. The helical spring rotates the molar by a couple that moves the crown distally and roots mesially (Fig. 10.48B).

The forces that operate in the buccolingual plane are illustrated in Figure 10.48, C and D. The vertical force on the molar extrudes it and rolls its crown lingually and its roots labially as the tooth rotates around its center of resistance (Fig. 10.48C). The upward force also translates the tooth upward. The downward force rolls the crowns of the anchor teeth buccally and moves their roots lingually as the teeth rotate around their centers of resistance (Fig. 10.48D). The downward force also translates the anchor teeth downward slightly. The clockwise grand rotation of the anchor unit creates an upward vertical force on the second premolar that may roll the crown of this anchor tooth lingually and translate it upward slightly (Fig. 10.48B). To counteract the lingual movement of the molar crown, a bend is placed in the mesial arm of the helical spring wire so that the hook lies over the center of the occlusal surface of the first premolar, before engaging the hook (Fig. 10.48E) (Dr. John Casko, 1987, personal communication).

Patient Treated with a Helical Uprighting Spring

A 12-year 6-month-old boy with an impacted lower left second molar that was uprighted by a helical spring is shown in Figures 10.49 to 10.52. The impacted molar had caries on its mesial surface, a complication that can occur to a partially erupted and impacted molar. A full arch edgewise appliance held the anchor teeth together. The helical spring is shown at its initial activation in Figures 10.49 and 10.50. The molar was uprighted in about 1 month as shown in Figures 10.50 and 10.52. The carious lesion in the second molar is visible in Figure 10.52. By comparing the height of the mesial leg and helix of the spring in Figures 10.49 and 10.51, it is obvious that the spring moved upward in

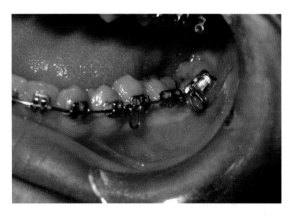

Figure 10.49. Activated helical uprighting spring to upright a lower left second molar is shown.

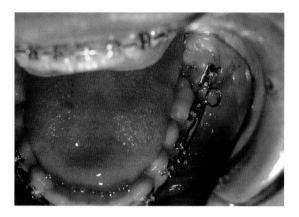

Figure 10.50. Activated helical spring is part of a full lower arch wire.

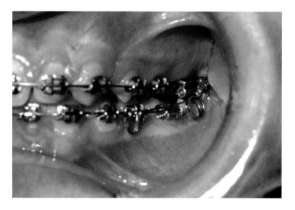

Figure 10.51. Appliance is shown after the lower second molar was uprighted.

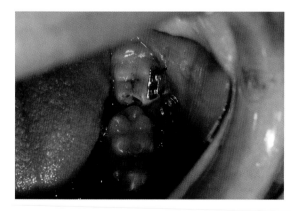

Figure 10.52. Carious lesion on the mesial surface of the impacted lower left second molar is visible.

comparison to the bracket on the lower first molar. The vertical forces on the uprighted second molar were counteracted by the opposing upper teeth. Also, the movement of the anchor teeth, which included the lower left first molar and all other erupted lower teeth, was minimized. To make room for the uprighting of the second molar in this patient, the lower first molar was bonded rather than banded.

Other Appliances Used to Upright Molars

Shellhart and Oesterle (1999) developed a pair of up righting springs that minimize the extent to which the up righted molar will move vertically. Roberts et al. (1982) designed an uprighting spring with the same goal. A flexible nickel titanium arch wire can be used to engage impacted molars to upright them. A temporary anchorage device (TAD) can be used to stabilize the movement of the anchor teeth while a nickel-titanium arch wire uprights the tipped molar. A flexible wire used in combination with a coil spring can also effectively upright a molar under circumstances that permit some extrusion of the molar.

Repositioning of Teeth Prior to Prosthetic Restoration

A 26-year 8-month-old woman received orthodontic treatment with a fixed edgewise appliance to position abutment teeth for a bridge (Figs. 10.53 to 10.58). Her upper right second premolar was missing and the adjacent first premolar required repositioning for the construction of a composite resin bridge. Figures 10.53 and 10.54 show the patient prior to orthodontic treatment. Figures 10.55 and 10.56 show the patient after orthodontic treatment. Figures 10.57 and 10.58 show the patient after she received her bridge.

A 32-year-old man who was missing his upper left first premolar presented for orthodontic treatment to align abutment teeth prior to prosthetic replacement (Figs. 10.59 to 10.64). The

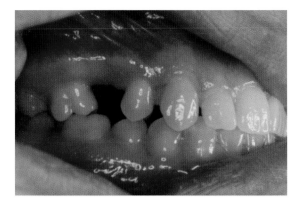

Figure 10.53. Missing upper right second premolar has allowed tipping of the first molar and first premolar.

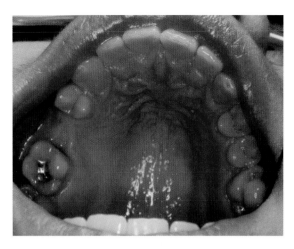

Figure 10.56. Occlusal view of the arch after removal of the fixed appliance is shown.

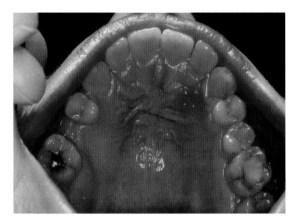

Figure 10.54. Occlusal view of the upper arch is shown before treatment.

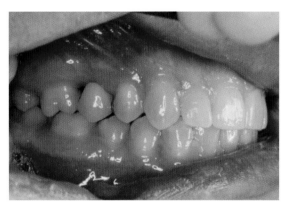

Figure 10.57. Composite resin bridge replaced the missing upper second premolar.

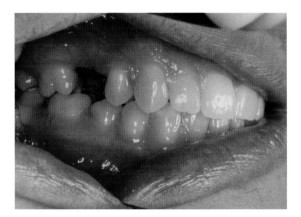

Figure 10.55. Molar and first premolar are shown after a edgewise fixed appliance aligned the teeth.

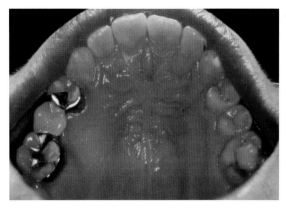

Figure 10.58. Occlusal view of the bridge.

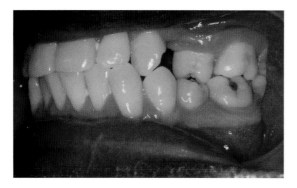

Figure 10.59. Patient with a missing upper left first premolar is shown.

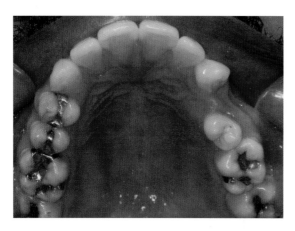

Figure 10.60. Occlusal view prior to treatment shows the rotated canine and second premolar adjacent to the extraction site.

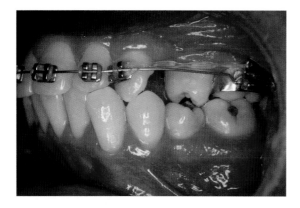

Figure 10.61. Lateral view of the edgewise fixed appliance showing a bend in the arch wire mesial to the upper first molars to maintain arch length while rotating the canine and premolar.

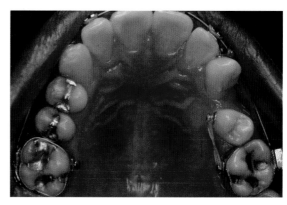

Figure 10.62. Occlusal view shows an elastic chain between lingual buttons on the premolar and molar.

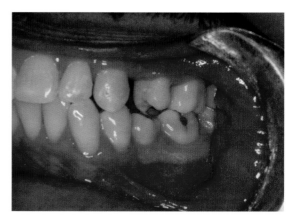

Figure 10.63. After orthodontic treatment, the abutment teeth are rotated to normal position.

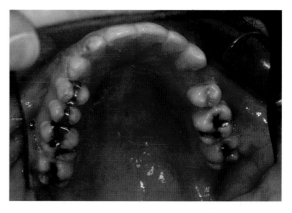

Figure 10.64. Occlusal view after treatment shows the aligned teeth ready for prosthetic replacement of the upper left first premolar.

teeth are shown before orthodontic treatment in Figures 10.59 and 10.60. The orthodontic appliance is shown in Figures 10.61 and 10.62. His left canine and second premolar were considerably rotated. An elastic chain was used between a buccal hook on the molar and the bracket on the canine to rotate the canine. The use of lingual buttons on the second premolar and molar is illustrated in Figure 10.62. The forces on the molar at the lingual button and the buccal hook counteract one another, keeping the molar from rotating. The teeth are shown after orthodontic treatment in Figures 10.63 and 10.64.

Additional examples of molar uprighting are illustrated by Staley and Reske (2001).

REFERENCES

Adams, C. P. 1984. The design, construction and use of removable orthodontic appliances. 5th ed. Bristol, England: John Wright & Sons Ltd, pp. 173–182.

Barberia-Leache, E., Suarez-Clua, M. C., and Saavedra-Ontiveros, D. 2005. Ectopic eruption of the maxillary first permanent molar: characteristics and occurrence in growing children. Angle Orthod. 75:610–615.

Bjerklin, K., and Kurol, J. 1981. Prevalence of ectopic eruption of the maxillary first permanent molar. Swed. Dent. J. 5:29–34.

Bjerklin, K., and Kurol, J. 1983. Ectopic eruption of the maxillary first permanent molar: etiologic factors. Am J. Orthod. 84:147–155.

Canut, J. A., and Raga, C. 1983. Morphological analysis of cases with ectopic eruption of the maxillary first permanent molar. Eur. J. Orthod. 5:248–253.

Carr, G. E., and Mink, J. R. 1965. Ectopic eruption of the first permanent maxillary molar in cleft lip and palate children. J. Dent. Child. 32:179–188.

Garcia-Fernandez, A. 2000. Two easy ways to solve spaces when the bone has a sand clock shape. Book of Abstracts, p. 52. Presented at the 100th Annual Session of the American Association of Orthodontists, Chicago, Illinois.

Iwasaki, L. R., Crouch, L. D., Reinhardt, R. A., and Nickel, J. C. 2004. The velocity of human orthodontic tooth movement is related to stress magnitude, growth status, and the ratio of cytokines in gingival crevicular fluid. In Harvard Society for the Advancement of Orthodontics, eds. Z. Davidovitch and J. Mah, pp. 133–143, Boston: Harvard Society for the Advancement of Orthodontics.

Kennedy, D. B., and Turley, P. K. 1987. The clinical management of ectopically erupting first permanent molars. Am. J. Orthod. Dentofac. Orthop. 92:336–345.

Kimmel, N. A., Gellin, M. E., Bohannan, H. M., and Kaplan, A. L. 1982. Ectopic eruption of maxillary first permanent molars in different areas of the United States. J. Dent. Children 4:294–296.

Kurol, J., and Bjerklin, K. 1982. Resorption of maxillary second primary molars caused by ectopic eruption of the maxillary first permanent molar: a longitudinal and histological study. ASDC J. Dent. Child. 49:273–279.

Kurol, J., and Bjerklin, K. 1986. Ectopic eruption of maxillary first permanent molars: a review. ASDC J. Dent. Child. 53:209–214.

O'Meara, W. F. 1962. Ectopic eruption pattern in selected permanent teeth. J. Dent. Res. 41:607–616.

Pulver, F. 1968. The etiology and prevalence of ectopic eruption of the maxillary first permanent molar. ASDC J. Dent. Child. 35:138–146.

Roberts, W. E., Marshall, K. J., and Mozsary, P. G. 1990. Rigid endosseous implant utilized as anchorage to protract molars and close an atrophic extraction site. Angle Orthod. 60:135–152.

Roberts, W. E., Nelson, C. L., and Goodacre, C. J. 1994. Rigid implant anchorage to close a mandibular first molar extraction site: a viable alternative to a fixed partial denture (FPD) or a single tooth replacement (STR) implant. J. Clin. Orthod. 28:693–704.

Roberts, W. W., Chacker, F. M., and Burstone, C. J. 1982. A segmental approach to mandibular molar uprighting. Am. J. Orthod. 81:177–184.

Shamy, F. E. 1972. Retraction of maxillary bicuspids and molars with a removable appliance. N. Z. Orthod. J. 1(Dec):17–24.

Shellhart, W. C., and Oesterle, L. J. 1999. Uprighting molars without extrusion. J. Am. Dent. Assoc. 130:381–385.

Staley, R. N., and Reske, N. T. 2001. Treatment of Class I non-extraction problems, principles of Appliance construction and retention appliances. In Text Book of Orthodontics, ed. S. E. Bishara, pp. 307–312, Philadelphia: W. B. Saunders Company.

Young, D. H. 1957. Ectopic eruption of the first permanent molar. J. Dent. Child. 24:153–162.

Orthodontic Examination and Decision Making for the Family Dentist

11

Introduction

The purpose of this chapter is to use the basic principles and clinical examples (potentiality) given in the preceding chapters to help individual dentists make decisions about malocclusions encountered in their patients (actuality). Learning is the actualization of potentiality. Learning is self-activity, a process of self-development (Mayer 1928). The teacher is an extrinsic proximate agent. Knowledge is acquired in two ways: (1) when natural reason itself comes to knowledge of the unknown which is discovery, and (2) when a teacher leads another to knowledge of the unknown in the same way he, as the learner, would lead himself (Mayer 1928).

Benjamin Bloom (1976), a leader in educational research, created mastery learning as a method of teaching that enables most students in a class room to reach high levels of achievement. The basic premise of mastery learning is that a student must master one learning task before learning the next task:

What any person in the world can learn, *almost all persons can learn if* provided with appropriate prior and current conditions of learning. This generalization does not appear to apply to the 2% or 3% of individuals who have severe emotional and physical difficulties that impair their learning. At the other extreme there are about 1% or 2% of individuals who appear to learn in such unusually capable ways that they *may* be exceptions to the theory. At this stage of the research it applies most clearly to the middle 95% of a school population.

The middle 95% of school students become very similar in terms of their measured achievement, learning ability, rate of learning, and motivation for further learning when provided with *favorable learning conditions*. One example of such favorable learning conditions is mastery learning where the students are helped to master

Essentials of Orthodontics: Diagnosis and Treatment by Robert N. Staley and Neil T. Reske © 2011 Blackwell Publishing Ltd.

each learning unit before proceeding to a more advanced learning task. In general, the average student taught under mastery-learning procedures achieves at a level above 85% of students taught under conventional instructional conditions. An even more extreme result has been obtained when tutoring was used as the primary method on instruction. Under tutoring, the average student performs better than 98% of students taught by conventional group instruction, even though both groups of students performed at similar levels in terms of relevant aptitude and achievement before the instruction began (Bloom 1976).

On the basis of his extensive educational research, Bloom (1976, 1985) determined that favorable learning conditions include (1) cues, instruction about what is to be learned, and directions for what the learner must do in the learning process; (2) reinforcement, the use of approval or disapproval by a teacher to help a student learn; (3) participation, the learner must do something with the cues to actually learn; and (4) feedback/correctives, a teacher adapting the cues, the use of reinforcement, and the amount of participation or practice to the characteristics and needs of an individual learner.

An American Dental Education Association Commission (2006) presented educational strategies for developing problem solving, critical thinking, and self-directed learning in dentists. The Commission recommended giving students opportunities to use the following reflective judgment process to analyze the diagnosis and treatment of a dental patient: (1) identify the facts and issues in a problem, (2) identify and explore causal factors, (3) retrieve and assess knowledge needed to appraise response and guide actions, (4) compare the strengths and limitations of options, (5) implement the best option to solve the problem, (6) monitor treatment and outcomes and modify treatment as needed, and

(7) appraise the outcomes of treatment, positively and negatively. Following these steps routinely with patients will help a novice acquire the skills observed in experts.

Orthodontic Screening

The orthodontic screening form shown in Figure 11.1 is completed at a chair-side examination of a patient. The diagnostic information gathered on the form is used to make a decision concerning the orthodontic treatment disposition of the patient. Three dispositions are listed on the form:

1. The patient has normal occlusion (normal dental and skeletal relationships) for the primary, mixed, or permanent dentition (**circle the letter Q**). The decision made for these patients is to monitor the patient's occlusion at future appointments.
2. The patient has a significant malocclusion problem requiring comprehensive orthodontic treatment (**circle the letter R**). The decisions made for these patients are: (a) inform the patient or parents of minors that the patient has a significant malocclusion, and (b) refer the patient to an orthodontist.
3. The patient has a malocclusion problem not requiring comprehensive orthodontic treatment, or a young patient has a condition requiring either interceptive orthodontic treatment or intervention to prevent the development of a malocclusion (**circle the letter S**). The decisions required for these patients are: (a) inform the patient or parents of minors that the patient has a malocclusion that needs to be treated, or that the patient needs a preventive interceptive treatment, and (b) that you can either deliver the required treatment, or refer the patient to a pediatric dentist or orthodontist.

Orthodontic Screening Form

Name_____   Date_____
Birth Date_____ Age_____ Phone_____
Address_____

Circle appropriate letters:

Face frontal	**Profile**	**Dentition Stage**
A1. Normal	B1. Normal/Sraight	C1. primary
A2. Long Anterior	B2. Convex	C2. early mixed
A3. Asymmetry	B3. Concave	C3. late mixed
		C4. permanent

Right Molar	**Right Canine**	**Left Canine**	**Left Molar**
D1. Class I	E1. Class I	F1. Class I	G1. Class I
D2. Class II	E2. Class II	F2. Class II	G2. Class II
D3. Class III	E3. Class III	F3. Class III	G3. Class III

Overjet	**Overbite**	**Post Cross Bite**	**Functional Shift**
H1. normal	I1. normal	J1. 2 teeth	
H2. >4mm	I2. >50%	J2. unilateral	K1. A-P
H3. 0 mm	I3. 0%	J3. bilateral	K2. lateral
H4. **Ant. Cross Bite**	I4. open-bite		

Max.TSALD	**Mand. TSALD**	**Other Factors**	
L.1 normal	M1. normal	N1. missing teeth	N5.habit
L2. spacing	M2. spacing	N2. supernumerary	N6.caries
L3. 1-3 mm	M3. 1-3 mm	N3. impacted tooth	N7.plaque
L4. >3 mm	M4. >3 mm	N4. poor hygiene	N8.filling

Radiographic Findings

O1. Missing teeth _____	O5. Root resorption primary
O2. Supernumerary _____	O6. Root resorption permanent
O3. Caries depth _____	O7. Ectopic eruption
O4. root length _____	O8. Eruption order C,Pm1_____

TMJ Symptoms

P1. Click	P4. Lock	P7. Limited opening
P2. Crepitus	P5. Pain	P8. Limited motion
P3. Popping	P6. Headache	P9. Bruxism

Orthodontic Disposition of Patient
Q. Normal occlusion, observe occlusal development.
R. Comprehensive orthodontic treatment, refer to orthodontist.
S. Limited orthodontic treatment appropriate.

Provisional treatment plan_____
Fee_____
Patient response: accept_____will think about it_____ no_____

Figure 11.1. Orthodontic screening form.

Guidelines for Orthodontic Decision Making

Guidelines for orthodontic decision making are shown in Figure 11.2. These guidelines help a family dentist to differentiate malocclusions requiring comprehensive orthodontic treatment from malocclusion problems that can be treated by the family dentist. Guidelines for factors such as crowding, spacing, overbite, and overjet, anterior crossbite, posterior crossbite, and space regaining are given in Figure 11.2.

When an upper or lower permanent first molar tips forward after the premature loss of a primary molar, the molar occlusion in that quadrant of the arch will be Class II in the upper arch or

Observed Condition	Decision/Management
Normal Occlusion (Class I molars and canines), no crowding, normal overbite and over jet.	Periodic observation in growing patients
Class I malocclusion, crowding in excess of 4mm in one arch	Refer to an orthodontist
Class I malocclusion, crowding minimal between 1 and 3mm, overbite < 50%, over jet < 4 mm	Appropriate for a family dentist to treat
Class I malocclusion, spacing in excess of 4mm in one arch	Refer to an orthodontist
Class I malocclusion, spacing 1 to 3mm in one arch	Appropriate for a family dentist to treat
Class I malocclusion, anterior or posterior open bite	Refer to an orthodontist
Class I malocclusion, deep overbite (greater than 50%)	Refer to an orthodontist
Class I malocclusion, overbite 10-50%	Appropriate for a family dentist to treat
Class I malocclusion, anterior cross bite involving 3 or more upper anterior teeth	Refer to an orthodontist
Class I malocclusion, anterior cross bite involving 1 to 2 upper anterior teeth	Appropriate for a family dentist to treat
Class I malocclusion, unilateral or bilateral posterior cross bite requiring more than 6 mm of upper arch expansion.	Refer to an orthodontist
Class I malocclusion, unilateral or bilateral posterior cross bite requiring up to 6 mm of upper arch expansion.	Appropriate for a family dentist to treat
Class I occlusion, congenitally absent teeth, impacted tooth, ankylosed primary molar	Refer to an orthodontist
Class I occlusion in the mixed dentition involving space maintenance, space regaining, and finger habits	Appropriate for a family dentist to treat
Class II malocclusion	Refer to an orthodontist
Class III malocclusion	Refer to an orthodontist

Figure 11.2. Guidelines for orthodontic decision making.

Class III in the lower arch. In these patients, family dentists can correct the problem in those patients who have a Class I relation in the molars on the unaffected side of the arch and an otherwise normal occlusion.

In the mixed-dentition patient, premature asymmetric loss of primary molars should be followed by the delivery of a space maintainer to avoid the complications associated with asymmetry and impaction of nonerupted teeth. This recommendation is appropriate for patients with Class I, Class II, and Class III malocclusions. In the permanent dentition patient, the loss of a tooth should be followed by appropriate intervention (implant, bridge, removable partial denture) to avoid the development of a malocclusion.

Differentiating Class I Problems Suitable for Limited Orthodontic Treatment from More Complex Class I Problems

Pretreatment Records

The pretreatment records of patients with Class I malocclusions are presented with additional diagnostic information in the text. The challenge to the reader is to (1) identify the malocclusion problem, (2) assess the difficulty of the problem (s), (3) differentiate the Class I limited problems from those requiring more extensive treatment, and (4) develop a treatment and appliance plan for the patient suitable for limited orthodontic treatment.

Patient 1. An 8-year 7-month-old boy presented with a chief concern that his upper incisors were in crossbite. In centric occlusion all four of his upper incisors were in crossbite (Figs. 11.3 to 11.6). In centric occlusion his permanent first molars and canines were in Super Class I occlusion (Figs. 11.4 and 11.5). When asked if he could move his lower incisors back into contact with his upper incisors (to determine the existence of an anteroposterior shift from centric relation to centric occlusion), he produced the centric relation occlusion shown in Figures 11.7

to 11.10. In centric relation, only his upper left central incisor was in crossbite and his molars were Class I. He had a 3.5-mm functional shift between centric relation and centric occlusion (Figs. 11.7 to 11.10). His upper left central incisor in crossbite was inclined (tipped) lingually. His lower left central incisor was rotated and had labial gingival recession as a result of its traumatic occlusion. Adequate arch length was available to move the upper left central incisor into the line of arch. Overbite and overjet measured in centric relation were 37% and 1.3 mm, respectively.

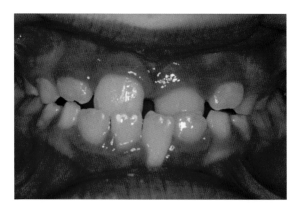

Figure 11.3. Front view of a patient in centric occlusion with an anterior crossbite of the upper right lateral incisor and both upper central incisors. Note the gingival recession on the labial root surface of the lower left central incisor.

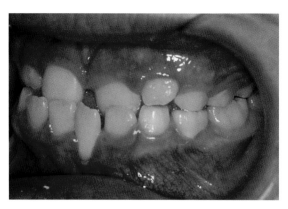

Figure 11.5. Left lateral view of the anterior crossbite in centric occlusion.

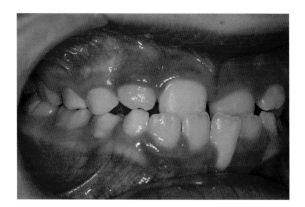

Figure 11.4. Right lateral view of the anterior crossbite in centric occlusion.

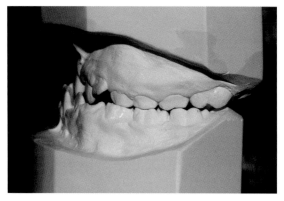

Figure 11.6. Left lateral view of the casts in centric occlusion showing canine and molar relations as Class III.

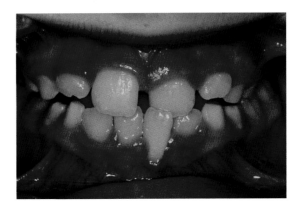

Figure 11.7. Front view of the patient in centric relation. Only the upper left central incisor is in crossbite. Note the traumatic occlusion involving the upper and lower left central incisors.

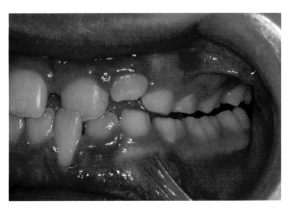

Figure 11.9. Left lateral view of the occlusion in centric relation.

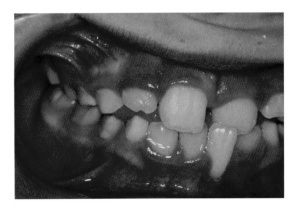

Figure 11.8. Right lateral view of the patient's occlusion in centric relation.

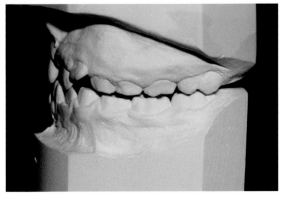

Figure 11.10. Left lateral view of the casts in centric relation showing canine and molar relations as Class I.

Patient 2. A 13-year 9-month-old boy in the permanent dentition presented with the chief concern that his upper lateral incisors were in anterior crossbite (Figs. 11.11 to 11.18). His first molars and canines were Class I (Figs. 11.14 and 11.15). He had 4.4 mm of upper arch crowding, normal upper intercanine width, an upper intermolar width of 49.1 mm that was 2 standard deviations narrower than the male mean, a lower intercanine width of 28.6 mm that was one standard deviation narrower than the norm, and a lower intermolar width of 50.1 mm that was 2 standard deviations narrower than the norm. The center of the incisal edges of the upper lateral incisors were about 5 mm lingual to the upper line of arch. He had an overbite of 20% and an overjet of 2 mm. There was no evidence of an anteroposterior functional shift.

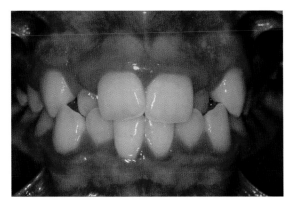

Figure 11.11. Front view of a patient in centric occlusion with the upper lateral incisors in crossbite.

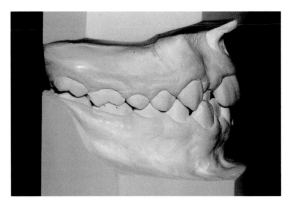

Figure 11.14. Right lateral view of the casts in centric occlusion showing canines and molars in Class I.

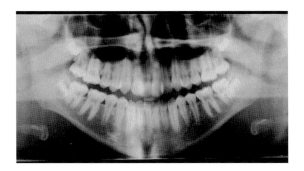

Figure 11.12. Panoramic radiograph of the teeth.

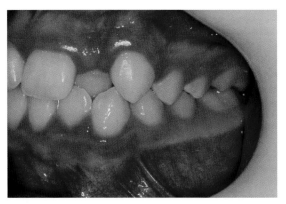

Figure 11.15. Left lateral view of the teeth in centric occlusion.

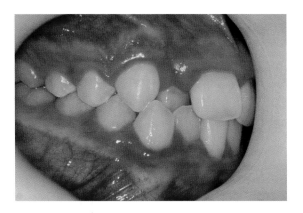

Figure 11.13. Right lateral view of the teeth in centric occlusion.

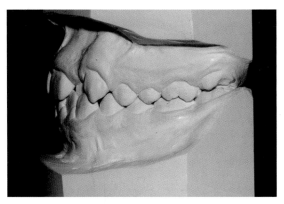

Figure 11.16. Left lateral view of the casts in centric occlusion showing canines and molars in Class I.

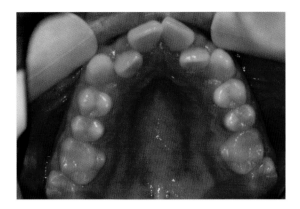

Figure 11.17. Occlusal view of the upper teeth.

Patient 3. A 6-year 4-month-old girl presented with a unilateral posterior crossbite diagnosed by her family dentist. The crossbite was on her right side and she had an associated lateral shift of 2 mm from centric relation to centric occlusion (Figs. 11.19 to 11.26). The panoramic radiograph depicts her early mixed-dentition stage of development (Fig. 11.20). Her maxillary intermolar width was 46.1 mm and that was normal for the mixed dentition (Table 8.2). Her mandibular intermolar width was 49.1 mm, 1 standard deviation wider than normal. She needed to

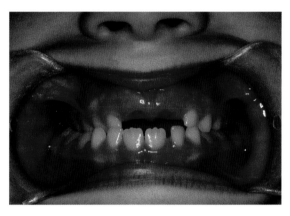

Figure 11.19. Front view of a patient with a unilateral posterior crossbite on the right side. The upper primary incisors have exfoliated.

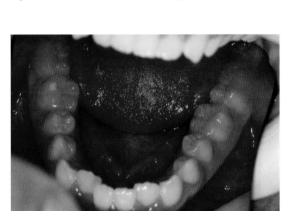

Figure 11.18. Occlusal view of the lower teeth.

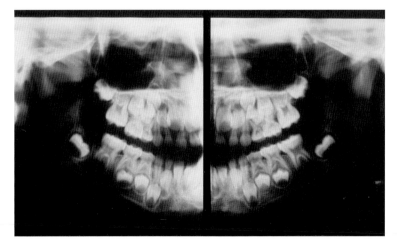

Figure 11.20. Panoramic radiograph of the patient.

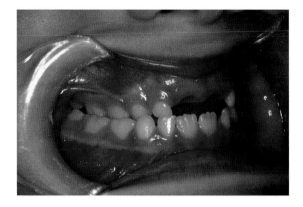

Figure 11.21. Right lateral view of the teeth in centric occlusion.

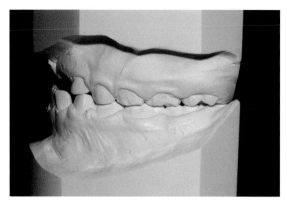

Figure 11.24. Left lateral view of the casts in centric occlusion showing the canines in Class I and the first permanent molars in Super Class I.

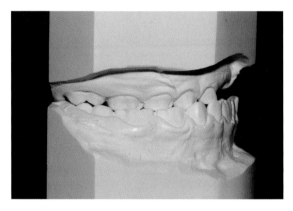

Figure 11.22. Right lateral view of the casts in centric occlusion showing canines and molars in Class I.

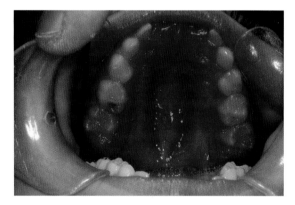

Figure 11.25. Occlusal view of the upper teeth.

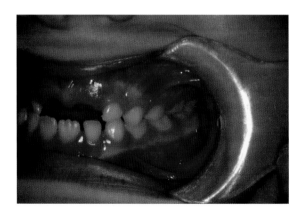

Figure 11.23. Left lateral view of the teeth in centric occlusion.

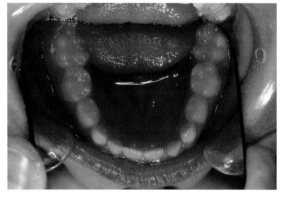

Figure 11.26. Occlusal view of the lower teeth.

widen her upper arch to 49.1 mm and an additional 1.2 mm for adequate buccal overjet for a total of 4.2 mm. Her Angle notation was E, E, I, SI. Overbite and overjet were not measurable because of the missing upper incisors.

Patient 4. A 6-year 2-month-old boy presented with anterior and unilateral crossbites (Figs. 11.27 to 11.34). He was in the early mixed dentition with only three erupted permanent teeth, the lower central incisors and lower left first molar. His upper right primary central and lateral incisors were in edge to edge (zero overbite and

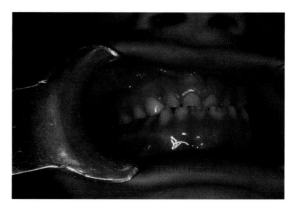

Figure 11.29. Right lateral view of the teeth in centric occlusion.

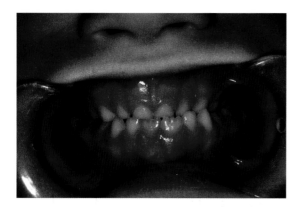

Figure 11.27. Frontal view of the teeth in centric occlusion with the incisors in anterior crossbite and a unilateral left posterior crossbite.

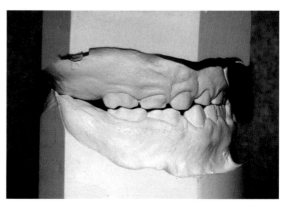

Figure 11.30. Right lateral view of the casts in centric occlusion showing Class I relationships in the primary canines and molars.

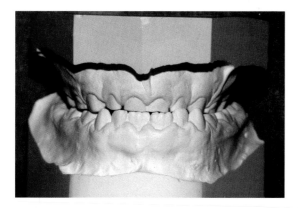

Figure 11.28. Frontal view of the casts in centric occlusion.

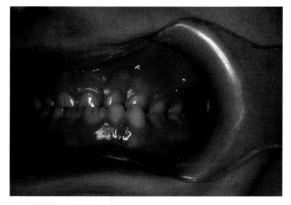

Figure 11.31. Left lateral view of the teeth in centric occlusion.

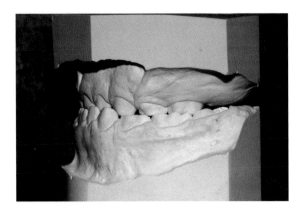

Figure 11.32. Left lateral view of the casts in centric occlusion showing canines in Class I and the primary molars in Super Class I.

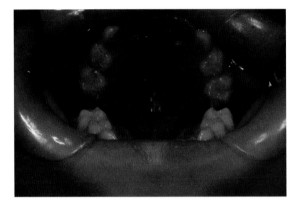

Figure 11.33. Occlusal view of the upper teeth.

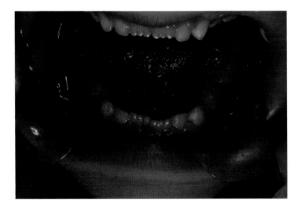

Figure 11.34. Occlusal view of the lower teeth.

overjet) with the lower incisors. His upper left primary central and lateral incisors and canines were in anterior crossbite. The patient had an anteroposterior functional shift of about 1 to 2 mm. His upper left primary molars were in crossbite (Figs. 11.31 and 11.32). He had a lateral functional shift of about 2 mm toward the left side. His upper intermolar width (between I and J) was 41.4 mm, within normal limits (Table 8.3). His lower intermolar width was 43.4, 1 standard deviation wider than normal. The etiology of his posterior crossbite was a wider-than-normal lower posterior arch width. The intermolar width difference was −2.0 mm. Adding the difference observed between the mean norms for upper and lower intermolar widths (2.7 mm, Table 8.3), gives a goal for expansion of 4.7 mm. His Angle notation was I, I, E, SI. The anterior crossbite involved upper primary incisors that had partially resorbed roots.

Patient 5. A 15-year 9-month-old adolescent girl presented with a 2.5 mm diastema between her upper central incisors (Figs. 11.35 to 11.42). She had an overjet of 2.4 mm and overbite of 44.9%. The Bolton overall ratio predicted 4 mm of mandibular excess, and the anterior ratio predicted 1 mm of mandibular excess. Her lower incisors were mildly crowded, less than 1 mm.

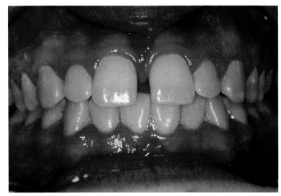

Figure 11.35. Front view of the teeth in centric occlusion. The patient was concerned about the diastema between her upper central incisors.

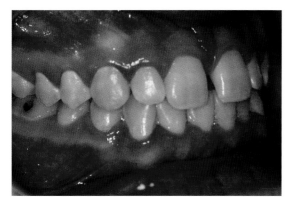

Figure 11.36. Right lateral view of the teeth in centric occlusion.

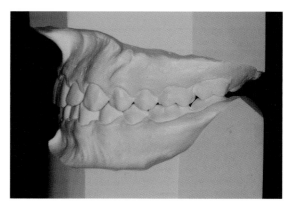

Figure 11.39. Left lateral view of the casts in centric occlusion showing canines and molars in Class I.

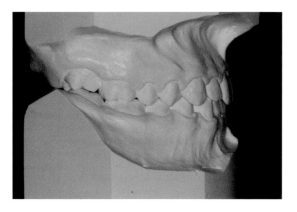

Figure 11.37. Right lateral view of the casts in centric occlusion showing canines and molars in Class I.

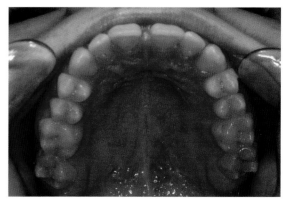

Figure 11.40. Occlusal view of the upper teeth.

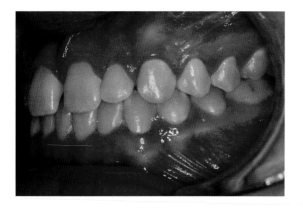

Figure 11.38. Left lateral view of the teeth in centric occlusion.

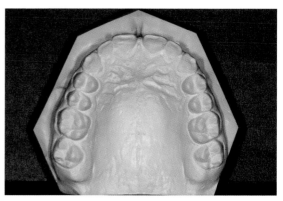

Figure 11.41. Occlusal view of the upper cast.

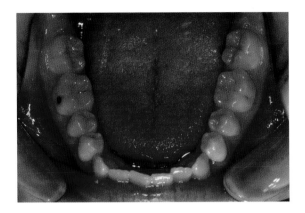

Figure 11.42. Occlusal view of the lower teeth.

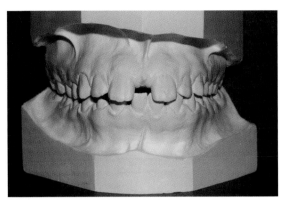

Figure 11.44. Front view of the casts in centric occlusion.

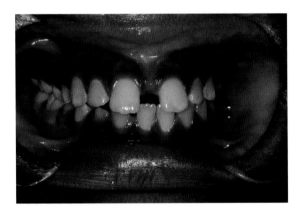

Figure 11.43. Front view of the teeth in centric occlusion. The patient was concerned about the diastema between her upper central incisors.

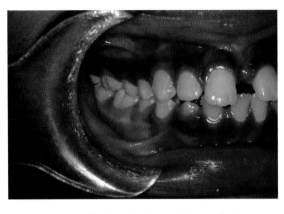

Figure 11.45. Right lateral view of the teeth in centric occlusion.

Patient 6. A 12-year 11-month-old adolescent girl presented with a 6.3 mm diastema between her upper central incisors (Figs. 11.43 to 11.50). She had an overjet of 3.6 mm and overbite of 44%. The Bolton overall ratio predicted a good fit for her teeth (zero excess). She had 8.6 mm of spaces in her upper arch and 7.9 mm of spaces in her lower arch.

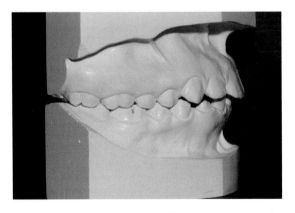

Figure 11.46. Right lateral view of the casts in centric occlusion showing the canines and molars in Class I.

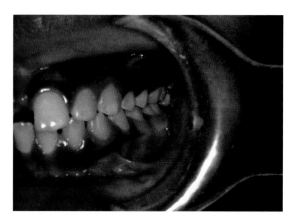

Figure 11.47. Left lateral view of the teeth in centric occlusion.

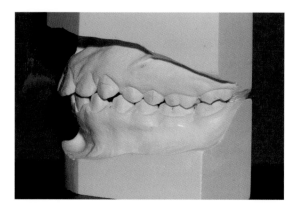

Figure 11.48. Left lateral view of the casts in centric occlusion showing the canines end to end (E) and the molars in Class I.

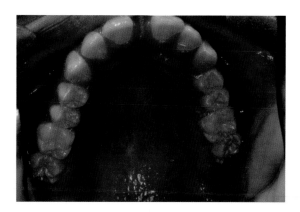

Figure 11.49. Occlusal view of the upper teeth.

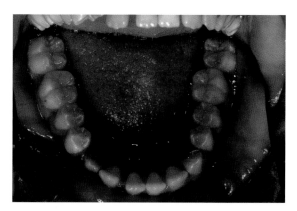

Figure 11.50. Occlusal view of the lower teeth.

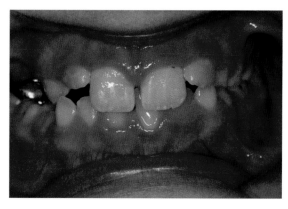

Figure 11.51. Front view of the teeth in centric occlusion.

Patient 7. An 8-year 5-month-old boy presented with an ectopically erupting lower right lateral incisor (Figs. 11.51 to 11.58). His Angle notation was I, I, E, I. He had 60% overbite and 2.5 mm of overjet. His upper dental midline was 1 mm to the right side and his lower dental midline was 2 mm to the right. The mixed dentition analysis predicted a 1 mm arch length excess in the lower arch. The ectopically erupting lower right lateral incisor was distal and lingual to its normal position (Fig. 11.58). The lower right primary canine and lateral incisor were still present in the lower arch (Fig. 11.57). It appears that the lower right primary first molar is ankylosed (Fig. 11.57).

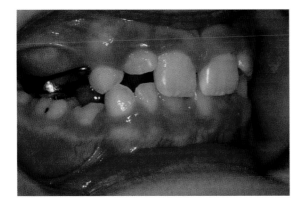

Figure 11.52. Right lateral view of the teeth in centric occlusion.

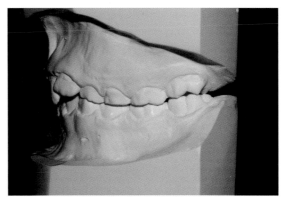

Figure 11.55. Left lateral view of the casts in centric occlusion showing the canines and permanent first molars end to end.

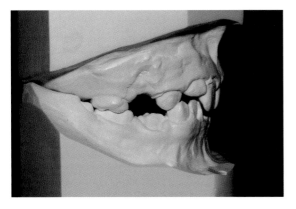

Figure 11.53. Right lateral view of the casts in centric occlusion showing the primary canines and molars in Class I.

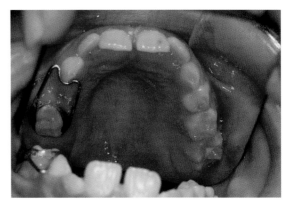

Figure 11.56. Occlusal view of the upper teeth.

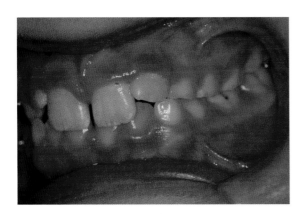

Figure 11.54. Left lateral view of the teeth in centric occlusion.

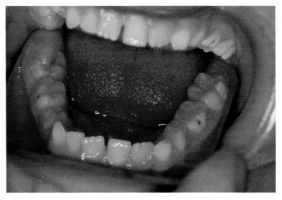

Figure 11.57. Occlusal view of the lower teeth.

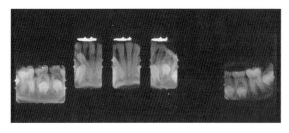

Figure 11.58. Periapical radiographs of the lower teeth showing the ectopic eruption of the lower right permanent lateral incisor.

Patient 8. An 8-year-old girl presented with an ectopically erupted upper right first molar (Figs. 11.59 to 11.66). Her Angle notation was II, I, I, I. She had an overjet of 2 mm and overbite of 50%. Primary molar A was lost either by the ectopic eruption of her upper right first molar or by caries.

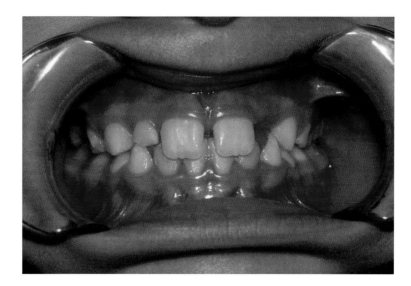

Figure 11.59. Front view of the teeth in centric occlusion.

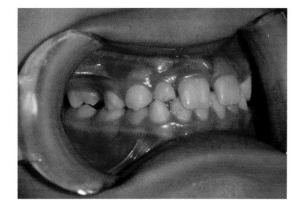

Figure 11.60. Right lateral view of the teeth in centric occlusion.

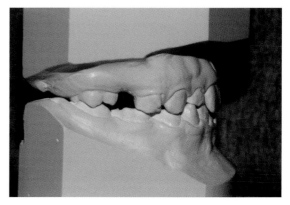

Figure 11.61. Right lateral view of the casts showing the primary canines in Class I and the permanent first molars in Class II.

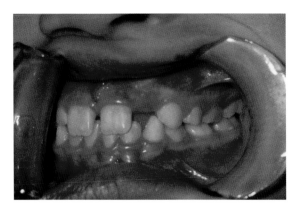

Figure 11.62. Left lateral view of the teeth in centric occlusion.

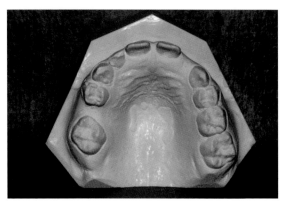

Figure 11.65. Occlusal view of the upper cast.

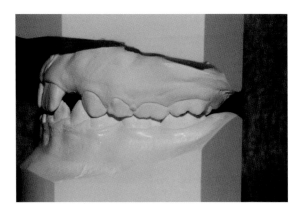

Figure 11.63. Left lateral view of the casts in centric occlusion showing the primary canines and permanent first molars in Class I.

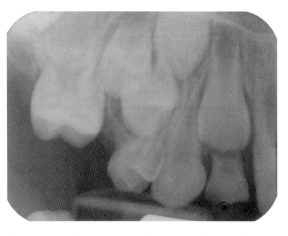

Figure 11.66. A periapical radiograph of the ectopic upper right first molar and impacted upper right second premolar.

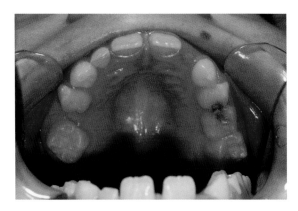

Figure 11.64. Occlusal view of the upper teeth.

Patient 9. A 9-year 2-month-old girl presented with lingually inclined permanent upper central incisors in anterior crossbite, an upper left lateral incisor erupting lingual to the line of arch, and both lower permanent lateral incisors erupted lingual to the erupted permanent central incisors (Figs. 11.67 to 11.74). She had an overbite of 44%. The Iowa Mixed Dentition Analysis predicted −0.8 mm of crowding in the upper arch and an excess of 2.8 mm space in the lower arch. Her occlusion was Class I. The panoramic radiograph shows an early mixed dentition with many developing nonerupted permanent teeth (Fig. 11.74).

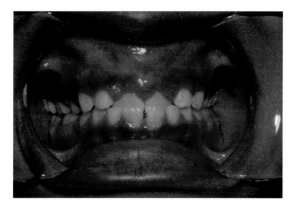

Figure 11.67. Front view of the teeth in centric occlusion. The upper central incisors were in anterior crossbite.

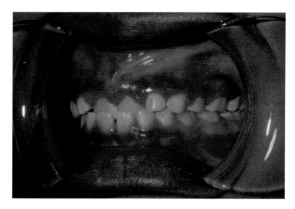

Figure 11.70. Left lateral view of the teeth in centric occlusion.

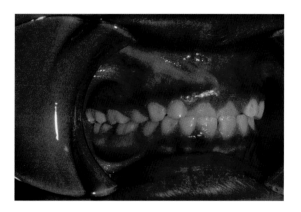

Figure 11.68. Right lateral view of the teeth in centric occlusion.

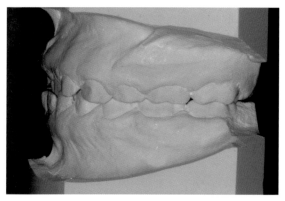

Figure 11.71. Left lateral view of the casts in centric occlusion showing the primary canines and the permanent first molars end to end.

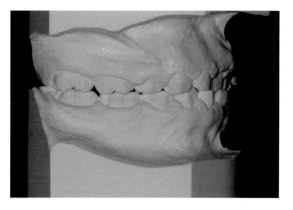

Figure 11.69. Right lateral view of the casts in centric occlusion showing the primary canines and the permanent first molars end to end.

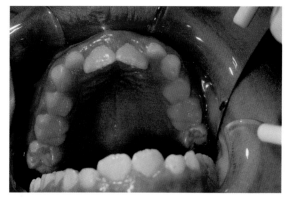

Figure 11.72. Occlusal view of the upper teeth.

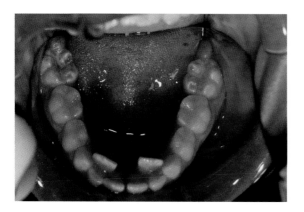

Figure 11.73. Occlusal view of the lower teeth.

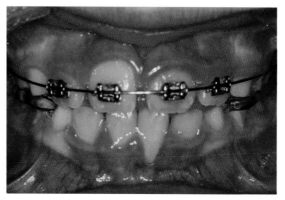

Figure 11.75. Front view of the upper fixed appliance and lower removable acrylic bite plate.

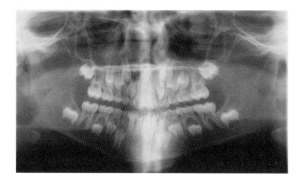

Figure 11.74. Panoramic radiograph of the teeth.

Treatment Records

The diagnoses and treatments given to the preceding patients are discussed in the following paragraphs. For most patients, photographs describe the appliance used to correct the malocclusion and show the occlusion at the end of treatment. The difficulty of the treatment and whether the malocclusion was appropriate for limited orthodontic treatment are also discussed.

Patient 1. The anteroposterior functional shift is a key diagnostic factor in the diagnosis of this patient's malocclusion. In centric relation, only the upper left central incisor is in crossbite (Fig. 11.7). The crossbite of the upper left central with the lower left central incisor in centric relation explains the forward position of the lower left central incisor and the marked recession of gingiva on the labial surface of its root. To avoid the traumatic occlusion, the patient moves his

mandible into the centric occlusion position (Figs. 11.3, 11.4, and 11.5). The Angle classification of the molars in centric occlusion (Super 1, Fig. 11.6) and centric relation (Class I, Fig. 11.10) predict that correction of the crossbite of the upper left central incisor will result in a molar relation of Class I after the functional shift has been eliminated. After an anteroposterior functional shift is eliminated, the mandible will move posteriorly from centric occlusion to centric relation. This patient had the ideal Angle molar relations in centric occlusion and centric relation for an anterior crossbite associated with an anteroposterior functional shift. The lingual inclination of the upper left central incisor and the more than adequate arch length available are most favorable for moving the tooth labially out of crossbite. **He was a good candidate for limited orthodontic treatment.**

His treatment is shown in Figures 11.75 to 11.80. A fixed appliance comprised of bands on the upper first molars and edgewise brackets on the upper incisors (2X4 appliance) and a lower posterior acrylic bite plate to open the bite were used to treat the patient (Fig. 11.75). After his treatment, the incisors were in a much better functional relationship. The recession on his lower left central incisor was not changed, but this problem can be observed and treated at an older age (Fig. 11.76). The buccal occlusion was Class I as shown in the photographs of his casts (Figs. 11.78 and 11.79). He was given an upper Hawley retainer.

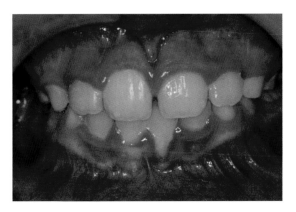

Figure 11.76. Front view after the crossbite was corrected.

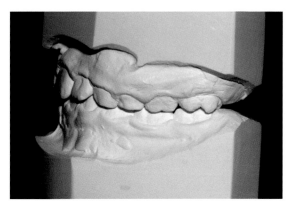

Figure 11.79. Left lateral view of the casts after treatment showing Class I primary canines and permanent first molars.

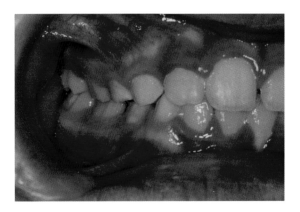

Figure 11.77. Right lateral view after treatment.

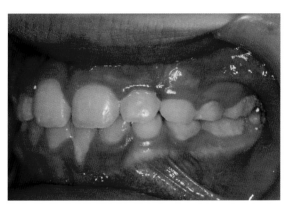

Figure 11.80. Left lateral view of the teeth after treatment.

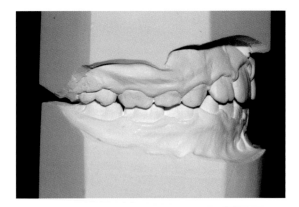

Figure 11.78. Right lateral view of the casts after treatment showing Class I primary canines and permanent first molars.

Patient 2. The key diagnostic factors for this patient were (1) inadequate arch length to move the upper lateral incisors out of crossbite, (2) the large distance from the crowns of the lateral incisors to the crest of the alveolar ridge, and (3) the absence of an anteroposterior functional shift. To create adequate arch length for the upper lateral incisors, the upper and lower arches must be made wider and longer. The palatal position of the lateral incisors unfavorably affects the inclination of the teeth. Movement of the lateral incisors out of crossbite and into the arch will give them too much inclination. After moving the lateral incisors out of crossbite, a rectangular

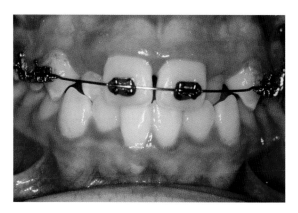

Figure 11.81. Front view of the initial upper fixed appliance.

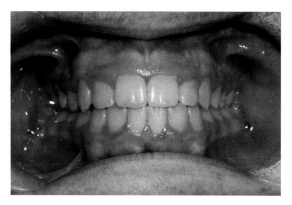

Figure 11.83. Front view of the teeth after treatment with full upper and lower edgewise fixed appliances.

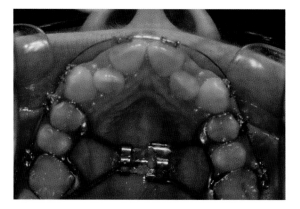

Figure 11.82. Occlusal view of the rapid maxillary expander and initial upper fixed appliance.

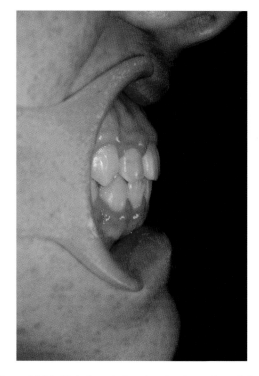

Figure 11.84. Right lateral view showing the canine relation, the inclination of the incisors, and the overjet.

upper arch wire will be needed to torque their roots to a more normal inclination. Failure to do this part of the treatment will expose the teeth to increased probability for relapse after treatment. Finally, the absence of an anteroposterior functional shift means that the upper lateral incisors must move the full distance forward to achieve normal overjet. Because of the above considerations, **this patient was not a candidate for limited orthodontic treatment.**

The treatment and final occlusion of this patient are shown in Figures 11.81 to 11.86. Treatment involved expansion of the upper arch with a Hyrax expander appliance (Fig. 11.82) in

order to create arch length for the lateral incisors. A fixed appliance was used with the expander (Fig. 11.81), and later on full edgewise appliances were placed in both arches to finish treatment. An 18 × 25-mil upper arch wire in

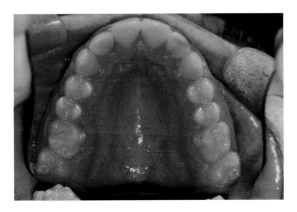

Figure 11.85. Occlusal view of the upper teeth after treatment.

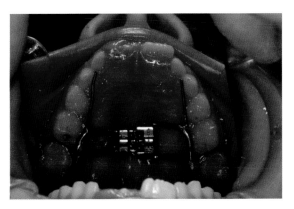

Figure 11.87. Occlusal view of the modified rapid expander shortly after it was cemented to the molars.

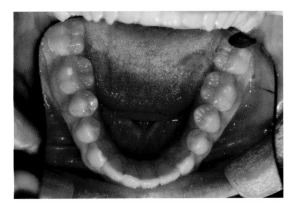

Figure 11.86. Occlusal view of the lower teeth after treatment.

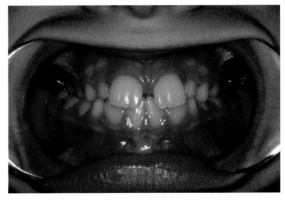

Figure 11.88. Front view of the occlusion after correction of the right unilateral posterior crossbite.

a 22 × 26-mil bracket slot were used to bring the roots of the lateral incisors to normal inclination (Figs. 11.83, 11.84, and 11.85). The occlusion was Class I at the end of treatment. The patient was given upper and lower Hawley retainers after removal of the orthodontic appliances.

Patient 3. The key diagnostic factors for the patient were (1) her normal upper arch, (2) lower arch wider than normal, and (3) a lateral shift toward the side of the crossbite. She needed a modest expansion of approximately 4 to 5 mm. **She was a good candidate for limited orthodontic treatment.**

A number of appliances could have successfully expanded her upper arch. A split acrylic expander with a jackscrew and Adams clasps was given to the patient. She refused to wear and activate the removable appliance. Her eventual treatment with a modified rapid maxillary appliance (Hyrax) is shown in Figures 11.87 to 11.94. Her occlusion after treatment was I, I, I, I (Figs. 11.97 and 11.98). This change in Angle notation from beginning to end of treatment is most likely related to the affect of the elimination of the lateral functional shift. Her treatment was retained with a fixed-removable trans-palatal arch (Fig. 11.93). Her lower arch was not treated.

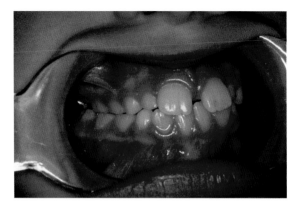

Figure 11.89. Right lateral view of the teeth after treatment.

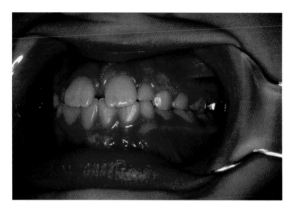

Figure 11.92. Left lateral view of the teeth after treatment.

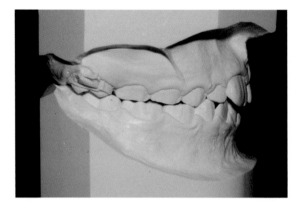

Figure 11.90. Right lateral view of the casts after treatment showing Class I primary canines and permanent first molars.

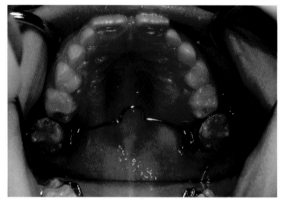

Figure 11.93. Occlusal view of the upper arch showing the trans-palatal arch used to retain the expander treatment.

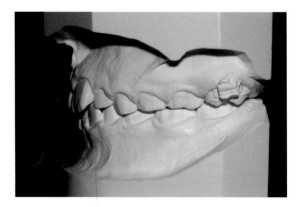

Figure 11.91. Left lateral view of the casts after treatment showing Class I primary canines and permanent first molars.

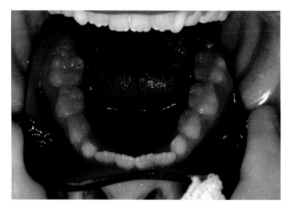

Figure 11.94. Occlusal view of the untreated lower arch after treatment.

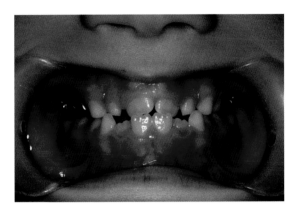

Figure 11.95. Front view of the teeth after correction of the left unilateral posterior crossbite.

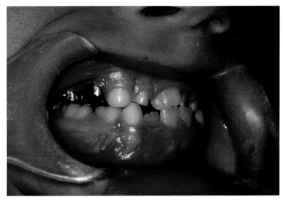

Figure 11.97. Right lateral view of the teeth after treatment.

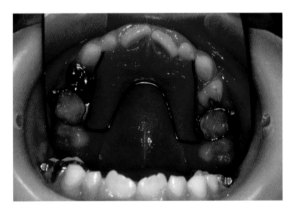

Figure 11.96. Occlusal view of the upper arch after treatment showing the W spring expander used to correct the crossbite.

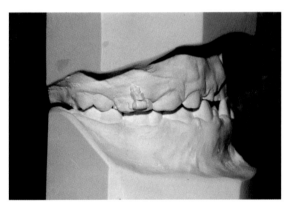

Figure 11.98. Right lateral view of the casts after treatment showing Class I primary canines and permanent first molars.

Patient 4. The important factors in the diagnosis of this patient were (1) a unilateral posterior crossbite on the left side with an associated lateral functional shift and (2) that the upper arch needs to be widened about 4.7 mm, even though the lower arch has an abnormally wide intermolar width. Constriction of a lower arch width only to correct a posterior crossbite is not usually wise or possible. If the lower posterior teeth in a wider-than-normal arch are inclined buccally, the clinician can consider the possibility of moving the teeth to a more normal inclination. The lower posterior teeth of this patient were

inclined normally. In all posterior crossbite treatments, the width of the lower arch must be coordinated with the upper arch, and widening of the lower arch requires even greater widening of the upper arch; (3) an anterior crossbite exists in association with an anteroposterior functional shift. The Angle notation for this patient was I, I, E, SI. The timing of the start of treatment should be considered in all mixed-dentition patients. Treatment at this time will involve only primary teeth. Elimination of the lateral shift in the primary dentition does not guarantee that the permanent molars will erupt without being in

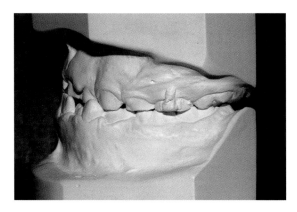

Figure 11.99. Left lateral view of the casts after treatment showing Class I primary canines and permanent first molars.

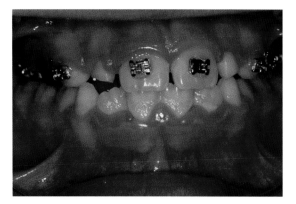

Figure 11.101. Front view of the teeth after the correction of the anterior crossbite of the upper central incisors with a fixed appliance added to the W spring expander.

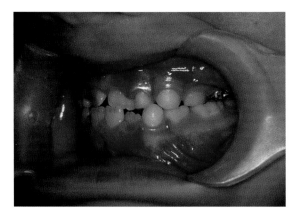

Figure 11.100. Left lateral view of the teeth after correction of the unilateral posterior crossbite.

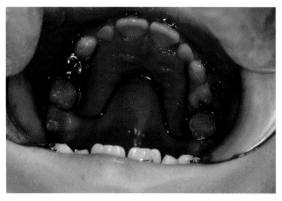

Figure 11.102. Occlusal view of the appliances.

crossbite. Movement of the upper primary incisors out of anterior crossbite was not possible considering the resorption of the primary incisor roots. **This was a patient suitable for limited orthodontic treatment who required a longer treatment time.**

Treatment was started in the primary dentition to correct the posterior crossbite (Figs. 11.95 to 11.100). A fixed W spring appliance was used to expand the upper arch (Fig. 11.96). The upper and lower first molars had erupted out of crossbite (Figs. 11.98 and 11.99). His Angle notation after correction of the unilateral posterior cross-

bite was I, I, I, SI (Figs. 11.97 to 11.100). After the posterior crossbite was corrected, the upper and lower dental midlines were coincident, an indication that the lateral functional shift had been eliminated (Fig. 11.95). After correctiin of the posterior crossbite, the permanent upper central incisors erupted into anterior crossbite (Figs. 11.95, 11.97, and 11.100).

A simple edgewise fixed appliance from the upper molar bands of the W spring appliance to the upper central incisors and three of the primary teeth was used to correct the anterior crossbite (Figs. 11.101 and 11.102). Correction of the

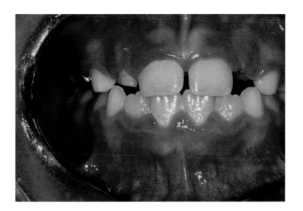

Figure 11.103. Front view of the teeth after the appliances were removed from the mouth.

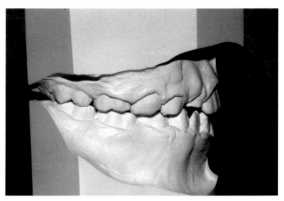

Figure 11.106. Right lateral view of the casts after treatment.

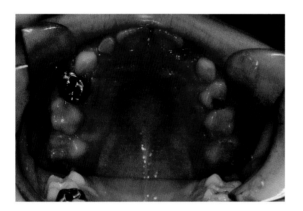

Figure 11.104. Occlusal view after the treatment.

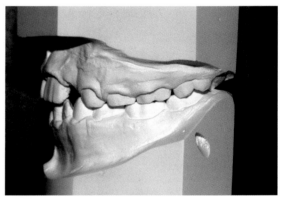

Figure 11.107. Left lateral view of the casts after correction of the anterior crossbite.

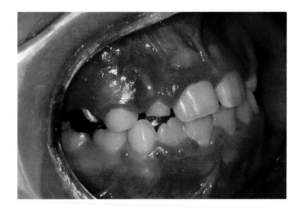

Figure 11.105. Right lateral view of the teeth after treatment.

anterior crossbite eliminated the anteroposterior functional shift (Figs. 11.103 to 11.108). The Angle notation after the anterior crossbite was corrected was E, E, I, I (Figs. 11.106 and 11.107). The change in Angle notation indicated that an anteroposterior functional shift had been eliminated. The patient was given an upper Hawley retainer with instructions to wear it for 1 year.

Patient 5. Because the spaces in this patient are located only between her upper incisors, the Bolton analysis predicts a mandibular tooth size excess, and the molars and canines are Class I, orthodontic treatment can be limited to the upper

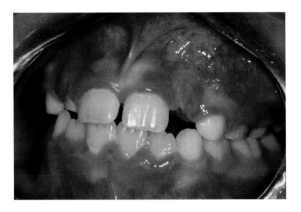

Figure 11.108. Right lateral view of the teeth after treatment.

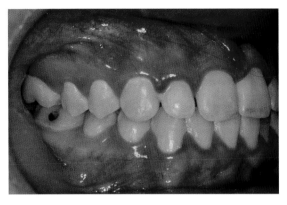

Figure 11.110. Right lateral view of the teeth after treatment showing small spaces around the upper lateral incisor.

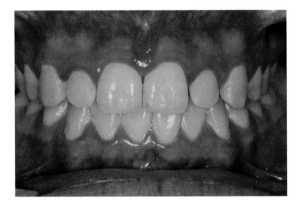

Figure 11.109. Front view of the teeth after treatment.

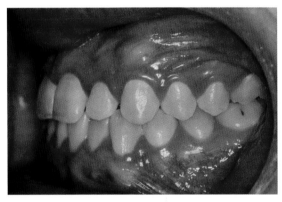

Figure 11.111. Left lateral view of the teeth after treatment showing the space distal to the upper left lateral incisor.

arch. If the patient were interested in aligning the lower incisors, the mandibular tooth size excess would be fully realized at the end of treatment. She was not concerned about the mild crowding of her lower incisors. The orthodontic treatment goal for this patient is to distribute the space between the upper canines to achieve the best aesthetic acid-etch composite resin build-up of the anterior teeth. A consultation with the dentist who is responsible for the aesthetic restorations, whether acid-etch build-ups or other aesthetic treatment, is mandatory before starting the orthodontic treatment. The size of the patient's upper central and lateral incisors dictated closure

of the midline diastema and build-up of the smaller lateral incisors. **The patient had a malocclusion problem suitable for limited orthodontic treatment.**

An upper fixed edgewise appliance was placed on the first molars and six anterior teeth, a 2 × 6 appliance. The diastema was closed with reciprocal forces acting on the central incisors (a two-link plastic chain and an 18-mil cylindrical arch wire). The lateral incisors were then centered in the spaces around them. At the end of treatment, spaces were found only in the lateral incisor region of the upper arch (Figs. 11.109 to 11.113). It is important to retain the teeth until the

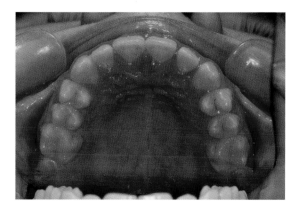

Figure 11.112. Occlusal view of the upper teeth after treatment.

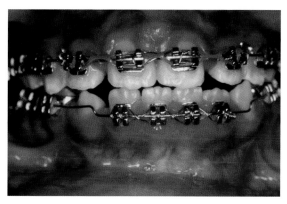

Figure 11.114. Front view of the upper and lower edgewise fixed appliances used to treat the spacing problem.

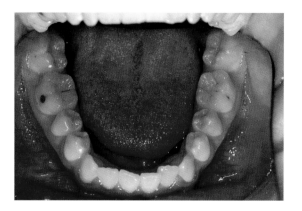

Figure 11.113. Occlusal view of the lower teeth that were not treated.

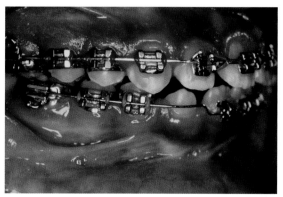

Figure 11.115. Right lateral view of the teeth and fixed appliance.

aesthetic dentistry is completed. A vacuum-formed clear plastic retainer was made for this patient after the removal of the fixed appliance. When the restorative treatment was completed, a Hawley retainer was made for the patient.

Patient 6. This patient had a Class I malocclusion involving excess spaces in both arches. Two important diagnostic findings have an impact on the difficulty of treatment and the final outcome of treatment. First, closure of the spaces distal to the upper left canine and both lower canines require full fixed edgewise appliances in both arches. Second, the Bolton overall ratio at 91.1%

is very close to Bolton's mean of 91.3%, which predicts that after all spaces are closed, the patient's upper and lower teeth will fit together very well. **Although the patient's treatment prognosis was excellent, her orthodontic treatment was not suitable for limited treatment.**

The treatment of this patient is illustrated in Figures 11.114 to 11.121. The full fixed edgewise appliance is shown in Figures 11.114 and 11.115. He occlusion after treatment is shown in Figures 11.116 to 11.121. Her teeth fit together very nicely as predicted by the Bolton analysis. A fixed lingual retainer was placed between her upper central incisors, a wise precaution. The

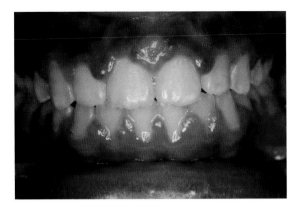

Figure 11.116. Front view of the teeth after treatment.

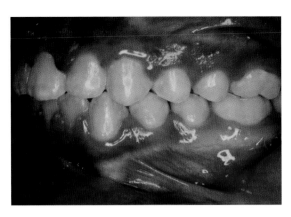

Figure 11.119. Left lateral view of the teeth after treatment.

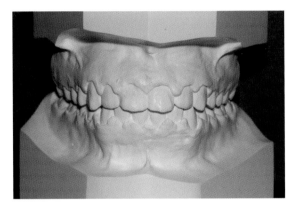

Figure 11.117. Front view of the casts after treatment.

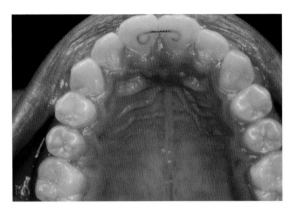

Figure 11.120. Occlusal view of the upper teeth and fixed bonded retainer between the upper central incisors.

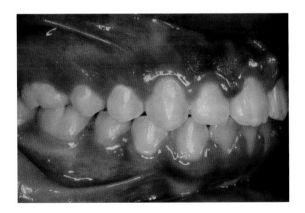

Figure 11.118. Right lateral view of the teeth after treatment.

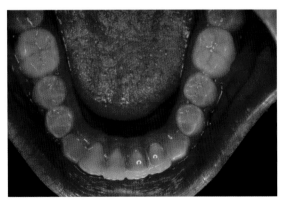

Figure 11.121. Occlusal view of the lower teeth after treatment.

fixed retainer is only expected to last for a few years, but without it a reopening of the diastema between the incisors is very probable, even when the patient is wearing a Hawley retainer. Hawley retainers in both arches were also given to the patient with instructions to wear them full-time for 6 to 9 months and at night for an indefinite period of time.

Patient 7. The features of this malocclusion that made it difficult to treat were the deeper than normal over bite, the ankylosis of a primary molar, and the ectopic eruption of the lower right lateral incisor. **For these reasons, this patient was not a good candidate for limited orthodontic treatment.**

The treatment of the ectopic eruption of this patient's lower right lateral incisor involved the use of fixed edgewise appliances in both arches (Figs. 11.122 to 11.126). The upper fixed edgewise 2 × 4 was used to create overjet for the bonding of the lower anterior teeth. Note that the primary second molars were used in both arches for the most posterior teeth in the fixed appliances. Vertical loops mesial to the primary lower second molars were used to maintain arch

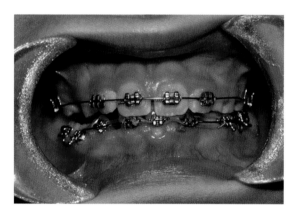

Figure 11.122. Front view of the fixed appliance used in this patient.

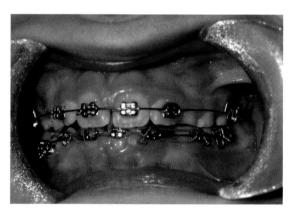

Figure 11.124. Left lateral view of the teeth and appliance.

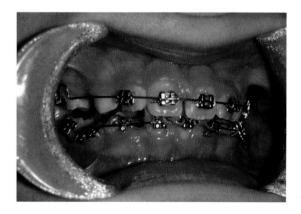

Figure 11.123. Right lateral view of the teeth and appliance.

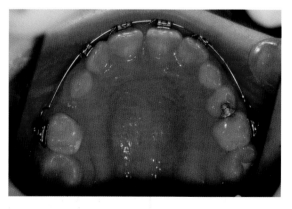

Figure 11.125. Occlusal view of the upper teeth. The upper incisors were moved forward to increase overjet to allow the lower incisors to move forward to accommodate the ectopic incisor.

length and give anchorage support for the mesial movement of the ectopic lateral incisor. The ankylosed lower right primary first molar provided anchorage with a vertical step in the arch wire just mesial to its bracket (Fig. 11.123). At the removal of the fixed appliances, ankylosis of all the lower primary molars was obvious (Figs. 11.127 to 11.132). The patient was retained with a lower lingual holding arch with spurs soldered on the wire at the distal surfaces of the lower lateral incisors (Fig. 6.7).

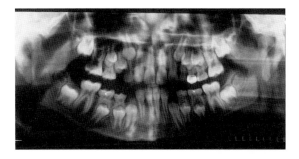

Figure 11.128. Panoramic radiograph taken after the removal of the orthodontic appliance.

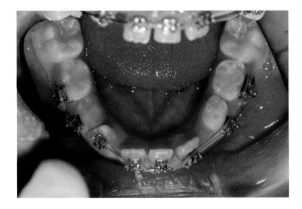

Figure 11.126. Occlusal view of the lower teeth. The lower incisors were moved to the left side on an arch wire with vertical loop stops mesial to the primary second molar tubes. The stopped wire maintained arch length.

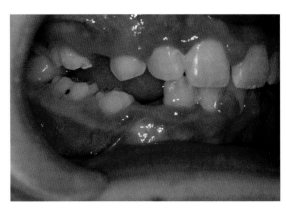

Figure 11.129. Right lateral view of the teeth after treatment.

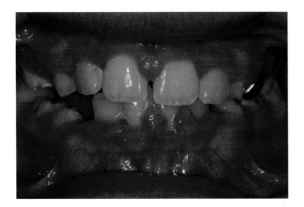

Figure 11.127. Front view of the teeth after the appliance was removed.

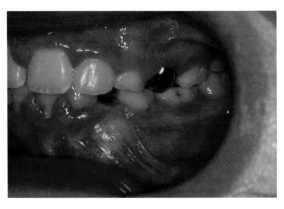

Figure 11.130. Left lateral view of the teeth after treatment.

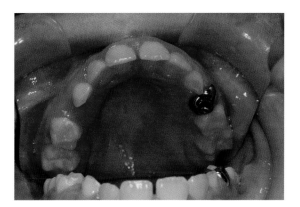

Figure 11.131. Occlusal view of the upper teeth after treatment.

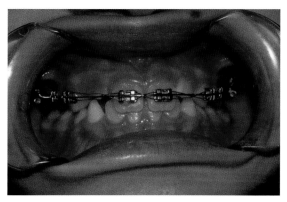

Figure 11.133. Front view of the teeth and appliance.

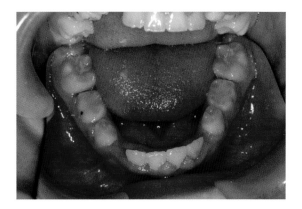

Figure 11.132. Occlusal view of the lower teeth after treatment. A lower lingual holding arch with spurs distal to the lateral incisors retained the treatment.

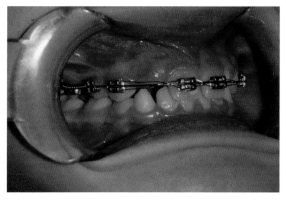

Figure 11.134. Right lateral view of the teeth and appliance.

Patient 8. The forward position of the upper right molar following the premature loss of the upper right primary second molar in an otherwise Class I occlusion is a problem that can be corrected with fixed or removable orthodontic appliances. **This patient has a malocclusion suitable for limited orthodontic treatment.**

The treatment of this patient is illustrated in Figures 11.133 to 11.136. An upper fixed edgewise appliance was used with coil spring retraction of the molar. The coil spring force was kept low with 18-mil stainless steel arch wires that allowed the mesially tipped upper first to move

with controlled tipping to a Class I occlusion. The upper arch wire distal to the upper right first molar extended beyond the molar tube a few millimeters to control movement of the molar and was bent toward the palate to eliminate irritation to the cheek (Fig. 11.136). A late stage in the treatment after the unexpected loss of the upper left primary second molar is shown in Figures 11.137 and 11.138. The occlusion is shown after removal the fixed appliance in Figure 11.139. She was given a Nance palatal holding arch as a retainer until the eruption of the second premolars (Fig. 11.140).

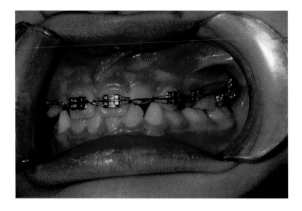

Figure 11.135. Left lateral view of the teeth and appliance. The anchor teeth are tied together with ligature wire.

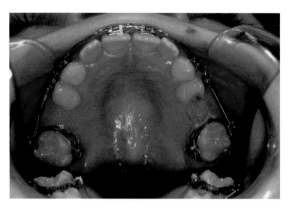

Figure 11.138. Occlusal view of the upper teeth late in treatment. The upper left primary second molar exfoliated during treatment.

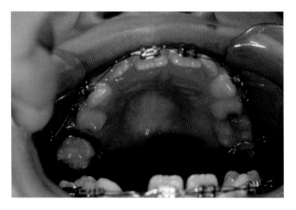

Figure 11.136. Occlusal view of the upper teeth and appliance.

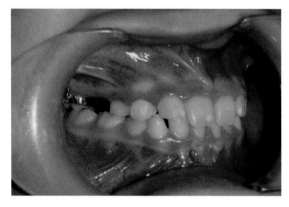

Figure 11.139. Right lateral view of the teeth after the appliance was removed.

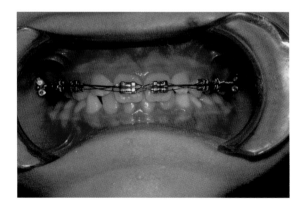

Figure 11.137. Front view of the teeth and appliance one month before removal of the appliance.

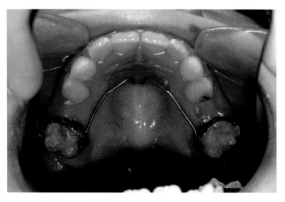

Figure 11.140. Occlusal view of the upper teeth showing the Nance palatal holding arch used as a retainer.

Patient 9. This patient has several problems: anterior crossbite of her upper central incisors, eruption of the upper lateral incisors lingual to the line of arch, and lower lateral incisors erupted 6 mm lingual to the line of arch. After moving the lower lateral incisor crowns into the arch, the teeth will need some labial root movement with a fixed edgewise appliance and rectangular arch wire. This patient had anterior crowding in both arches with almost adequate arch length pre-

dicted by the mixed dentition analysis. She may yet have further crowding difficulties after the permanent canines and premolars have erupted. **Because this patient had a combination of difficult problems, her malocclusion is not suitable for limited orthodontic treatment.**

Fixed edgewise appliances in both arches were used to achieve the occlusion shown in Figures 11.141 to 11.148. At the removal of the fixed appliances, the patient was given clear plastic

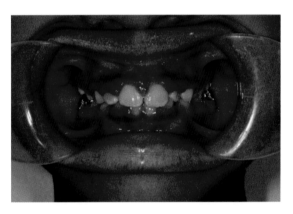

Figure 11.141. Front view of the teeth after removal of the appliance.

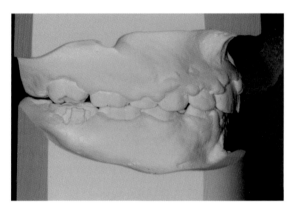

Figure 11.143. Right lateral view of the casts showing a Class I permanent molar relation.

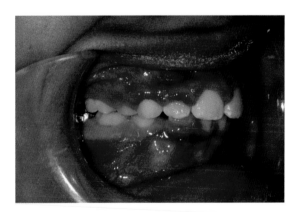

Figure 11.142. Right lateral view of the teeth after treatment.

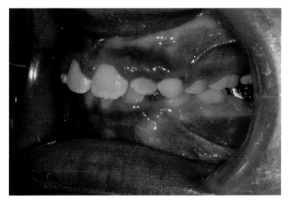

Figure 11.144. Left lateral view of the teeth after treatment.

retainers until more permanent retainers were constructed. The photographs show some relapse of the upper and lower incisors when the Hawley and a lower lingual holding arch were given to the patient (Figs. 11.146, 11.147, and 11.148).

If the patient does not wear the retainers, relapse of the anterior crowding is highly probable. Periodic observation of this patient must continue until the upper and lower canines and premolars have erupted.

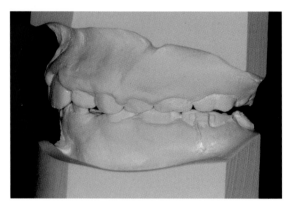

Figure 11.145. Left lateral view of the casts showing a Class I permanent molar relation.

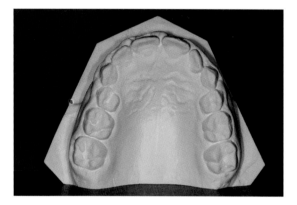

Figure 11.147. Occlusal view of the upper cast after treatment.

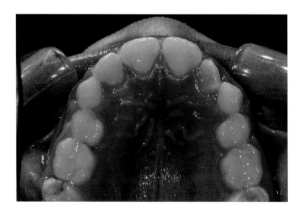

Figure 11.146. Occlusal view of the upper arch after treatment. Lack of retainer compliance resulted in slight opening of the midline diastema and rotation of the left lateral incisor.

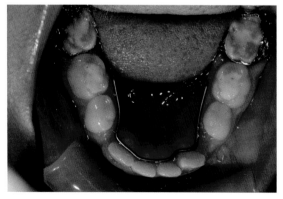

Figure 11.148. Occlusal view of the lower teeth after treatment. Failure of the patient to wear a temporary retainer resulted in the malalignment of the lower incisors. A lower lingual arch retained the treatment.

REFERENCES

ADEA Commission on Change and Innovation in Dental Education. 2006. Educational strategies associated with development of problem-solving, critical thinking, and self-directed learning. J. Dent. Educ. 70:925–936. (http:www.adea.org/cci/)

Bloom, B. S. 1976. Human characteristics and school Learning. New York: McGraw-Hill Book Company.

Bloom, B. S. 1985. Developing talent in young people. New York: Ballantine Books.

Mayer, M. H. 1928. The philosophy of teaching of Saint Thomas Acquinas. Harrison, NY: Roman Catholic Books.

How Orthodontic Appliances Move Teeth

12

Introduction

When an orthodontic appliance delivers a force of sufficient magnitude to a tooth, the tooth will move, if its root is surrounded by healthy periodontal tissues and alveolar bone. An orthodontic force compresses the periodontal ligament and alveolar bone adjacent to the advancing root, stimulating resorption of alveolar bone by osteoclasts. The root surface opposite to the compression side stretches the periodontal ligament and, in turn, stimulates the activity of osteoblasts to form new alveolar bone in the wake of a moving tooth. A healthy periodontal ligament is essential for tooth movement. When the root of a tooth is directly connected to the alveolar bone with no intervening periodontal ligament, a condition called **ankylosis,** the tooth will not respond to orthodontic forces. For a similar reason, it is not possible to move an osseous integrated dental implant with an orthodontic appliance.

An orthodontic force produces different cellular responses on the compression and tension sides of the root during tooth movement (Foster 1982). On the compression side, lower orthodon-

Essentials of Orthodontics: Diagnosis and Treatment
by Robert N. Staley and Neil T. Reske
© 2011 Blackwell Publishing Ltd.

tic forces that do not occlude the blood vessels of the periodontal ligament stimulate osteoclasts to resorb the alveolar bone facing the compressed periodontal ligament. On the tension side, blood vessels dilate, osteoid tissue (new bone) is created by osteoblasts on the surface of the alveolar bone facing the stretched periodontal ligament, and the fibers in the periodontal ligament connected to the alveolar bone reorganize. High orthodontic forces on the compression side of the root that occlude blood vessels and create cell-free areas (hyaline-like) in the periodontal ligament prevent osteoclastic resorption of the alveolar bone surface. Without bone resorption, the tooth cannot move in the direction of the force. Under these conditions, increased blood flow to internal spaces in the alveolar bone on the pressure side eventually stimulates osteoclasts from within the bone to resorb the alveolar bone in a process called **undermining resorption.** Excessively high forces can kill cells in the periodontal ligament, cause pain to the patient, result in root resorption, and will delay movement of a tooth.

Schwarz (1932) demonstrated in a histologic study the rotation of the premolars in a dog around a point approximately in the middle of the root after the teeth were moved in a buccal direction by a finger spring. He named the center of rotation the **tilt axis.** On the side of the root opposite to the finger spring between the tilt axis

213

and the alveolar crest, the periodontal ligament was compressed and the surface of the alveolar bone facing the periodontal ligament was undergoing resorption. On the opposite side of the root between the tilt axis and the crest of the alveolar bone, the periodontal ligament was stretched and new alveolar bone was developed on the surface of the bone facing the stretched periodontal ligament.

This pattern was reversed on the sides of the root between the axis of rotation and apex. Schwarz placed lingual arches with finger springs in the mandibular and maxillary arches of a young dog. He moved a lower right fourth premolar buccally with a 0.5-mm (0.020-inch) diameter spring that delivered 3 to 5 grams of force for 5 weeks, adjusting the spring twice, at the beginning and after 2.5 weeks. The tooth

moved 1 mm. Drawings were made of Schwarz's histologic photomicrographs. Two histologic drawings of the tooth after 5 weeks of movement are shown in Figure 12.1. A low-magnification view of the tooth, its axis of rotation, and surrounding tissues is shown in Figure 12.1A. A high-magnification view of the compression side of the tooth near the alveolar crest is shown in Figure 12.1B. This view shows the old bone with its haversian systems, a line of resorption at the surface of the alveolar bone facing the compressed periodontal ligament, and some individual osteoclasts near the resorption line. Schwarz moved an upper right second premolar buccally with a 0.35-mm (0.014-inch) diameter spring that delivered 20 grams of force for 2.5 weeks. Two histological drawings of this tooth are shown in Figure 12.2. A low-magnification view

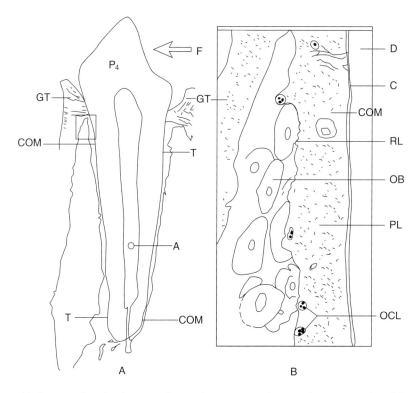

Figure 12.1. A mandibular premolar of a dog moved 1 mm by a 0.5-mm-diameter finger spring that delivered 3 to 5 grams of force for 5 weeks. (**A**) Low-magnification section. A, Axis of rotation; F, force; GT, gingival tissue; COM, compression; T, tension. (**B**) High magnification of compression side. C, Cementum; D, dentin; OB, old bone with haversian systems; OCL, osteoclast; RL, resorption line; PL, periodontal ligament. (Redrawn after Schwarz 1932.)

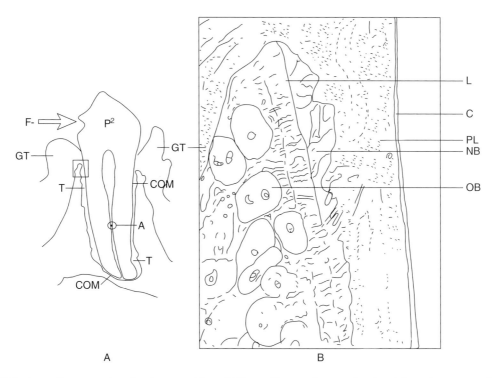

Figure 12.2. A maxillary premolar of a dog moved by a 0.35-mm-diameter finger spring that delivered 20 grams of force for 2.5 weeks. (**A**) Low-magnification section. A, Axis of rotation; F, force; GT, gingival tissue; COM, compression; T, tension. (**B**) High magnification of tension side. C, Cementum; D, dentin; L, line of demarcation between old and new bone; NB, new bone; OB, old bone with haversian systems. (Redrawn after Schwarz 1932.)

of the tooth, its axis of rotation, and the surrounding tissues is seen in Figure 12.2A. A high-resolution view of the tension side of the tooth near the cervix of the crown is shown in Figure 12.2B. This view shows new bone developed adjacent to the stretched periodontal ligament, a line of demarcation between the new, and old bone with its haversian systems.

On the basis of his histologic evidence, Schwarz concluded that the 3- to 5-gram and 20-gram finger spring forces resulted in biologically favorable orthodontic tooth movement. Schwarz also moved a lower right second premolar buccally with a 0.5-mm (0.20-inch) diameter spring that delivered 67 grams of force for 5 weeks, adjusting the spring twice, at the beginning and after 2.5 weeks. At 2.5 weeks after starting the spring force, the tooth stopped moving; after the second

activation, the tooth moved again. Two histologic drawings of this tooth are shown in Figure 12.3. A low-magnification view of the tooth, its axis of rotation, and the surrounding tissues is seen in Figure 12.3A. A high-magnification view of the compression side of the tooth near the alveolar crest is shown in Figure 12.3B. In the high-magnification slide, the periodontal ligament is compressed, and a line of resorption is seen on the alveolar bone facing the periodontal ligament. According to Schwarz the force from the spring had decreased to zero, the resorption line is densely covered by osteoblasts, and the initial resorption has quickly changed to apposition. A resorption cavity reached into the dentin of the root. Schwarz (1932) concluded that a force of 67 grams was fairly strong and caused root resorption.

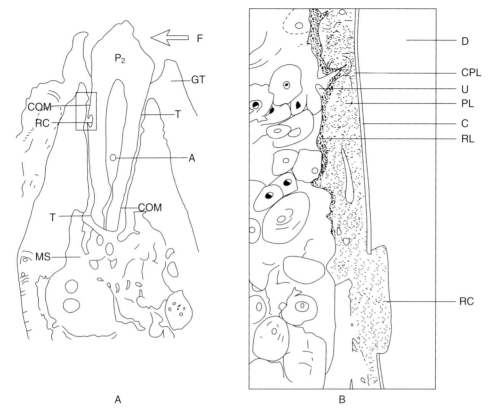

A   B

Figure 12.3. A mandibular premolar of a dog moved by a 0.5-mm-diameter finger spring that delivered 67 grams of force for 5 weeks. (**A**) Low-magnification section. A, Axis of rotation; F, force; GT, gingival tissue; COM, compression; RC, resorption cavity; T, tension; MS, marrow space. (**B**) High magnification of compression side. C, Cementum; CPL, compressed periodontal ligament; D, dentin; PL, periodontal ligament; RC, resorption cavity; RL, resorption line covered with osteoblasts; U, undermining resorption (may be a Howship's lacunae). (Redrawn after Schwarz 1932.)

Buck and Church (1972) moved human maxillary first premolars buccally with 70 ± 7 grams of force using 18-mil (0.45-mm) diameter stainless steel finger springs soldered to a stainless steel palatal arch soldered to bands on the maxillary first molars. At this level of force, they observed osteoclasts within the alveolar bone on the compression side participating in undermining resorption and loss of cells in the compressed periodontal ligament.

From this brief evidence in animal and human studies, we conclude that finger spring forces from 5 to 20 grams produce biologically favorable tooth movement. Finger spring forces of 70 grams and higher will cause biologically unfavorable events in the tooth root, periodontal ligament, and alveolar bone.

Biomechanics

The material in this Chapter is an updated version of a previous publication (Staley 1987). Orthodontic appliances move teeth in three planes of space (Badawi et al. 2009). For this discussion, the three planes of space associated

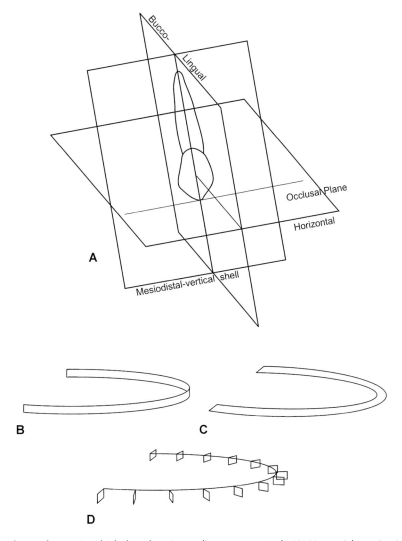

Figure 12.4. Three planes of space in which the edgewise appliance moves teeth. (**A**) Upper right canine is shown in relation to the three planes of space. (**B**) Mesiodistal-vertical parabolic shell. (**C**) Horizontal plane at the middle of the buccal or facial surface of the crown. (**D**) Buccolingual planes that bisect the crowns around the dental arch.

with the dental arches are (1) a parabolic-shaped mesiodistal vertical (MDV) shell that passes through the long axis of each tooth [Dempster, Adams, and Duddles (1963)]; (2) buccolingual planes that pass through the long axis of each tooth at right angles to the MDV shell for each tooth; and (3) a horizontal plane that passes through the midpoints of the buccal and facial surfaces of the clinical crowns at a right angle to the buccolingual and parabolic MDV shell (Fig. 12.4). The MDV shell may have a curvature in the anteroposterior direction (curve of Spee). The horizontal plane may have a curvature from the right side of the arch to the left (curve of Wilson).

Because orthodontic appliances move a tooth in all three planes of space simultaneously, none of the movements of a tooth are expressed wholly in only one of these planes. Andrews (1972, 1989) described the terms *angulation* and *inclination* in ideal occlusions. In the parabolic-shaped **MDV** parabolic shell that extends around the arch, an orthodontic appliance can alter the **angulations** of the long axes of teeth and move them along the long axis of the arch wire (Fig. 12.4B). Teeth also move vertically up and down in this plane (or shell). In the **horizontal plane**, an orthodontic appliance moves a tooth buccally, labially, or lingually (Fig. 12.4C). The appliance rotates the crown and root of an abnormally rotated tooth in the horizontal plane. The **buccolingual planes** bisect the teeth from the facial to lingual, are unique for each tooth, and extend around the parabolic arch (Fig. 12.4D). In the **buccolingual planes**, orthodontic appliances can change the **inclination** of the long axis of a tooth. In the edgewise appliance, change in the inclination of the long axis of a tooth is called "torquing," because, the edgewise wire is twisted (torqued) by a clinician so that when the arch wire is engaged in the rectangular slot of a bracket or tube, it will rotate the tooth around the center of the arch wire in the rectangular slot of the edgewise bracket (Fig. 12.5C).

Isaac Newton (1952), an English mathematician and physicist, proposed a theory containing three basic assumptions that describe the motions of bodies or particles that travel great distances in comparison to their mass. He was interested in describing the motions of the planets and their satellites in the solar system. He considered the earth a particle, because for its mass the earth travels a great distance around the sun. Newton's three "laws" of motion accurately describe the motions of bodies on earth. Scientists have analyzed the motions of rigid and deformable bodies composed of many particles. We assume that a tooth is a rigid body having a center of mass that corresponds to the particle that Newton described. A tooth is embedded in alveolar bone; therefore, its center of mass for our purposes is the center of mass of the embedded part of the root, not the center of mass for the entire tooth. The center of mass of the embedded part of the root is called the **center of resistance**. The roots of most single-rooted teeth are similar to the geometric form called a semiellipsoid. The center of mass of a semiellipsoid is located three-eighths the distance from its base to its apex on its long axis (Ginsberg and Genin 1984).

The upper central incisors have roots that resemble a cone. The center of mass of a cone is located one-fourth the distance from its base to its apex on its long axis. The center of resistance of a tooth was located in the illustrations of this chapter halfway between the cervix of the tooth and the apex of its root(s) on the long axis of the root, as an approximation.

Newton described two different forces that act on a body: a surface traction and a body force. An orthodontic appliance delivers a surface traction to a tooth. Gravity is an example of a body force, because it pulls on all the particles of a body.

Newton's First Law

Newton's first law of motion states that a particle that is free of all forces will remain at rest or in a state of moving forward uniformly unless an impressed force compels it to change. This is known as the *law of inertia*. Teeth are not bodies free of all forces. Occlusal, eruptive, growth, muscular, and habitual forces impress on the teeth of patients with a malocclusion. In patients with normal occlusion, intraoral forces exist in an equilibrium that stabilizes the teeth during growth, adulthood, and aging. Orthodontic appliances overcome the forces of inertia and move the teeth of patients with malocclusion into new, more normal positions to establish a new and hopefully more stable equilibrium of intraoral forces. Appliances must apply sufficient force to a tooth to overcome its innate resistance to movement; its inertia that comes from its mass; the gingival, periodontal, and bony tissues surrounding its root; and the forces that impact its crown. The tooth-moving force must also overcome the force of friction that is associated with the edgewise fixed appliance (Andreasen and Quevedo 1970). In addition, the force must overcome any impressed forces, such as those arising from occlusion, if these forces oppose the force delivered by the orthodontic appliance.

Newton's Second Law

Newton's second law states that the acceleration of a particle is proportional to the impressed force and inversely proportional to the mass of the particle, and the particle accelerates in the same direction as the force. Clinicians have two major concerns: (1) that the force delivered to the tooth is of sufficient magnitude to move the tooth in a biologically sound manner and (2) that the force will move the tooth in the desired direction. The brackets, tubes, bands, and cementing materials of a fixed appliance become part of the tooth. The strength of the bonds between the fixed appliance and the teeth must be great enough to resist the forces delivered by the appliance when it moves the teeth and moderate enough to not damage the enamel surface when the appliance is removed.

Newton summarized his second law of motion in the equation: $F = MA$, where F is force, M is mass, and A is acceleration. Engineers define *force* in terms of dynes and newtons. One dyne is the force required to accelerate a mass of 1 gram 1 centimeter per second squared. One Newton is the force required to accelerate a mass of 1 kilogram 1 meter per second squared. Clinicians usually measure force in units of mass or weight such as grams or ounces. One Newton is equivalent to 102.8 grams or 3.6 ounces.

Keys to Understanding the Delivery of Orthodontic Forces

To explain how teeth move in removable and fixed edgewise appliances, the following assumptions are made: (1) that a tooth is a rigid body partly embedded in an adaptable, flexible, biologically active matrix; (2) that a tooth, when subjected to a force of sufficient and appropriate magnitude, moves in the responsive matrix; (3) that the motions of a tooth in the appliance are described by rotations; and (4) that the forces delivered to the tooth by the appliance conform to the principles of a lever.

Crabb and Wilson (1972) retracted maxillary canines in 20 human patients with finger springs on removable appliances that delivered 30 grams (6 patients), 40 grams (7 patients), and 50 grams (7 patients). They found that the canines moved at an equal rate for the three groups, about 1 mm in a month. In the 50-gram force group, three patients initially experienced pain, the finger springs displaced to the distal side of the tooth, and the canines appeared to tilt distally more than in the other two groups. This study indicates that finger spring forces of 30 and 40 grams move canines and premolars in a biologically sound manner. The experiments of Schwarz (1932) in dogs point to the possibility that finger spring forces much lower than 30 grams could also be effective in moving human teeth.

Hixon et al. (1969) studied the retraction of canines along 21.5 × 25 mil arch wires in edgewise fixed appliances with 0.022 × 0.028 mil slots during the treatment of orthodontic patients. The canines were retracted along the arch wire with forces up to 1500 grams.

Why do the optimum forces shown to be effective in the finger springs of removable appliances differ so much from the forces used in fixed edgewise appliances with large wires? The **keys** to orthodontic force delivery are found in (1) the principle of the lever, (2) the size of the edgewise bracket, and (3) the size and alloy composition of the arch wire used in the edgewise rectangular bracket slot. The lever arm of the finger spring is much longer than the three lever arms of the edgewise appliance. The lever arm of the finger spring extends from where the finger spring contacts the crown of the canine to the center of resistance of the canine (Fig. 12.5A). The length of the lever arm for a human maxillary canine was estimated by measuring the distance with calipers from the height of contour on the mesial crown surface to a point on the middle of the

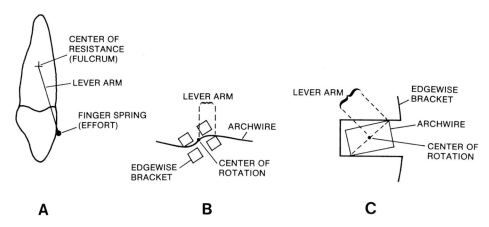

Figure 12.5. Lever arms in (**A**) a finger spring delivering force in the mesiodistal-vertical parabolic shell, (**B**) an arch wire rotating an edgewise bracket slot in the mesiodistal-vertical parabolic shell, and (**C**) a rectangular arch wire delivering a torque force in the buccolingual plane.

mesial surface of the root located apical to the cementoenamel junction (CEJ) three-eighths of the distance between the CEJ and the apical tip of the root. The mean estimated length of the lever arm measured in 13 randomly selected extracted Caucasian adult maxillary canines was 10.98 ± 1.3 mm. Let us assume that the average length of the finger spring lever arms used by Crabb and Wilson (1972) to retract canines was approximately 11 mm. The most favorable forces were 30 and 40 grams, with a mean of 35 grams. A finger spring force of 35 grams would produce a moment of 385 gram-millimeters.

A **moment** is the product of the force (35 grams) times the length of the lever arm (11 mm). The principle of the balanced beam (Thurow 1966) enables us to convert the moment estimated from Crabb and Wilson (1972) to a moment in the edgewise fixed appliance. Using this approach, we can estimate the force required in the edgewise appliance to deliver a 35-gram force to a tooth. This will demonstrate why forces differ so much for finger springs and fixed appliances. The edgewise rectangular bracket slot creates levers in the MVD shell, the buccolingual planes, and in the horizontal plane. The lever arms for the MVD shell and horizontal planes extend from the center of rotation of the canine bracket to the outer edge of the bracket

slot (Fig. 12.5B and 12.9A). The length of these lever arm will vary with the size and design of the bracket.

For this discussion, the length of the lever arms will be 2 mm. To produce a moment equal to the finger spring (385 gram-millimeters), a clinician would need to apply a force of 192.5 grams (192.5 grams times 2 mm equals 385 gram-millimeters). This amount of impressed force would overpower a small cylindrical stainless steel arch wire, causing distal tipping and undesirable rotation of the canine. On the other hand, this force may not be sufficient to retract or rotate the canine on a very large rectangular arch wire with its increased friction and binding (Burrow 2009). The length of the lever arm for torquing teeth in the buccolingual plane of space is very short in an edgewise fixed bracket (Fig. 12.5C). The lever arm extends from the center of the arch wire to the edge of the wire in contact with the bracket slot. In a 21 × 25 mil rectangular steel arch wire, this lever arm is approximately 0.4 mm. To produce a moment equal to the finger spring (385 gram-millimeters), a force of 962.5 grams must be delivered by the arch wire (962.5 grams times 0.4 mm equals 385 gram-millimeters). A large rectangular stainless steel arch wire can generate the force needed to torque a tooth. In the 22-mil slot size, stainless steel arch wires with effective torque have dimensions of approximately 18×25 mil and larger.

Friction within the edgewise appliance consumes some impressed force and should be increased if possible on teeth used for anchorage and decreased for teeth that must move.

General Displacements of Rigid Bodies: Euler and Chasles

After Newton, who lived from 1642 to 1727, scientists have learned more about the motions of rigid bodies. Knowledge was advanced by Leonhard Euler, a Swiss mathematician who lived from 1707 to 1783. He discovered a theorem that described the pure rotation of a rigid body around one point: *The most general rotation of a rigid body about a point is equivalent to a rotation about some axis through that point.* Theoretically, rigid bodies can be purely rotated about a fixed axis, during which particles of the body located on the axis of rotation remain fixed and all other particles travel circular paths around the axis of rotation (Yeh and Abrams 1960). In the edgewise appliance, the arch wire and bracket slot can produce a pair of forces called a couple, which are equal in magnitude, are opposite in direction, and act in the same plane to rotate a tooth around a point located in the center of the bracket (Fig. 12.2B). Because the edgewise appliance is not absolutely rigid, it cannot purely rotate a tooth. The tooth is free to wobble slightly in the buccolingual plane as a couple rotates it.

Michel Chasles, a French mathematician who lived from 1793 to 1880, greatly advanced knowledge when he discovered a theorem that describes the most general displacement of a rigid body: *The most general finite displacement of a rigid body is equivalent to a translation of some point called base point plus a rotation about an axis through that point* (Yeh and Abrams 1960).

Chasles' theorem describes how a finger spring from a removable appliance moves a tooth (Fig. 12.5A). When the finger spring moves a tooth, it translates the tooth a short distance by

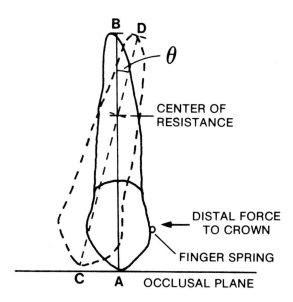

Figure 12.6. Movement of a tooth in response to a force delivered by a finger spring in the mesiodistal-vertical parabolic shell. The tooth primarily rotates around its center of resistance and is translated a small distance.

moving all the particles in the tooth including the particle at the center of resistance (base point) in the direction of the force. The tooth also rotates around an axis going through the center of resistance (base point) in the root. The finger spring moves the crown in the direction of the force and the root apex moves in a direction opposite to that of the crown (Fig. 12.6). As the location of the impressed force on the tooth crown moves nearer to the center of resistance, it will translate the tooth more and rotate it less, and vice versa. Clinicians describe the rotation of a tooth primarily about its center of resistance as a tipping motion.

Limitations of Illustrating Three-Dimensional Tooth Movements in Two-Dimensional Figures

In the figures illustrating orthodontic tooth movement, the small translation that occurs in the direction of each impressed force is ignored.

Furthermore, the motions of the tooth are simplified by illustrating the movement in only one plane, when in fact a tooth simultaneously moves in all three planes of space (Badawi et al. 2009). Depicting the motions of teeth as strictly planar, rather than three-dimensional is not ideal, but it helps to explain tooth movements with two-dimensional illustrations.

Translation of a Tooth in the Edgewise Fixed Appliance

Theoretically, rigid bodies can be purely translated, during which each particle of the body undergoes the same displacement (Yeh and Abrams 1960). To purely translate a rigid body, the impressed force must pass through the center of mass of the body and not rotate the body. If we construct a three-dimensional coordinate system for the rigid body and use six restraints to stop the body from displacing and rotating in the *x*, *y*, and *z* planes (two restraints for each plane), we can theoretically push or pull a rigid body without rotating it. Because orthodontic fixed appliances deliver forces to the surface of the tooth crown, rather than through the center of resistance in the root, and because orthodontic appliances are not absolutely rigid, they cannot purely translate a tooth. The center of resistance in the root is very small, similar to the size of an atom. The position of the center of resistance in the root varies during orthodontic treatment according to the amount of root surface in contact with the periodontal ligament supported by alveolar bone.

Angle (1928, 1929) invented the edgewise appliance to achieve improved control of the movements of teeth. Orthodontists have appreciated the ability of the edgewise appliance to move teeth bodily and to finish the occlusion with precision in all three planes of space. The largest rectangular wires are not generally used to move teeth along the arch wire but are used to level the curve of Spee and improve the inclination (torque) of the teeth during the finishing stage of treatment. To move a tooth along the arch wire, clinicians use smaller rectangular wires and larger cylindrical wires with reduced friction and binding.

How a Tooth Is Translated in the Edgewise Fixed Appliance

How, then, does the edgewise appliance translate a tooth along an arch wire? Bishop (1964) showed that if a rigid body is rotated about one axis and then is rotated equally and oppositely about a parallel axis, the body will translate.

He illustrated the concept with a line drawing (Fig. 12.7). Let line 1 in Figure 12.7 be rotated by angle θ about the axis, which intersects the plane at A; the line is brought to position 2. An equal and opposite rotation θ about axis B brings the line to position 3. Now line 3 is parallel to line 1 so that the two rotations restore the line's original direction but not its position. You will notice that the successively equal and opposite rotations of line 1 resulted in its vertical repositioning. Bishop (1964), a professor of mechanical engineering at the University of London, basically explained how the edgewise appliance translates a tooth when it is moved along an edgewise arch wire. According to Bishop (1964), the finite rotations, illustrated in Figure 12.7, are not vector quantities since they do not follow the parallelogram law.

When a maxillary canine is retracted distally along an arch wire in the edgewise appliance, a force impressed on the mesial surface of the bracket and directed distally toward the molar tube translates the tooth a short distance and rotates the tooth about its center of resistance until the bracket slot binds against the arch wire (Fig. 12.8A). The lines AB, CD, and EF in Figure 12.8 represent the long axis of the crown. The angle theta formed by the lines AB and CD represents the rotation caused by the distal force around the center of resistance. If the distal force is sufficiently great, the bracket will flex the wire

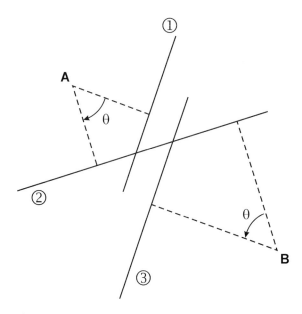

Figure 12.7. Illustration of the long axis of a body that undergoes successive equal and opposite rotations about parallel axes. Line 1 is first rotated through angle θ at axis A; an equal and opposite rotation θ about axis B brings the line to 3. Now line 3 is parallel to line 1 but not in the same position. This principle explains how a tooth is translated in the edgewise appliance. (Redrawn from Bishop 1964.)

and the bracket and the arch wire will create a force known as a couple. A couple is composed of two forces acting in the same plane that are equal in magnitude and opposite in direction (Fig. 12.5B). If the distal force is of appropriate magnitude, it will allow the arch wire to initiate a couple that will rotate the tooth around the center of the bracket, moving the root backward and moving the tip of the crown slightly forward. The angle alpha formed by the lines CD and EF represents the rotation caused by the couple at the bracket (Fig. 12.8A). When the angles theta and alpha are equal, the tooth translates distally along the arch wire (Fig. 12.8A).

If an arch wire produces a couple of less magnitude than the distal force, the crown of the tooth will rotate backward around the center of resistance more than the couple at the bracket

can rotate the root distally (Fig. 12.8B). This is known as *controlled tipping*. If the force delivered from the couple exceeds the distal force, the root will increase its angulation (Fig. 12.8C). Figure 12.8D shows the torque of an incisor when a rectangular arch wire creates a couple centered in the wire that operates in the buccolingual plane.

A distal force, depending on its strength, direction, and location on the bracket and the size and alloy of the wire, translates a tooth in the edgewise appliance by using four levers. The lever arm rotating around the center of resistance in the MDV shell is long (10–11 mm) and is started by small forces. The lever arms rotating around the bracket in the MDV shell and the long axis of the tooth are short (2 mm) and are started by large forces. The lever arm rotating in the buccolingual plane is very short, is started by large forces, and operates with large rectangular arch wires. With round and smaller rectangular wires, a distal force translates a tooth in a recurring sequence by purely translating it a short distance and, depending on the direction and location of the force at the bracket, rotating it around its center of resistance and the center of the bracket in the MDV shell and rotating it around its long axis.

The following reports of Hixon et al. (1970) and Andreasen (1976) support the preceding explanation of how the edgewise appliance translates teeth along the mesiodistal-vertical shell. Hixon et al. (1970) concluded from their study of canine retraction:

The deflection of an 0.0215 by 0.028 inch arch with a 7 mm span between the brackets is especially worth noting. With this steel arch, which is 'heavy' by clinical standards, there was a 1 mm deflection when 200 gram forces were applied. While these findings illustrate one reason that only two thirds of the canines and one fourth of the mandibular molar units moved bodily, they also indicate that retraction, even with conventional arches, probably consists of initial tipping movements as the arch bends, followed by a certain amount of uprighting as the activating

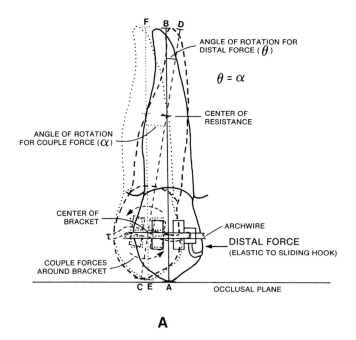

A

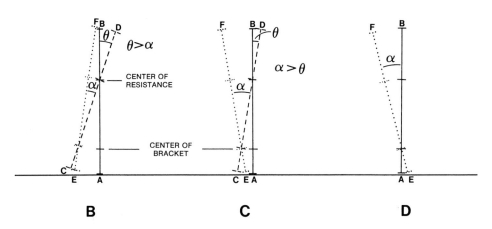

B　　　　　　　　**C**　　　　　　　　**D**

Figure 12.8. Tooth movement in the mesiodistal-vertical parabolic shell with the edgewise appliance. (**A**) Translation of a canine in response to a distal force first rotates the tooth about its center of resistance and then the arch wire rotates the tooth about the center of the bracket, resulting in a slightly different vertical position of the tooth. (**B**) Controlled tipping when the distal force predominates. (**C**) Distal root movement when the force of the bracket couple predominates. (**D**) Rotation around the center of the rectangular arch wire during torque in the buccolingual plane. Lines AB, CD, and EF represent the long axis of crown: (AB) before movement, (CD) after the tooth rotates around the center of resistance, and (EF) after rotating around the bracket.

force exhausts itself before reactivation. With the Begg technique there is but one large 'tipping' and one 'uprighting' movement, as compared to a series of such movements with conventional arches.

Andreasen (1976) described the "walking" of the bracket distally along an edgewise arch wire:

> Tooth movement produced by translating a bracket over a wire, therefore, will undergo the following changes in position: (1) first, the tooth will tip according to the freedom allowed by the size of the bracket slot and size of wire inserted by the operator; (2) next, the diagonally opposite ears of the bracket will touch the arch wire, and as the applied force continues to translate the tooth, the wire will tend to bend in an s-shaped configuration due to the vertical forces produced by the bracket ears against the deforming wire; tooth movement at this time will stop until (3) lastly, the root uprights enough so the vertical forces are small enough to allow the horizontal force to once again slide the bracket and tooth over the wire.

Rotation of a Tooth in the Edgewise Fixed Appliance

When a force translates a tooth along an arch wire in the mesiodistal-vertical shell, it tends to rotate the tooth around its long axis, because the force acts on a bracket that is located buccal to the center of resistance and the long axis of the tooth (Fig. 12.9). The tooth will rotate around its axis depending on the location of the force on the bracket, the size and flexibility of the arch wire, and the buccolingual freedom of the wire within the bracket slot. The sliding hook acting along the arch wire on the mesial surface of the bracket will rotate a tooth as shown in Figure 12.9A. In comparison, a force placed on a vertical post located on the distal-gingival ear of an edgewise bracket has a reduced potential for rotating the tooth during translation. If a lingual button is placed on the tooth with a sliding hook, a distal force on the button will counteract

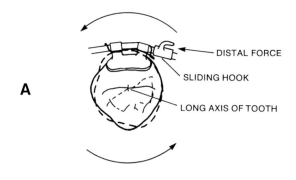

A

DISTAL FORCE
SLIDING HOOK
LONG AXIS OF TOOTH

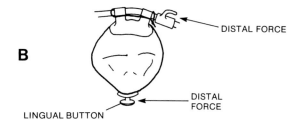

B

DISTAL FORCE
DISTAL FORCE
LINGUAL BUTTON

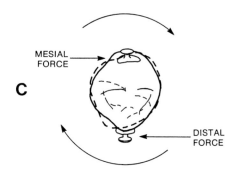

C

MESIAL FORCE
DISTAL FORCE

Figure 12.9. Rotating a canine around its long axis in the horizontal plane: (**A**) a distal force applied on the mesiobuccal surface of the bracket rotates a tooth, (**B**) equal distal forces on both the mesiobuccal and lingual surfaces of the tooth prevent rotation, and (**C**) equal mesial and distal forces in opposite directions (a couple) rotate a tooth.

the rotation potential of the sliding hook (Fig. 12.9B). If a tooth is rotated abnormally, it can be rotated by placing buccal and lingual forces that create a couple in the horizontal plane (Fig. 12.9C).

Newton's Third Law

Newton's third law of motion states that to every action there is always opposed an equal reaction, or the mutual actions of two bodies upon each other are always equal and opposite in direction. All the illustrations in this book that show a force as an arrow should have included in them an arrow opposing that force (Dr. George F. Andreasen, 1987, personal communication). As a tooth moves in response to forces from an orthodontic appliance, the periodontal ligament, alveolar bone, and gingiva surrounding the tooth resist this force. The gingiva stretched by a tooth moved by an orthodontic appliance can pull an adjacent tooth in the same direction if the adjacent tooth is free to move. The tissues supporting the teeth must be considered adaptable, flexible, and responsive to biologically favorable orthodontic forces.

The concept of anchorage in orthodontics is related to Newton's third law. When an orthodontic appliance delivers a force that pushes or pulls a tooth, it also pushes or pulls other teeth. In a removable Hawley appliance, all of the teeth other than the tooth to be moved are joined together in an anchorage unit to resist the force from the finger spring. Removable appliances also use palatal and lingual tissues as part of the anchor unit.

Edgewise fixed appliances challenge us with complex anchorage problems. Because all of the teeth included in an edgewise appliance can move individually, numerous action-reaction movements occur simultaneously among all of the teeth in an upper or lower arch. Various mechanical tactics are used to join teeth together in a fixed appliance anchorage unit. If two teeth or groups of teeth must move in opposite directions, such as upper central incisors with a diastema between them, the impressed force from a plastic chain can reciprocally bring the teeth together (Fig. 12.10A). Anchorage units are created with continuous and figure-eight wire ligatures that join several teeth together. A stopped arch wire can also be used to join teeth together in an anchorage unit to oppose the movement of one

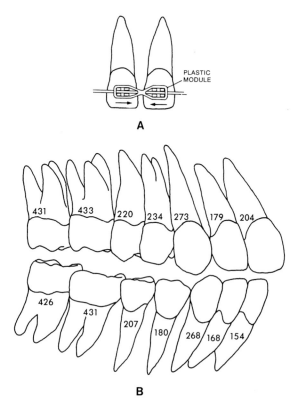

Figure 12.10. Anchorage in the edgewise appliance: (**A**) reciprocal anchorage to close a diastema and (**B**) root surface areas. (From Jepsen 1963.)

or two teeth. Palatal holding arches, trans-palatal arches, lingual arches, head gear, chin cups, and ankylosed teeth are used as sources of anchorage. Mini-screws and bone plates have been introduced for the purpose of creating an anchor unit in alveolar bone.

The surface areas of the roots have been measured to evaluate the anchorage values of teeth. The mean surface areas of the roots are shown in Figure 12.10B (Jepsen 1963). The molars have the greatest root surface areas followed by the canines with the next largest surface areas. Clinicians using the edgewise fixed appliance will pit a canine against as many other anchor teeth as possible when the canine must be moved farther than the anchor teeth (Quinn and Yoshikawa 1985).

REFERENCES

Andreasen, G. F., and Quevedo, F. R. 1970. Evaluation of friction forces in the 0.022×0.028 edgewise bracket in vitro. J. Biomechan. 3:151–160.

Andreasen, G. F. 1976. Biomechanical rudiments. Iowa City: University of Iowa.

Andrews, L. F. 1972. The six keys to normal occlusion. Am. J. Orthod. 62:296–309.

Andrews, L. F. 1989. Straight wire, the concept and appliance. San Diego: L. A. Wells Company.

Angle, E. H. 1928. The latest and best in orthodontic mechanism. Dent. Cosmos. 70:1143–1158.

Angle, E. H. 1929. The latest and best in orthodontic mechanism. Dent. Cosmos. 71:164–174, 260–270, 409–421.

Badawi, H. M., Toogood, R. W., Carey, J. P. R., Heo, G., and Major, P. W. 2009. Three-dimensional orthodontic force measurements. Am. J. Orthod. Dentofac. Orthop. 136:518–528.

Bishop, R. E. D. 1964. Dynamics. Encyclopedia Britannica. 7:822–825.

Buck, D. L., and Church, D. H. 1972. A histologic study of tooth movement. Am. J. Orthod. 62:507–516.

Burrow, S. J. 2009. Friction and resistance to sliding in orthodontics: a critical review. Am. J. Orthod. Dentofac. Orthop. 135:442–447.

Crabb, J. J., and Wilson, H. J. 1972. The relation between orthodontic spring force and space closure. Dent. Pract. 22:233–240.

Dempster, W. T., Adams, W. J., and Duddles, R. A. 1963. Arrangement in the jaws of the roots of the teeth. J. Am. Dent. Assoc. 67:779–797.

Foster, T. D. 1982. A textbook of orthodontics. 2nd ed. Oxford: Blackwell Scientific Publications.

Ginsberg, J. H., and Genin, J. 1984. Statics. 2nd ed. New York: John Wiley and Sons.

Hixon, E. H., Aasen, T. O., Arango, J., Clark, R. A., Klosterman, R., Miller, S. S., and Odom, W. M. 1970. On force and tooth movement. Am. J. Orthod. 57:476–489.

Hixon, E. H., Atikian, H., Callow, G. E., McDonald, H. W., and Tacy, R. J. 1969. Optimal force, differential force, and anchorage. Am. J. Orthod. 55:437–457.

Jepsen, A. 1963. Root surface measurement and a method for x-ray determination of root surface area. Acta Odontol. Scand. 21:35–46.

Newton, I. 1952. Mathematical principles of natural philosophy. Chicago: Encyclopedia Britannica, Inc. Great Books of the Western World, Volume 34.

Quinn, R. S., and Yoshikawa, D. K. 1985. A reassessment of force magnitude in orthodontics. Am. J. Orthod. 88:252–260.

Schwarz, A. M. 1932. Tissue changes incidental to orthodontic tooth movement. Int. J. Orthod. 18:331–352.

Staley, R. N. 1987. Orthodontic laboratory manual. Iowa City: University of Iowa Campus Stores, pp. 129–167.

Thurow, R. C. 1966. Edgewise orthodontics. St. Louis: The C. V. Mosby, pp. 3–9.

Yeh, H., and Abrams, J. I. 1960. Principles of mechanics of solids and fluids. Volume 1: Particle and rigid-body mechanics. New York: McGraw-Hill Book Company.

The Edgewise Fixed Appliance

13

Introduction

A fixed appliance is attached to the teeth unlike a removable appliance. Because a fixed appliance cannot be easily removed or altered by a patient, treatment progress is usually dependable. In many patients who require limited orthodontic treatment, the malocclusion can be treated more quickly with a fixed appliance than with a removable appliance. The greatest disadvantage of the multibracketed fixed appliance compared to removable appliances is the difficulty some patients experience with poor oral hygiene and cariogenic diets that expose them to the development of enamel white spot lesions during treatment.

The Edgewise Appliance

E. H. Angle (1928, 1929) invented the edgewise appliance near the end of his life. Angle invented several other fixed appliances earlier, but he thought that the edgewise appliance had the

Essentials of Orthodontics: Diagnosis and Treatment
by Robert N. Staley and Neil T. Reske
© 2011 Blackwell Publishing Ltd.

greatest promise. Angle invented brackets with rectangular slots and tubes with 22×28-mil dimensions. His appliance was made of nickel alloys. He used rectangular arch wires to move a tooth in all three planes of space with the edgewise appliance.

Since its invention, the edgewise appliance has undergone numerous modifications in the design of brackets, tubes, arch wires, and auxiliary devices. Examples of modern bands and brackets are illustrated in Figure 13.1. The appliance has rectangular tubes on the most distal teeth in each arch, usually the first or second molars, and brackets on the other teeth. Arch wires with ideal arch form are put into the appliance to align the teeth. Arch wires are made from wire having two basic cross sections: cylindrical (round) and rectangular. The arch wire is held in each bracket slot with a small-diameter (10 mil) annealed stainless steel wire or an elastomeric (plastic) module. A variety of edgewise appliances not requiring arch wire ligation have been developed (Fig. 13.1C). Arch wires generate forces that move the teeth. Teeth also move mesially and distally along an arch wire in response to impressed forces from latex modules (rubber bands), plastic modules, coil springs, and extraoral devices such as headgear.

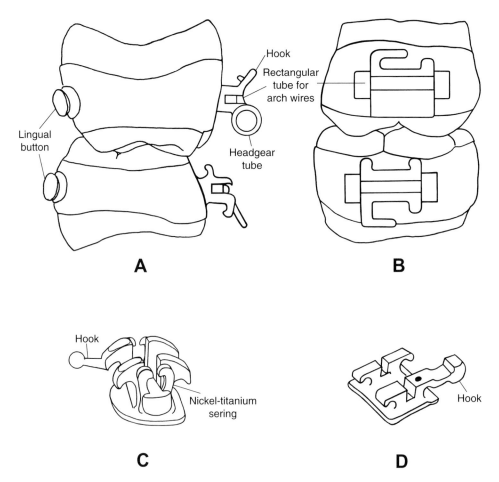

Figure 13.1. The modern edgewise appliance: (**A**) the left first molar bands viewed from the mesial surface, (**B**) the left molar bands viewed from the buccal surface, (**C**) a self-ligating bracket with a power arm, and (**D**) a premolar bracket with a power arm. (Drawn from the appliance, 3M Unitek Corporation, Monrovia, CA.)

Arch Wires

In the 1930s, manufacturers began making arch wires with stainless steel, a less costly material than gold. Stainless steel arch wires were much stiffer than similar sized gold wires. Smaller stainless steel wires with reduced stiffness were made for the initial alignment of the teeth. A smaller slot and tube appliance (18 × 25) was introduced to use smaller steel wires and deliver less force to the teeth. Woven arch wires com-posed of several small-diameter steel wires bound together were developed to increase the flexibility of steel wire for the initial alignment of teeth. Andreasen and Morrow (1978) pioneered a major advance in orthodontic treatment when they introduced nickel-titanium alloy arch wires that had great flexibility, spring back, and delivery of lower forces. Burstone and Goldberg (1980) introduced titanium-molybdenum alloy arch wires with flexibility intermediate between nickel-titanium and stainless steel that further enhanced the use of the edgewise appliance. The larger stainless steel wires are still used in the 22 × 26-mil slot to level the curve of Spee and torque teeth in the latter stages of treatment. The larger wires deliver the forces needed to level arches and torque teeth.

Bands

Stainless steel bands were initially custom made by clinicians for each tooth. The band material was "pinched" on each tooth, removed, and welded before cementation. Manufacturers developed preformed bands for all of the teeth, with a variety of sizes for each tooth group. Banding of all the teeth occurred from the 1930s through the 1970s. Since then the bonding of brackets has replaced the banding of all the teeth except the first molars. Bands on molars have tubes for headgear to resist the forces delivered by the headgear. The first molars are also bonded in many patients.

Separators

Separators must be placed in most patients before bands can be fitted. Several types of separators are used, the most common being plastic rings. Special pliers stretch the plastic ring and help to push it through the contact point. Plastic rings separate the teeth in a few days after which they may loosen and be lost. Before fitting the band, a clinician must remove the separator from the embrasure. When the separator is missing, the clinician must check to see if it slipped subgingivally, and if it did, he or she must remove it.

Fitting a Band

The interproximal spaces created by the separators enable the clinician to fit a band properly. Before banding and bonding, the teeth must be cleaned. Teeth vary in size and shape, which makes the fitting with preformed bands a chal-

lenge for some teeth. A large cusp of Carabelli complicates the fitting of maxillary molar bands. The smallest band that fits the crown is best. The mesial and distal edges of the band should be located at the height of the marginal ridges. This position will usually place the molar buccal tube at the middle of the buccal surface. The molar buccal tube must be centered on the buccal surface of the crown when viewed from the occlusal surface. If a first molar is bonded, the tube should be directed toward the middle of the central incisor crowns.

When fitting a band on a tooth, ask the patient to push it down onto the tooth by biting on a plastic band- seater. Bands have a tendency to slip down too far on the mesial surface of a tooth crown. Begin by pushing the band down more on the distal half of the crown. Later on, push the band down fully on the mesial surface. The band is also pushed down on the buccal and lingual sides of the tooth crown. After the band is fully seated, the occlusal edges of the band are adapted to the grooves and crown contours with a metal instrument called a burnisher. Do not adapt the gingival end of the band to the tooth crown, because that would make removal of the band difficult. In younger patients who have not experienced sufficient passive eruption, a clinician may trim the gingival edge of a band with curved crown and bridge scissors to keep the band from injuring the gingival tissues (Guymon 2010). A cut edge is sharp and should be ground smooth to avoid injury to the gingival tissues. If a preformed band is trimmed too much, it will not have enough contact with the tooth crown to stay cemented very long. All bands irritate the gingival tissues; the goal is to minimize this irritation as much as possible.

Cementing a Band

After adapting the band, remove it from the tooth with band removal pliers. Clean and dry the band and tooth crown. Mix enough cement to either fill the band or liberally cover the inner surface of the band. Seat the band fully on the tooth and clean off excess cement from the crown and gingival tissues. Light cure the cement.

Band Cements

Bands are cemented on teeth with glass ionomer and hybrid-glass ionomer cements because the fluoride released from these materials protects the enamel from caries. The glass ionomer cements fail more frequently at the band-cement interface than at the cement-enamel interface, leaving the cement attached to and protecting the enamel (Norris et al. 1986). The glass ionomer cements disintegrate in saliva at a low rate, making them suitable for the longer treatment times encountered in orthodontic patients (Phillips et al. 1987). The glass ionomer cements can reduce enamel demineralization at orthodontic band margins (Donly et al. 1995). A failure rate for bands cemented with glass ionomer cement on 1,424 first permanent molars in 513 orthodontic patients was 15.6% (Millett and Gordon 1992). The mean survival time was 33.1 months. Treatment mechanics significantly influenced survival time, with extraction cases and Begg mechanics being associated with the shortest survival times.

Removal of Bands

Bands are removed after treatment with band removal pliers. The pliers have one beak that grips the band and another beak covered by a plastic pad that rests on the occlusal and incisal surfaces of the crown. In removing upper molar bands, the bond between the tooth and the band is broken by placing the gripper beak first on the lingual part of the band and then placing the pliers on the buccal part of the band. When the upper molar band is removed, the gripper beak is placed on the palatal side of the band to roll the band off the lingual crown surface. In removing lower molar bands, the bond between the band and tooth is broken first by placing the gripper beak on the buccal part of the band and then on the lingual part of the band.

Bonding of Brackets

The bonding of orthodontic brackets began in the 1960s after the discovery by Buonocore (1955) that acrylic filling materials could be attached to the enamel surface after etching the surface with phosphoric acid and the discovery of bis-GMA adhesives by Bowen (1962).

Newman (1964) was an early advocate of bonding brackets to the enamel surface. By 1980, most orthodontists were bonding brackets to the incisors, canines, and premolars in their patients. The typical bonding system consists of an unfilled sealant placed on the etched enamel surface and a filled resin (composite resin) that attaches to the sealed enamel surface and the base of the bracket. A dry-etched enamel surface is the ideal condition for bonding. Recently, a combination of sealant and acid called self-etching primer has reduced the steps needed to bond a bracket. Sealants and self-etching primers have been developed for use in moist as well as dry conditions.

The fillers added to acrylic resin to form composite resins help control dimensional change, increase hardness and chemical inertness, and give the material an appearance similar to teeth. The filler particles range from 1 to 40 micrometers in size and are made from a variety of materials such as fused silica, crystalline quartz, lithium aluminum silicate, and borosilicate glass.

The etch time for a 35% phosphoric acid gel is from 15 to 20 seconds. The self-etching primer is rubbed on the enamel surface for 3 to 5 seconds for teeth located mesial to the first molars. The primer is dried for 1 to 2 seconds with a gentle burst of air. Sealants and self-etching primers are light cured before the bracket with composite resin is pushed onto the enamel surface. Composite resin adhesive is either dispensed from tubes or precoated on bracket bases. The precoated brackets must not be removed from their containers until the time of bonding. Ambient light will cure the adhesive on the precoated bracket, if it is subjected to room light a few minutes. Current composite resins are mostly light cured for direct bonding, but some chemically cured composite resins are still available for bonding.

Anatomic Considerations

The teeth and arches of a 17-year-old male with a normal Class I occlusion never treated with an orthodontic appliance illustrate several features that influence the placement and use of an edgewise fixed appliance (Fig. 13.2). Occlusal views of his upper and lower arches show how arch wires must be bent in the horizontal plane to accommodate differences in the size and rotational position of the teeth in an arch (Fig. 13.2, A, B). The standard first order bends placed in the arch wires used in the edgewise appliance for the upper arch are (1) lateral inset, (2) canine offset, and (3) molar offset and toe-in; the standard bends in the lower arch wire are (1) canine

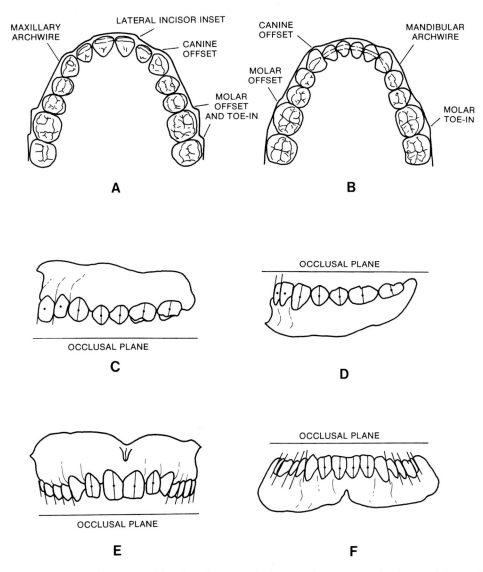

Figure 13.2. The occlusion of a 17-year-old male with a normal Class I occlusion: (**A**) occlusal view of the maxillary arch, (**B**) occlusal view of the mandibular arch, (**C**) buccal view of the maxillary left teeth, (**D**) a buccal view of the mandibular left teeth, (**E**) front view of the maxillary teeth, and (**F**) front view of the mandibular teeth.

offset, (2) first molar offset, and second molar toe-in (Tweed 1966).

When the casts are viewed from the buccal, the midpoints of the labial and buccal surfaces of his teeth vary in their vertical positions (Fig. 13.2, C and D). Arch wires without vertical bends (flat in the horizontal plane) will move the centers toward a common horizontal level if the brackets and bands were placed in the middle of the clinical crowns. The curve of Spee is most visible in the buccal view of his lower cast (Fig. 13.2D) and in the vertical step between the upper first and second molars (Fig. 13.2C). Level arch wires work to level the occlusal plane. Leveling of the curve of Spee, a common goal in comprehensive orthodontic treatment, will open his bite or decrease his overbite.

The vertical lines drawn through the centers of the facial and buccal surfaces of the crowns (the facial axis of the clinical crown, Andrews [1989]) show the angulations in the mesiodistal-vertical parabolic shell of the long axes of the crowns of the incisors, canines, and posterior teeth to the occlusal plane (Fig. 13.2, C–F).

The vertical lines drawn on the buccal surfaces of the crowns show the inclination in the buccolingual planes of the buccal crown surfaces of the upper and lower canines and posterior teeth in this normal occlusion (Fig. 13.2, E and F). The buccolingual inclinations of the upper and lower incisor crowns are shown in Figure 13.2, C and D.

To treat patients with the original edgewise appliance, Tweed (1966) placed first order bends, artistic bends to attain proper angulations of incisor crowns; second order tip back bends to prepare anchorage, reverse curves to level the curve of Spee; and third order bends in rectangular arch wires to torque teeth to achieve proper inclination in the buccolingual planes. The original appliance had rectangular bracket slots and molar tubes oriented at approximately 90 degrees to the buccal and facial surfaces of the tooth crowns and positioned similar distances buccally and facially from the crowns. This orientation of brackets and tubes required that a clinician place bends in the arch wires to move the teeth into their correct locations, inclination, angulations, and occlusion.

The Straight Wire Appliance™

In 1970, Andrews (1989) invented the Straight Wire Appliance™. After measuring and studying 120 nontreated ideal Class I occlusions, Andrews made brackets and tubes with rectangular slots oriented to the buccal and facial clinical crown surfaces that incorporated the average inclination, angulations, and buccolingual offsets observed in the sample of ideal occlusions. This important advance in the development of the edgewise appliance enabled clinicians to concentrate on other important aspects of treatment without having to spend an inordinate amount of time bending arch wires. Clinicians nevertheless need at times during treatment to place bends in arch wires of patients, especially during the finishing stage of treatment. The variability in arch form, tooth size, tooth shape, configuration of alveolar bone, and cephalometric relationships seen in patients often requires a customized straight arch appliance to obtain the best occlusion. The appliance is customized to the patient when a clinician places bends in the arch wires that move the teeth to their final positions and occlusion. Andrews' (1972) six keys to ideal occlusion are important goals for any clinician treating a malocclusion problem.

At this time, many versions of the straight arch appliance are available in the marketplace. The rectangular slots are offered in different "prescriptions." A clinician is responsible to know and understand the differences among the appliances and, in particular, to understand the straight arch appliance that he uses. Round arch wires are used in limited treatment patients. They effectively use the offset and angulation features of straight arch appliances.

Bracket and Molar Tube Placement

The correct placement of brackets and bands on the crowns of the teeth is very important

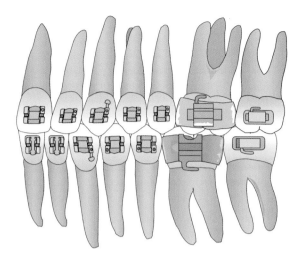

Figure 13.3. A facial-buccal view of edgewise bands and brackets on the left teeth. (Courtesy Orthoclipart by Michael L. Swartz.)

Table 13.1. Recommended Bracket Slot Heights (mm)

	Maxilla	Mandible
Central incisor	4.00	4.00
Lateral incisor	3.75	4.00
Canine	4.50	4.50
First premolar	4.25	4.25
Second premolar	4.00	4.00
First molar	3.75	3.75
Second molar	3.50	3.50

From White (1999).

to the success of the edgewise fixed appliance. Figure 13.3 illustrates the placement of brackets and molar tubes on the left-side teeth. The molar tubes and bracket slots are placed at the midpoint of the facial and buccal surfaces of the clinical crowns both vertically and mesiodistally (Andrews 1989). White (1999) recommended specific bracket slot heights (Table 13.1). Because teeth vary in size among patients, a specific measurement for slot height is not universally applicable to patients. The heights recommended by White make it possible in most patients to level the curve of Spee and achieve good inter-digitation of the teeth.

The slots of the upper incisor brackets are usually placed slightly closer to the gingiva on the distal compared to the mesial side of the bracket to ensure proper crown angulations. Based on his study of ideal occlusions, Andrews (1989) recommended angulations of 5 degrees for the central incisors and 9 degrees for the lateral incisors. Andrews (1989) recommended 2-degree angulations for the lower central and lateral incisors. Andrews recommended the following angulations for upper teeth: (1) canine 11 degrees, (2) first and second premolars 2 degrees, and (3) first and second molars 5 degrees. Andrews recommended the following angulations for lower teeth: (1) lower canines 5 degrees and (2) lower premolars and molars 2 degrees.

The brackets shown in Figure 13.1, C and D, and the canine brackets in Figure 13.3 have vertical extensions on the distal gingival bracket ears called hooks. Andrews (1989) put Power Arms™ on canines and posterior teeth, honoring Calvin Case (1921) who introduced them. The arms extended vertically to the level of the center of resistance on each tooth. The purpose of a canine Power Arm™ was to counteract the tipping caused by a distal force on the mesial surface of its bracket during translation.

The brackets and tubes are illustrated from the occlusal in Figure 13.4. The brackets are centered on the buccal and facial surfaces. Appropriate molar offsets are built into the molar tubes in each arch.

Andrews (1989) recommended the following inclinations based on his study of ideal occlusions: (1) upper central incisors 7 degrees, upper lateral incisors 3 degrees, upper canines and premolars –7 degrees, upper molars –9 degrees, and (2) lower incisors 1 degree, lower canines –11 degrees, lower first premolars –22 degrees, lower first molars –30 degrees, and lower second molars –35 degrees. Andrews was convinced that optimal functional occlusion requires that all crowns be properly inclined. Since about 1990 many different "prescriptions" for a variety of straight arch appliances have been marketed by companies manufacturing orthodontic bands

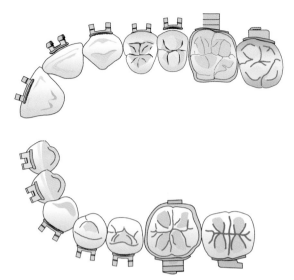

Figure 13.4. Occlusal views of edgewise bands and brackets on the maxillary and mandibular left teeth. (Courtesy Orthoclipart by Michael L. Swartz.)

and brackets. Each clinician must understand the straight arch appliance or hybrid between straight arch and non–straight arch fixed appliance that he or she uses to treat malocclusions.

Direct and Indirect Bonding

Bonding brackets directly to the teeth is very common in orthodontic treatment. This requires careful placement of the brackets and may require rebonding to correct poorly bonded brackets. Correct angulation of the slot can be difficult to attain in direct bonding. If the angulation is in error, a correction can be made by replacing bends in the arch wire or rebonding.

Indirect bonding is a technical challenge but the effort results in accurate positioning of the brackets in the mouth based on accurate placement of the brackets in the laboratory on a cast of the teeth. Many methods for doing indirect bonding have been developed (White 1999). If a bond fails during or after indirect bonding, it is usually replaced by direct bonding of the replacement bracket.

Removal of Brackets and Bonded Attachments from Teeth

The safest method of mechanical debonding is to use a cutter plier (No. 346) that creates a wedge at the base of the bracket to peel the bracket from the enamel (Powers and Messersmith 2001). Another method is to squeeze the ears of a metal bracket with utility pliers deforming the bracket and peeling the bracket off the tooth. Removal of brackets from ceramic veneers may cause damage to the veneer using using common debonding methods (Brantley and Eliades 2001).

Arch Form

The form of the arch, as viewed from the occlusal surfaces of the teeth, varies in patients. Choosing a preformed arch wire that has a form similar to the arch form of the patient prior to treatment is usually recommended. For that reason, manufacturers make wires with several different shapes. The Bonwill-Hawley (Hawley 1905) arch form was in use before the origin of the edgewise appliance. It is still used in orthodontic treatment. The Bonwill-Hawley arch form must be altered in the region of the molars in the non–straight wire appliances as illustrated in Figure 13.2, A and B. The molar adjustments of this form in straight wire appliances may also be necessary. Several other arch forms such as natural arch and broad arch forms are available. One manufacturer (3M Unitek Corporation, Monrovia, CA) has the following arch forms: (1) standard [Bonwill-Hawley], (2) Orthoform I tapered, (3) Orthoform II square, (3) Orthoform III ovoid, and (4) Orthoform LA. Wires in all of these arch forms may require adjustment bends to move the teeth to their appropriate positions and occlusion. The variety of wires in different arch forms makes it possible to give each patient an arch form appropriate for his or her alveolar processes. In general, respecting the patient's original arch form is best for most patients. Patients with posterior crossbites undergo width changes in the upper arch that alter the arch form. In these patients, arch wires after the widening should maintain the increased width of the arch.

REFERENCES

Andreasen, G. F., and Morrow, R. E. 1978. Laboratory and clinical analyses of Nitinol wire. Am. J. Orthod. 73:142–151.

Andrews, L. F. 1972. The six keys to normal occlusion. Am. J. Orthod. 62:296–309.

Andrews, L. F. 1989. Straight wire, the concept and appliance. San Diego, L. A. Wells Company.

Angle, E. H. 1928. The latest and best in orthodontic mechanism. Dent. Cosmos. 70:1143–1158.

Angle, E. H. 1929. The latest and best in orthodontic mechanism. Dent. Cosmos. 71:164–174, 260–270, 409–421.

Bowen, R. L. 1962. Dental filling material comprising vinyl silane treated silica and a binder consisting of the reaction product of bis phenol A and glycidyl acrylate. United States Patent 3,066,112.

Brantley, W. A., and Eliades, T. 2001. Orthodontic materials Scientific and clinical aspects. Stuttgart: Thieme, pp. 116–117.

Buonocore, M. G. 1955. A simple method of increasing the adhesion of acrylic filling materials to enamel surfaces. J. Dent. Res. 34:849–853.

Burstone, C. J., and Goldberg, A. J. 1980. Beta titanium: a new orthodontic alloy. Am. J. Orthod. 77:121–132.

Donly, K. J., Istre, S., and Istre, T. 1995. In vitro enamel remineralization at orthodontic band margins cemented with glass ionomer cement. Am. J. Orthod. Dentofac. Orthop. 107:461–464.

Case, C. S. 1921. Technics and principles of dental orthopedia and prosthetic correction of cleft palate. Chicago: C. S. Case Company.

Guymon, R. J. 2010. "Passive eruption patterns in central incisors." M.S. thesis, University of Iowa, pp. 8–9.

Hawley, C. A. 1905. Determination of the normal arch and its application to orthodontia. Dent. Cosmos. 47:541–552.

Millett, D. T., and Gordon, P. H. 1992. The performance of first molar orthodontic bands cemented with glass ionomer cement-a retrospective analysis. Br. J. Orthod. 19:215–220.

Newman, G. V. 1964. Bonding plastic orthodontic attachments to tooth enamel. NJ Dental Soc. J. 35:346–58.

Norris, D. S., McInnes-Ledoux, P., Schwaninger, B., and Weinberg, R. 1986. Retention of orthodontic bands with new fluoride-releasing cements. Am. J. Orthod. 89:206–211.

Phillips, R. W., Swartz, M. L., Lund, M. S., Moore, B. K., and Vickery, J. 1987. In vivo disintegration of luting cements. J. Am. Dent. Assoc. 114:489–492.

Powers, J. M., and Messersmith, M. L. 2001. Enamel etching and bond strength. In Orthodontic Materials, Scientific and Clinical Aspects. Brantley, W. A. and Eliades, T. eds. Stuttgart: Thieme.

Tweed, C. H. 1966. Clinical orthodontics, Vol. 1. St. Louis: The C. V. Mosby Company, pp. 102–116.

White, L. W. 1999. A new and improved indirect bonding technique. J. Clin. Orthod. 33:17–23.

Retention Appliances

14

Introduction

This chapter presents basic concepts and procedures essential to the making of retainers delivered at the end of active orthodontic treatment. Clinicians who ask a laboratory service to make an effective retainer must know how to properly design it and be able to judge the quality of the product, fit it into the mouth, and adjust it.

The purpose of retainers is to hold the teeth in their new positions until the soft and bony tissues have stabilized. After full edgewise appliance treatment, retainers are usually worn full-time for 6 months and at nights for an indefinite period of time. In mixed-dentition patients, retainers are worn for 1 year or until the beginning of the permanent dentition. The lower lingual and palatal holding arches are worn until the permanent canines and premolars have erupted.

Fixed Retainers and Tooth Positioners

Fixed retainers will be discussed in this chapter only in this brief introduction. Fixed bonded lingual retainers between upper central incisors

Essentials of Orthodontics: Diagnosis and Treatment
by Robert N. Staley and Neil T. Reske
© 2011 Blackwell Publishing Ltd.

(1 × 1) prevent the reopening of a diastema in the maxillary arch. Upper lingual fixed retainers require adequate overjet and smaller than normal overbite for successful placement. The patient must not bite on hard food with the anterior teeth because this can dislodge the retainer. Fixed bonded lingual retainers between the lower canines (3 × 3) help maintain intercanine width and canine positions and support alignment of the lower incisors. These fixed retainers have a limited life, usually about 10 years.

These fixed retainers collect food debris and make using floss between the teeth a chore. The lower fixed retainer will collect dental calculus, requiring periodic cleaning by a dental hygienist. The fixed retainers may come loose. In some situations, the retainer can be carefully rebonded to the tooth or teeth. In many cases, the best choice is to remove the remaining bonds and replace the fixed retainer with a Hawley or other removable retainer. Figure 14.1 shows a prescription for maxillary and mandibular fixed retainers. Figures 14.2 through 14.6 show different sizes and shapes of fixed bonded retainers.

Tooth positioners are used by orthodontists to improve the fit and occlusion of the teeth immediately after removal of the fixed appliance (Kesling 1946). The patient is usually asked to wear the tooth positioner for as many hours a day as possible for about 1 month. The teeth are

College of Dentistry
The University of Iowa
Department of Orthodontics

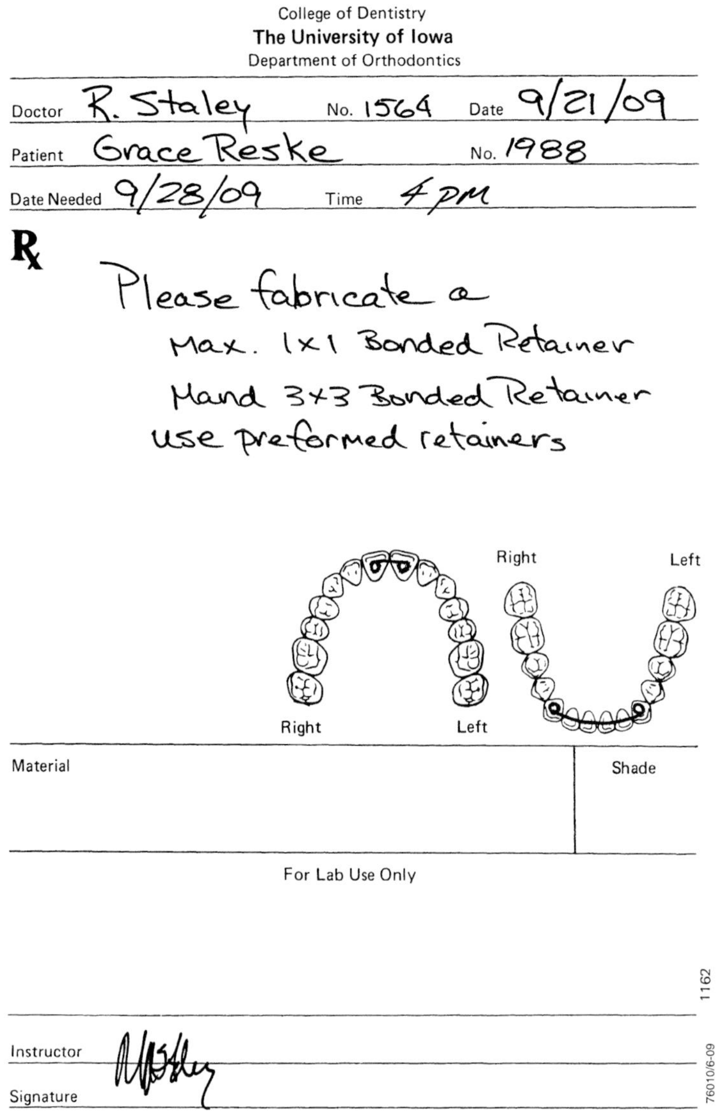

Doctor R. Staley No. 1564 Date 9/21/09

Patient Grace Reske No. 1988

Date Needed 9/28/09 Time 4pm

℞

Please fabricate a
Max. 1x1 Bonded Retainer
Mand 3x3 Bonded Retainer
use preformed retainers

Right
Left
Right
Left

Material

Shade

For Lab Use Only

1162

Instructor Signature

76010/6-09

Figure 14.1. Bonded retainers prescription.

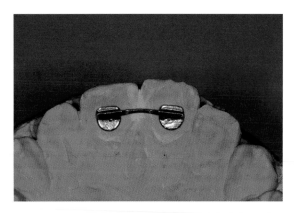

Figure 14.2. Bonded maxillary 1 × 1 retainer.

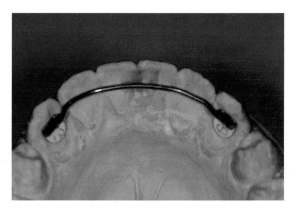

Figure 14.3. Bonded mandibular 3 × 3 retainer.

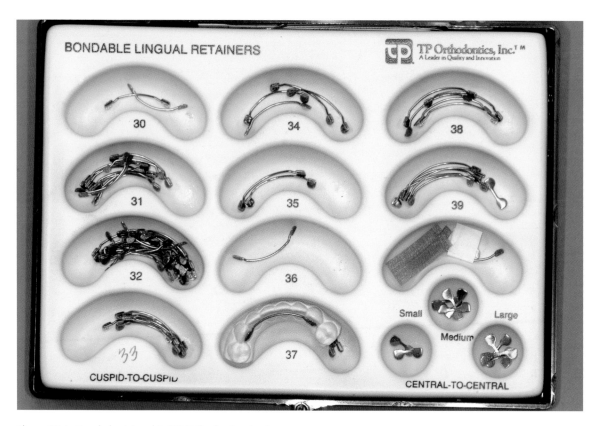

Figure 14.4. Bonded retainer kit (TP Orthodontics, Inc.).

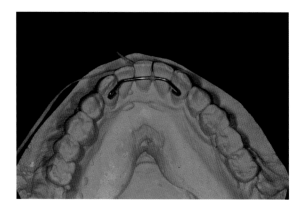

Figure 14.5. Bonded 0.030-inch round, stainless steel wire, canine to canine.

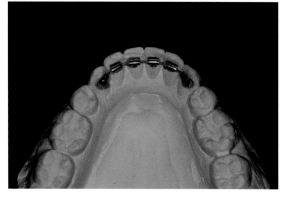

Figure 14.6. Bonded Krause bonded 3 × 3 retainer.

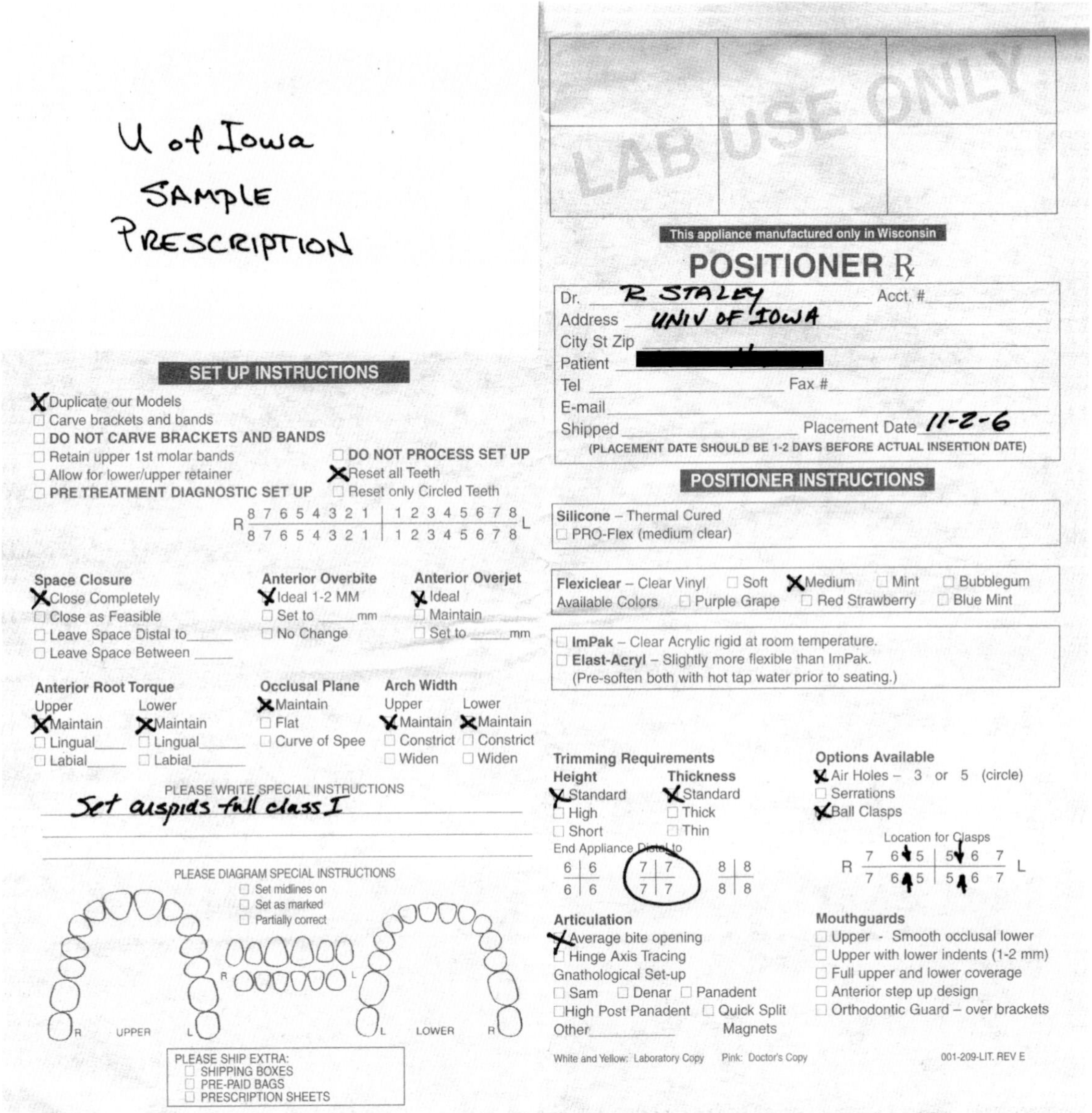

U of Iowa
SAMPLE
PRESCRIPTION

SET UP INSTRUCTIONS

☒ Duplicate our Models
☐ Carve brackets and bands
☐ **DO NOT CARVE BRACKETS AND BANDS**
☐ Retain upper 1st molar bands   ☐ **DO NOT PROCESS SET UP**
☐ Allow for lower/upper retainer   ☒ Reset all Teeth
☐ **PRE TREATMENT DIAGNOSTIC SET UP**   ☐ Reset only Circled Teeth

R
8 7 6 5 4 3 2 1 | 1 2 3 4 5 6 7 8
8 7 6 5 4 3 2 1 | 1 2 3 4 5 6 7 8
L

Space Closure
☒ Close Completely
☐ Close as Feasible
☐ Leave Space Distal to_____
☐ Leave Space Between _____

Anterior Overbite
☒ Ideal 1-2 MM
☐ Set to _____mm
☐ No Change

Anterior Overjet
☒ Ideal
☐ Maintain
☐ Set to _____mm

Anterior Root Torque
Upper   Lower
☒ Maintain   ☒ Maintain
☐ Lingual____ ☐ Lingual____
☐ Labial____   ☐ Labial____

Occlusal Plane
☒ Maintain
☐ Flat
☐ Curve of Spee

Arch Width
Upper   Lower
☒ Maintain   ☒ Maintain
☐ Constrict   ☐ Constrict
☐ Widen   ☐ Widen

PLEASE WRITE SPECIAL INSTRUCTIONS
Set cuspids full class I

PLEASE DIAGRAM SPECIAL INSTRUCTIONS
☐ Set midlines on
☐ Set as marked
☐ Partially correct

R   UPPER   L   L   LOWER   R

PLEASE SHIP EXTRA:
☐ SHIPPING BOXES
☐ PRE-PAID BAGS
☐ PRESCRIPTION SHEETS

This appliance manufactured only in Wisconsin

POSITIONER R

Dr. *R STALEY*   Acct. #_____
Address *UNIV OF IOWA*
City St Zip _____
Patient _____
Tel _____ Fax # _____
E-mail _____
Shipped _____ Placement Date *11-2-6*
(PLACEMENT DATE SHOULD BE 1-2 DAYS BEFORE ACTUAL INSERTION DATE)

POSITIONER INSTRUCTIONS

Silicone – Thermal Cured
☐ PRO-Flex (medium clear)

Flexiclear – Clear Vinyl ☐ Soft ☒ Medium ☐ Mint ☐ Bubblegum
Available Colors ☐ Purple Grape ☐ Red Strawberry ☐ Blue Mint

☐ ImPak – Clear Acrylic rigid at room temperature.
☐ Elast-Acryl – Slightly more flexible than ImPak.
(Pre-soften both with hot tap water prior to seating.)

Trimming Requirements
Height
☒ Standard
☐ High
☐ Short
End Appliance Distal to

6 | 6   7 | 7   8 | 8
6 | 6   7 | 7   8 | 8

Thickness
☒ Standard
☐ Thick
☐ Thin

Articulation
☒ Average bite opening
☐ Hinge Axis Tracing
Gnathological Set-up
☐ Sam ☐ Denar ☐ Panadent
☐ High Post Panadent ☐ Quick Split
Other _____ Magnets

Options Available
☒ Air Holes – 3 or 5 (circle)
☐ Serrations
☒ Ball Clasps

Location for Clasps
R
7 6 5 | 5 6 7
7 6 5 | 5 6 7
L

Mouthguards
☐ Upper - Smooth occlusal lower
☐ Upper with lower indents (1-2 mm)
☐ Full upper and lower coverage
☐ Anterior step up design
☐ Orthodontic Guard – over brackets

White and Yellow: Laboratory Copy   Pink: Doctor's Copy   001-209-LIT. REV E

Figure 14.7. Prescription for a tooth positioner.

somewhat mobile after the fixed appliance is removed and remain so for a few weeks. It is during this time that a cooperative patient can improve the occlusion of the teeth by wearing a tooth positioner. After wearing the tooth positioner, Hawley retainers are made for mainte-

nance of the occlusion. Figure 14.7 is a prescription form for requesting a laboratory to make a tooth positioner. Figures 14.8 through 14.10 are views of the tooth positioner and the casts with the teeth set in ideal occlusion used to make the tooth positioner.

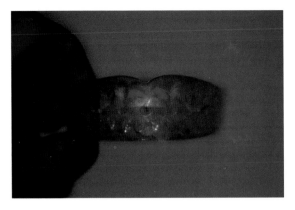

Figure 14.8. Clear tooth positioner, with air holes.

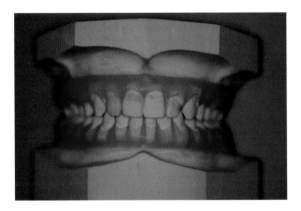

Figure 14.9. Tooth positioner cast setup.

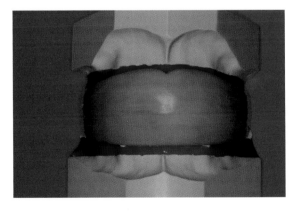

Figure 14.10. White rubber tooth positioner on casts.

Invisible Retainers

Invisible thermoplastic retainers have been in use since the 1970s and are made with clear thermo formed materials that range from 0.5-mm (0.020-inch) to 1.5-mm (0.060-inch) thickness. They should be formed and trimmed so that they maintain arch width and tooth rotations, are strong and not brittle, and are comfortable for the patient to wear 24 hours per day.

The invisible retainer has become more a part of permanent retention because of low cost, ease of fabrication, and high degree of stabilization of the dentition. However, for long-term use, wear and breakage are disadvantages compared to the Hawley retainer designs.

A laboratory prescription is shown for invisible retainer fabrication (Fig. 14.11). The fabrication of maxillary and mandibular invisible retainers is shown in Figures 14.12 through 14.35. Working casts are prepared for construction of the removable appliances by carefully removing positive defects and filling negative defects with stone or light curing resin. In the mandibular arch, remove the tongue to expose the lingual areas and allow access to create a lingual flange in the appliance. Also look for undesirable undercuts around all teeth and block-out as necessary, especially with patients with periodontal problems or missing teeth.

Since we attempt to use the same casts for the Hawley retainer construction, we prefer to have strong casts with flat, solid bases that are approximately 12 mm thick at the thinnest point. Apply silicone spray or liquid separating foil to the casts. Position the cast on the Biostar in the lead pellets cup so that the area 5 mm below the gingival margin of the cast is at the same height as the cup rim. Adapt the pellets from the cast to the cup's rim.

We prefer a full palatal coverage for invisible retainers, especially when maxillary expansion was part of the orthodontic treatment. Place a sheet of 0.75-mm (0.30-inch) clear retainer material on the chamber and secure it with the frame clamp. Heat the material according to the manufacturers directions for heating and cooling

College of Dentistry
The University of Iowa
Department of Orthodontics

Doctor N. Smith No. 1492 Date 5-14-08

Patient Sam Balogna No. 560

Date Needed 5-14-08 Time 4:30 pm

℞

Please fabricate maxillary and Mandibular invisible retainers with 3/4 mm clear thermoplastic. cut as per design. Delivery this afternoon please.

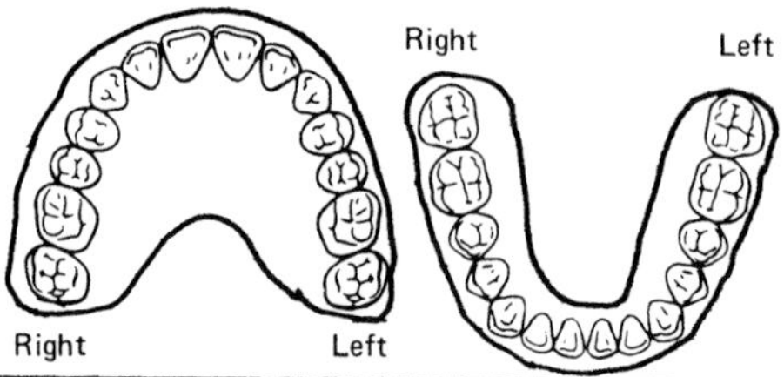
Right
Left
Right
Left

Material

Shade

For Lab Use Only

1162

Instructor

Signature

76010/6-09

Figure 14.11. Prescription for invisible retainers.

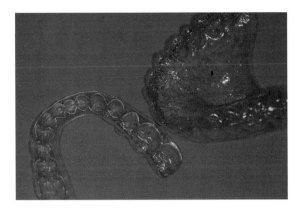

Figure 14.12. Invisible retainers, set.

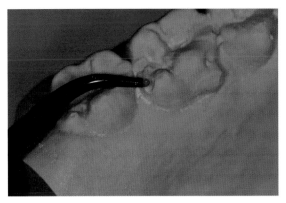

Figure 14.14. Fill voids with light-cure resin or stone.

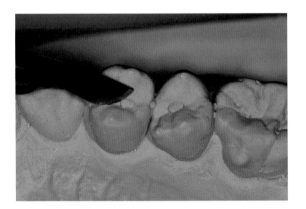

Figure 14.13. Remove positive bubbles.

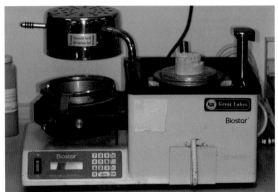

Figure 14.15. Biostar thermo forming machine.

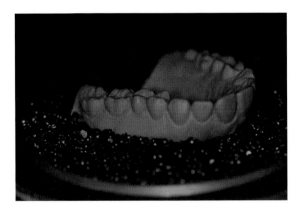

Figure 14.16. Maxillary cast set in lead pellets, with 5 mm between gingival margins and lead pellets.

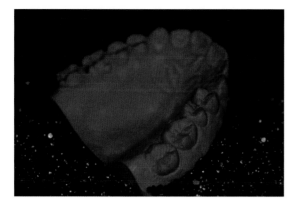

Figure 14.17. Maxillary cast in position; separator has been applied.

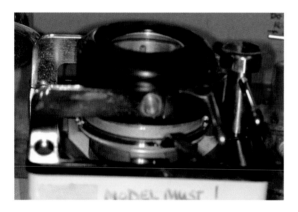

Figure 14.18. Biostar chamber closed with air pressure applied for 2 minutes.

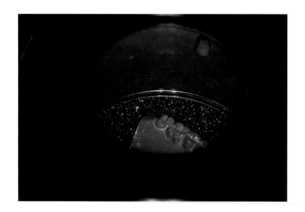

Figure 14.19. View inside chamber.

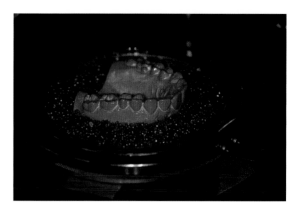

Figure 14.20. The ¾-inch or 1-mm material has been formed for invisible retainer.

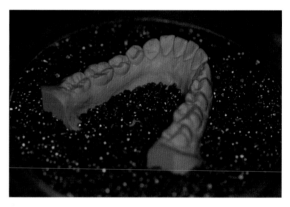

Figure 14.21. Mandibular cast positioned with lingual length of 6 mm accounted for.

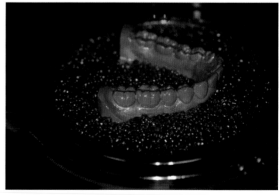

Figure 14.22. Material formed for mandibular invisible retainer.

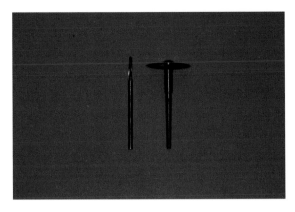

Figure 14.23. Carbide bur and safe-side disc used for removal of retainers from casts.

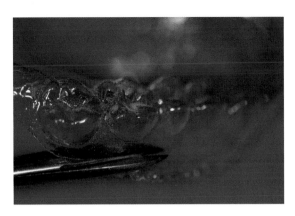

Figure 14.26. Trim to desired length with crown shears.

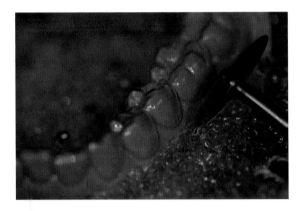

Figure 14.24. Safe-side disc used to rough cut retainer.

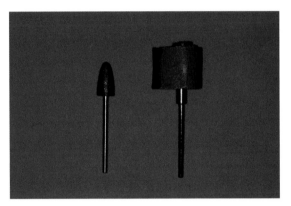

Figure 14.27. Ruby carver stone and sandpaper mandrel with 150 grit sandpaper.

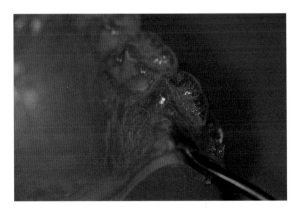

Figure 14.25. Carefully pry retainer from cast with a wax spatula.

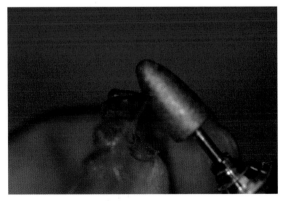

Figure 14.28. Ruby carver smoothing and trimming to length.

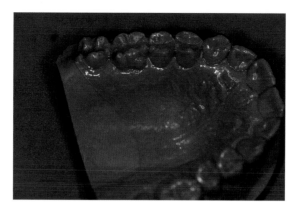

Figure 14.29. Maxillary invisible retainer with full palatal coverage.

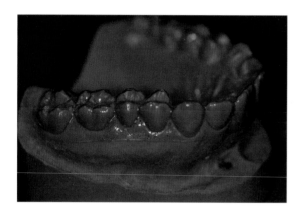

Figure 14.30. Facial length trimmed just below gingival margins.

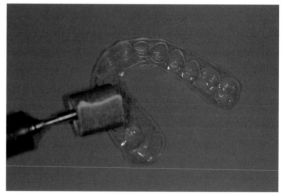

Figure 14.32. Smooth edges of both retainers with sandpaper.

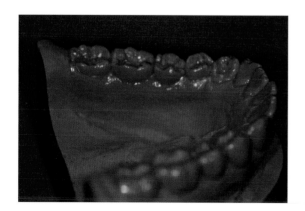

Figure 14.31. Mandibular posterior lingual length trimmed 5 to 6 mm below gingival margins.

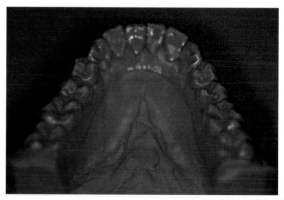

Figure 14.33. Mandibular anterior lingual 3 mm below gingival margins.

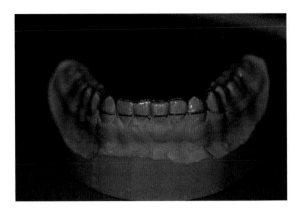

Figure 14.34. If undesirable undercuts exist, shorten facial to middle of teeth.

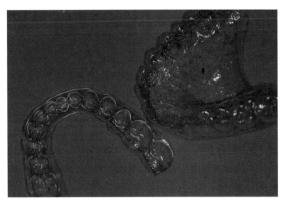

Figure 14.35. Finished set of invisible retainers.

times. After forming the material, cool for 2 minutes under pressure to avoid backpressure distortion. Remove the maxillary cast with the material still in place. Set aside. Now place the mandibular cast into the pellets, again so that the area 5 mm below the gingival margin is at the same height as the cup rim. Place pellets in the lingual area only to a height that will leave 6 to 8 mm below the gingival margin exposed. Adapt pellets to the cup's rim. Form the material for the mandibular cast. Cool for 2 minutes, and remove the cast and appliance from the machine.

Cut out the material from the casts by using a safe-side lightning disk for thin materials or a carbide bur for thicker materials. Cut across the back of the casts and around the facial surface just above the line where the lead pellets meet the cast, approximately 4 mm from the facial gingival margins. Remove the material from the casts carefully by prying with a wax spatula at the most distal points and in the anterior vestibule to avoid cast breakage. Thin materials may be trimmed with a pair of crown shears. Thicker materials must be trimmed with heavy plate shears or a carbide cutting bur. Reduce the material facially to 2 mm below the gingival margin and form a horseshoe shape in the palate distal

to the first molars terminating at the distal embrasure of the last tooth on both sides of the arch on a full coverage appliance. If palatal coverage is not desired, cut the palate of the invisible retainer 6 to 8 mm below the lingual gingival margin. Smooth the trimmed areas with a ruby carver and finish with 150 grit sandpaper on a sandpaper mandrel.

Essix Retainers

The Essix retainer (Sheridan et al. 1993) is another form of invisible retainer that covers only the anterior section of the dental arches canine to canine. This reduces the appliance bulk and allows posterior teeth to "settle" into full occlusal contact. Both maxillary and mandibular casts can be placed into the thermoplastic forming machine and formed at the same time, thus using only one sheet of 1-mm (0.040-inch) material to fabricate both appliances. Removal, trimming and smoothing are accomplished in the same manner as invisible retainers. Figure 14.36 shows a laboratory prescription for fabrication of Essix retainers. Figures 14.37 through 14.40 illustrate the laboratory fabrication steps for Essix retainers.

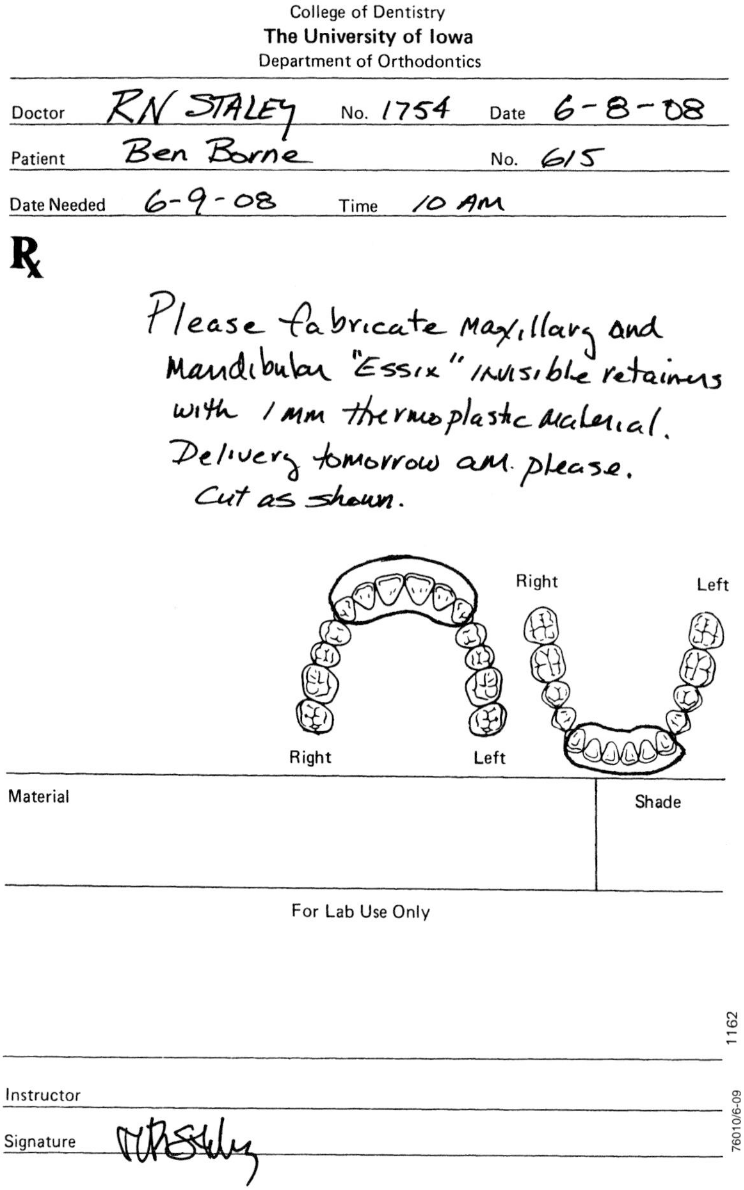
College of Dentistry
The University of Iowa
Department of Orthodontics

Doctor RN STALEY No. 1754 Date 6-8-08

Patient Ben Borne No. 615

Date Needed 6-9-08 Time 10 AM

℞

Please fabricate Maxillary and Mandibular "Essix" invisible retainers with 1 mm thermoplastic material. Delivery tomorrow am. please. Cut as shown.

Right
Left
Right
Left

Material

Shade

For Lab Use Only

1162

Instructor

Signature

76010/6-09

Figure 14.36. Prescription for an Essix retainer.

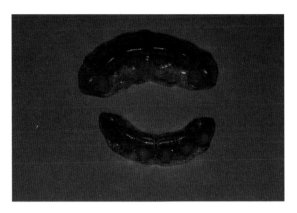

Figure 14.37. Maxillary and mandibular Essix retainers.

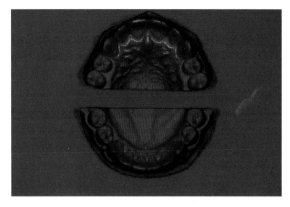

Figure 14.40. Finished Essix retainers. *Note:* Lingual length.

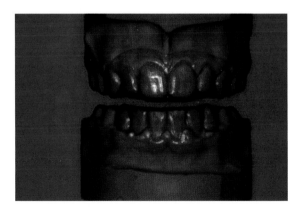

Figure 14.38. Casts ready for thermo-plastic application in Biostar.

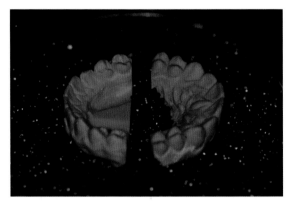

Figure 14.39. Finished Essix retainers trimmed to distal of canines.

Basic Retainer Design

The standard "Hawley retainer" is a removable appliance that was developed in the United States in the early 1900s by Dr. C. A. Hawley (1919). Dr. Hawley's design features a wire to maintain arch shape, wires for retention, and an acrylic body to hold the maxillary and mandibular teeth in place while the patient is wearing the retainer. This design also allows the patient to remove the appliance for eating and cleaning of the teeth and cleaning of the appliance.

A standard maxillary Hawley retainer consists of a labial bow that spans from the distal of one canine to the distal of the other canine and two clasps on posterior teeth on either side of the arch that are embedded into acrylic on the palatal side (Fig. 14.41). A standard mandibular Hawley retainer consists of a canine-to-canine labial bow and either two clasps or two occlusal rests on posterior teeth on either side of the arch that are embedded into a lingual body of acrylic (Fig. 14.42).

Variations of the Hawley retainer design are modifications to the original design usually requiring that the labial bow be extended and soldered to the clasps (Fig. 14.43). Another modification to the Hawley design is one creating a wraparound design, without clasping, that has

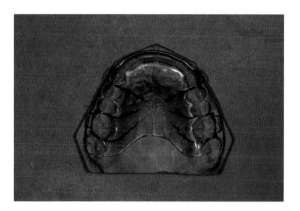

Figure 14.41. Standard maxillary Hawley retainer.

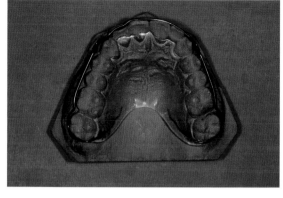

Figure 14.44. Modified Hawley wraparound retainer.

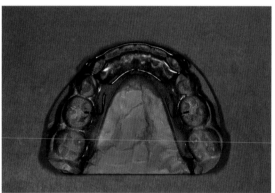

Figure 14.42. Standard mandibular Hawley retainer.

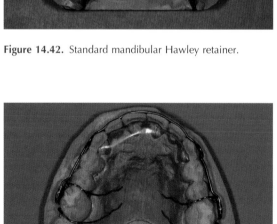

Figure 14.43. Modified Hawley labial bow soldered to Adams clasps.

the labial bow extending to the most distal posterior teeth before crossing to the lingual side to be embedded into acrylic (Fig. 14.44).

Clasping for removable Hawley appliances can be in the form of simple arrow, ball, buccal tube, or c-clasps or more complicated forms such as the Adams or ReSta clasps that aid in maintaining stability of the removable retainer and thus the stability and position of the teeth.

Wire-Bending Skills

Before the clinician/technician can start to fabricate or adjust removable retainers, some basic wire-bending skills must be learned. Wire-bending exercises are designed to teach techniques necessary to produce and make adjustments to quality orthodontic appliances. Tools used for bending and cutting wires in the laboratory consist of at least three pliers, a cutter, and a wire turret. Figure 14.45A shows bird beak pliers. Figure 14.45B shows a Hawley loop pliers. Figure 14.45C shows a three-prong pliers.

The bird beak No. 134 or 139 pliers (Fig. 14.46) are designed to make sharp, rounded bends in a wire. The pliers consist of a flat, triangular pad that opposes a conical beak. The wire is held between the beaks and finger pressure is applied to form bends around the conical

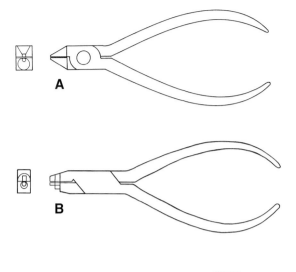

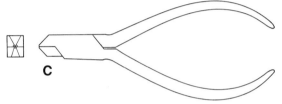

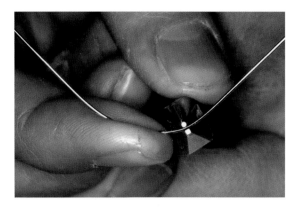

Figure 14.46. Bird beak pliers. Finger or thumb bends wire around round beak.

Figure 14.45. (A) Bird beak pliers. (B) Hawley loop pliers. (C) Three-prong pliers.

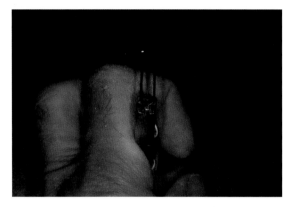

Figure 14.47. Hawley loop pliers. Finger or thumb bends wire around larger round beak for perfect adjustment loops.

beak. Sharp bends are made close to the tip of the cone, whereas rounded bends are formed toward the base of the cone. The conical beak design causes less stress on the wire compared to bending the wire over square edge pliers.

The second pliers used for rounded bends are Hawley loop bending pliers (Fig. 14.47). These pliers feature a small round tip, a step to a larger round section, and a step to a convex contouring section with square sides on one beak while the opposing beak has serrations and a small square section at the tip, a step to a larger square section, and a step to a concave section. The tip makes small helices, the middle section can make perfect adjustment loops or helices, and the third section can gently contour and form a labial bow.

The three-prong pliers (Fig. 14.48) are used with heavy 0.026- to 0.036-inch wire. Bends are

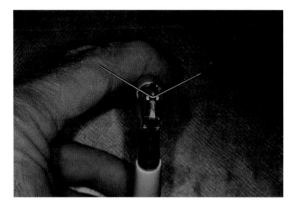

Figure 14.48. Three-prong pliers. Single beak pushes wire between the double beaks squeezing pliers.

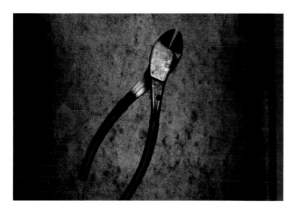

Figure 14.49. Hard wire cutter.

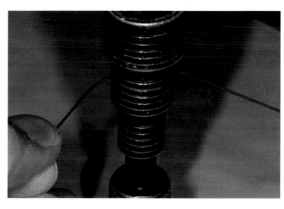

Figure 14.50. Easy parabolic wire bends made around a wire turret, which puts less stress into wire.

formed by squeezing the pliers. With the wire placed at the reference mark on the wire, the two prongs located on one side of the pliers push the wire around the opposing side single prong, creating a "V" bend. Three common uses of the three-prong pliers are to adapt the arch wire to tooth anatomy, to bend acrylic retaining zigzags, and to make wire adjustments. For bends greater than 45 degrees, do not use three-prong pliers as gouging of the wire may occur.

Many other pliers are available that produce different sizes and shapes of bends for clinical use, but the three mentioned here will be adequate for most laboratory wire bending.

A high-quality hard diagonal wire cutter (Fig. 14.49) is essential for cutting wires from 0.012 to 0.040 inch. In the operatory, ligature tie cutters are used for 0.009- to 0.011-inch soft wire ties and end cutters are used for clipping all sizes of hard arch wire from 0.012 to 0.028 inch.

The wire turret (Fig. 14.50) may be used to bend wires with perfect parabolic shape for labial bows and lingual arches without introducing stress inducing bends or nicks from pliers.

Figure 14.51A-C show three exercises for wire bending practice. For exercise 1, use the No. 134 bird beak pliers and a 7-inch piece of 0.030-inch round, stainless steel wire on the pattern. For exercise 2, use the three-prong pliers and a 7-inch piece of 0.030-inch round, stainless steel wire on the pattern. For exercise 3, use the No. 134 bird beak and/or the Hawley loop bending pliers and a 7-inch piece of 0.026-inch round, stainless steel wire on the pattern.

After you have successfully formed each of the exercise patterns and become comfortable with the pliers, you are ready to adapt labial bows, clasps and springs for retainer fabrication.

Maxillary Labial Bow Bending

The Hawley labial bow is a basic retainer design that can be used if no occlusal interferences exist at the distal occlusal margin of the canines. The labial bow aids in appliance retention and maintains the alignment of anterior teeth during this final phase of treatment. Many general dentists' request that the labial bow be formed into an average arch form. If done so, the bow will not always touch all the anterior teeth in a manner that would be necessary to maintain the tooth positions.

The orthodontist has carefully achieved ideal tooth positions with the fixed appliance and desires retainers that will maintain those positions. The use of tooth positioners to improve final positioning and invisible retainers to hold exact position suggests that the labial bow must

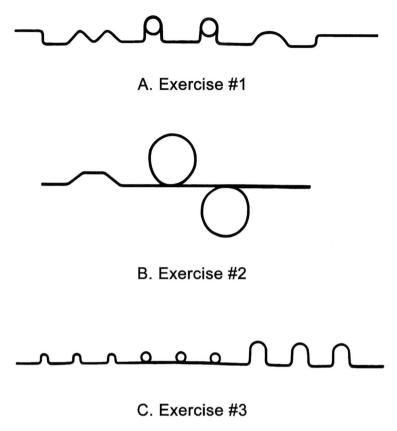

A. Exercise #1

B. Exercise #2

C. Exercise #3

Figure 14.51. (**A**) Exercise No. 1: Bend a 7-inch length of 0.030-inch round wire with bird beak pliers to match form. (**B**) Exercise No. 2: Bend a 7-inch length of 0.030-inch round wire with three-prong pliers to match form. (**C**) Exercise No. 3: Bend a 7-inch length of 0.026-inch round wire with bird beak and/or Hawley loop pliers to match form.

contact all of the anterior teeth intimately to prevent undesirable rotation recurrence.

Newcomers are advised to draw the desired position of the wire on the cast prior to bending. A 7-inch length of 0.030-inch round stainless steel wire is formed around a wire turret to produce a perfect parabolic curve relative to the patient's anterior tooth alignment. Place the wire on the cast and mark the midline on the wire with a permanent marker (fine point Sharpie). The wire should approximate the arch shape from canine to canine. Open or close the parabolic curve to match the arch shape. Carefully bend to maximum contact from mesial line angle to distal line angle on the centrals and laterals,

and from the mesial line angle to the center of the canines in order to maintain the exact positions of these teeth. Remember to always check bends by positioning the wire center mark in exactly the same place at the midline between the centrals. Also lay the wire flat on the tabletop to ensure you are bending each bend on the same horizontal plane. At the distal line angle of the center mark, bend the wire toward the mesial line angle of the lateral. Check the bend and increase or offset if desired. Then bend the wire to fit the lateral from mesial line angle to distal line angle. Check bends making sure wire maintains contact with both the central and lateral before proceeding. Next mark the wire at the distal line angle

College of Dentistry
The University of Iowa
Department of Orthodontics

Doctor *R. Greaves* No. *1004* Date *8-3-08*

Patient *Van Morgani* No. *290*

Date Needed *8-10-08* Time *11 AM*

Rx

Please fabricate a maxillary Hawley retainer with .030 rd labial bow and .026 adams clasps on 1st molars.
Clear acrylic please.

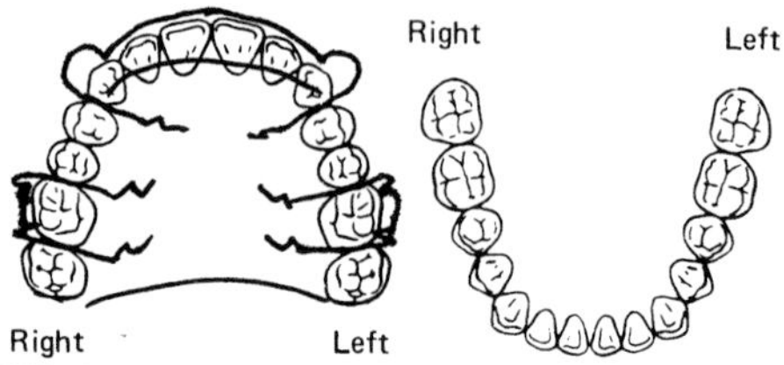

Material

Shade

For Lab Use Only

Instructor

Signature *R Greaves*

1162

76010/6-09

Figure 14.52. Prescription for a maxillary Hawley retainer with Adams clasps.

of the lateral and mark between the lateral and canine. Bend the wire toward the mesial line angle of the canine and bend a canine offset to achieve wire contact from the mesial line angle of the canine to the middle of the canine. Check bends again. The central, lateral, and canine should all have contacts and the wire should also lay flat on the tabletop. Now work from the midline to the opposite canine in the same manner. When completed, the wire should remain in intimate contact with the centrals, laterals, and the mesial half of the canines.

Do not proceed until you have passive contact with all six anterior teeth. Upon completion of the labial bow bending from canine to canine, the wire *must* be passive, lie on the drawn horizontal plane, and contact each central, lateral, and canine properly to maintain the ideally positioned teeth in their finished position.

Once satisfied, continue by marking the wire 1 mm mesial to the midpoint of the canine and make a 90-degree bend toward the gingiva and slightly out away from the tissue. Adjustment loops of 5 to 7 mm in width and length are located near the midpoints of the canines and terminate in the acrylic in the palate mesial to the first premolars. Use bird beak pliers or Hawley loop bending pliers to bend perfectly shaped adjustment loops in your labial bow wire. Adjust the loop so the loop is parallel to, but not touching, the tissue. Angle the distal side of the loop toward the occlusal embrasure and between the canine and first premolar. Bend the wire tightly through occlusal embrasure and downward toward the palatal tissue.

All wires crossing occlusal embrasures into lingual acrylic must be closely adapted to eliminate possible interference with opposing teeth. Maintain 0.5-mm space between the wire and the palatal tissue and make retention bends at the end of the wire. The wire should be 10 to 15 mm long from the point at which it crosses the occlusal embrasure to the end. Check the wire again to ensure each tooth is still in contact and the wire is on the drawn horizontal plane. If it is not ideal, adjust it until it is. Then proceed to bend the opposite adjustment loop. Mark the wire 1 mm mesial to the middle of the opposite canine and bend a 90-degree bend toward the gingival tissue. Make the adjustment loop again 5 to 7 mm wide and keep the top of the loop slightly off the tissue. Bend the distal of the loop toward the occlusal embrasure and bend it tightly through the occlusal embrasure. Bend the wire 0.5 mm above the tissue on the palatal side. Cut to 10 to 15 mm in length from the occlusal contact and make retention bends in the end of the wire.

Check the wire for fit again. The wire *must* be passive, lie on the drawn horizontal plane, and contact each central, lateral, and canine properly in order to be able to maintain the ideally positioned teeth in their finished position. Figure 14.52 shows a prescription for a maxillary Hawley retainer with labial bow and Adams clasps. Figure 14.53 shows a completed labial bow on a maxillary cast. Figures 14.54 through 14.109 illustrate the step-by-step bending of the maxillary labial bow. Figure 14.110 shows a completed maxillary Hawley retainer with labial bow and Adams clasps.

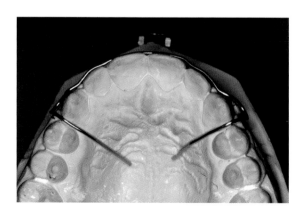

Figure 14.53. Maxillary labial bow.

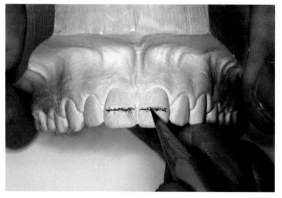

Figure 14.54. Mark the middle of centrals to position wire height on cast.

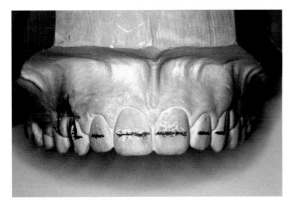

Figure 14.55. Continue line to laterals and canines on the horizontal plane.

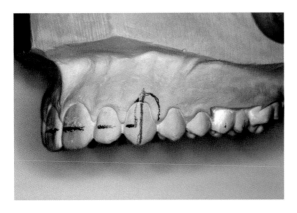

Figure 14.56. Mark long axis of canines. Draw 5- to 6-mm adjustment loops onto cast.

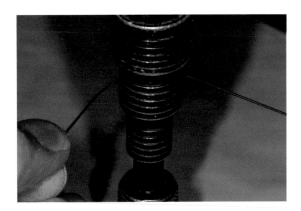

Figure 14.57. Bend a 7-inch length of 0.030-inch round wire around wire turret.

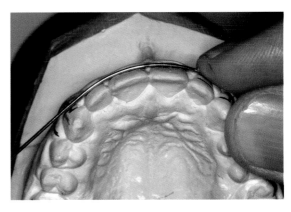

Figure 14.58. Check parabolic curve, open or close curve for shape across centrals. Mark wire at midline with a Sharpie pen for later wire checks.

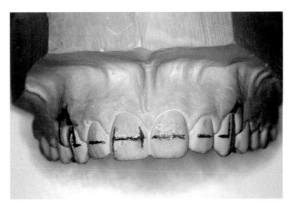

Figure 14.59. The goal is to contact each central and lateral, line angle to line angle.

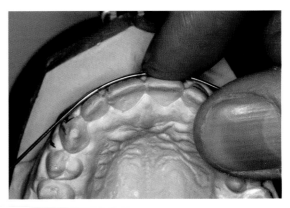

Figure 14.60. Check and mark wire for a lateral inset bend. Mark the wire directly between the central and lateral.

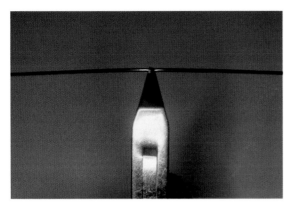

Figure 14.61. Always try to bend wire on the horizontal plane. Position wire perpendicular to the pliers.

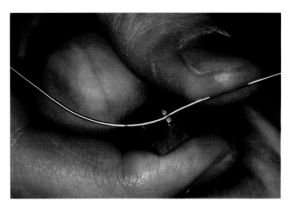

Figure 14.64. With thumb, push out on lateral side of wire.

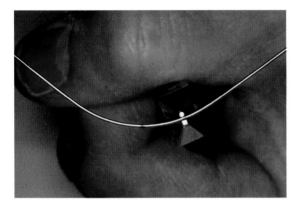

Figure 14.62. Place wire into pliers on the mark between the central and lateral.

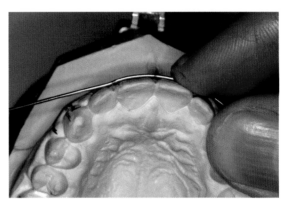

Figure 14.65. Check central and mesial contact on lateral.

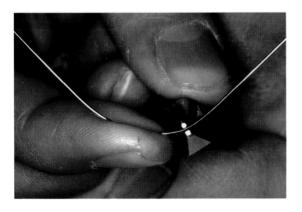

Figure 14.63. With finger, pull in on central side of wire.

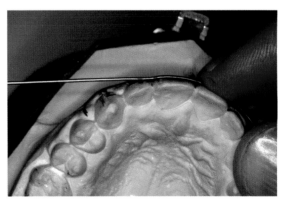

Figure 14.66. Mark last point of wire contact on lateral.

259

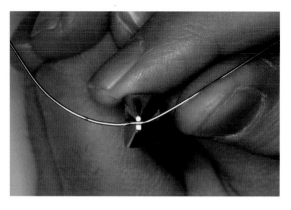

Figure 14.67. With mark just outside pliers, bend wire toward the lingual.

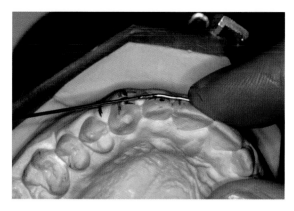

Figure 14.70. Also mark for canine offset between lateral and canine.

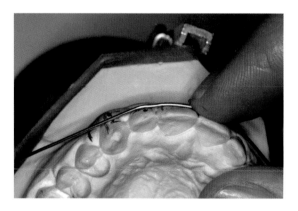

Figure 14.68. Check contacts on central and lateral.

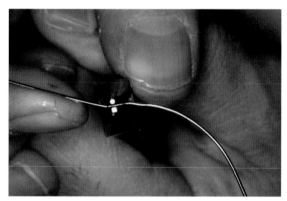

Figure 14.71. With the wire in pliers, place offset mark just outside of beak and bend wire facially.

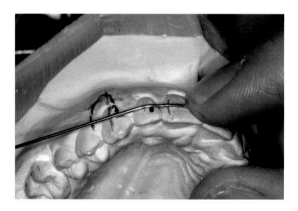

Figure 14.69. Mark last point of contact on lateral.

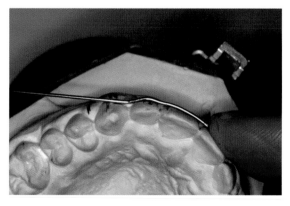

Figure 14.72. Check offset bend and wire contacts to lateral and central. Adjust where necessary.

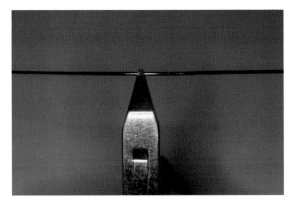

Figure 14.73. Check wire often to be sure wire is being bent parallel to horizontal plane.

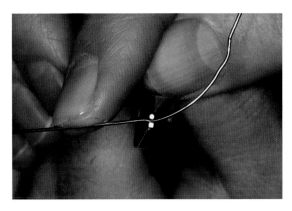

Figure 14.76. Also bend facially on lateral side of pliers.

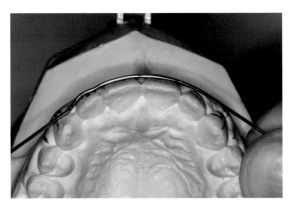

Figure 14.74. With the wire mark placed at midline check contacts on patients right central, lateral and canine, and left central. Mark between left central and lateral for the lateral inset bend.

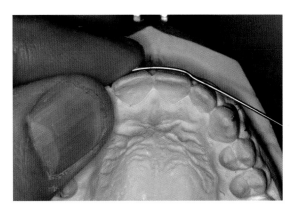

Figure 14.77. Check fit to left central and mesial of lateral. Mark last point of contact on lateral.

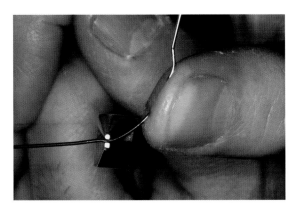

Figure 14.75. Place lateral bend mark between pliers beaks and bend wire to lingual on the central side.

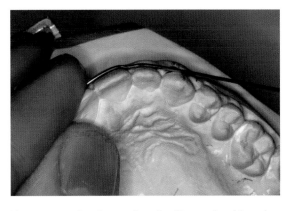

Figure 14.78. Bend around to distalline angle of lateral to make contact with canine. Mark canine offset bend between lateral and canine. Bend canine offset.

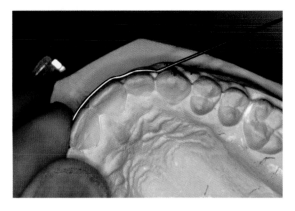

Figure 14.79. Check fit from midline to mesial of left canine.

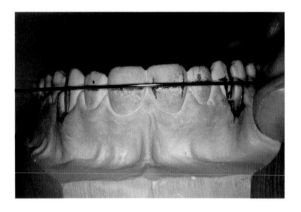

Figure 14.80. Check wire against line on casts' horizontal plane.

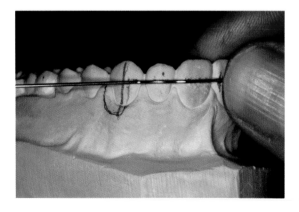

Figure 14.81. Adjustment loop 90-degree bends should be 1mm mesial to middle of canines.

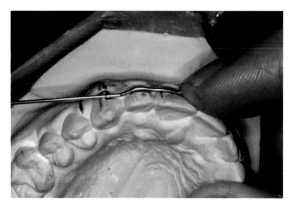

Figure 14.82. Mark wire for 90-degree adjustment loop bend.

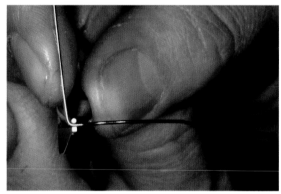

Figure 14.83. With mark just outside pliers beaks, make bend.

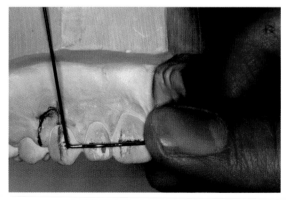

Figure 14.84. Check bend; it should be parallel to long axis of canine.

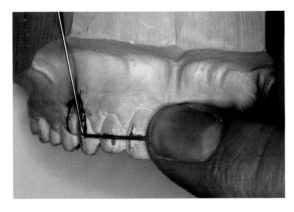

Figure 14.85. Adjustment loop bends must also slant out away from tissue contact above canine.

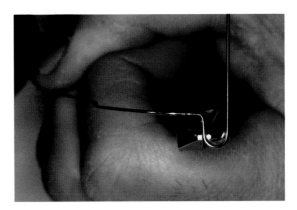

Figure 14.88. Make the adjustment loop bend.

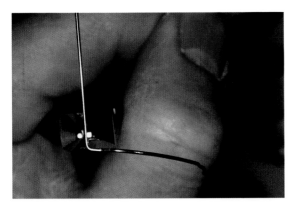

Figure 14.86. Place wire deep into pliers to bend around the middle of the conical beak to make a 5- to 7-mm adjustment loop.

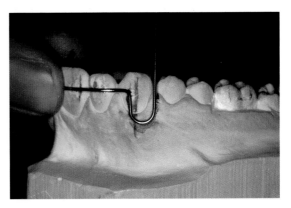

Figure 14.89. Check and adjust distal arm of loop to align with canine and premolar embrasure.

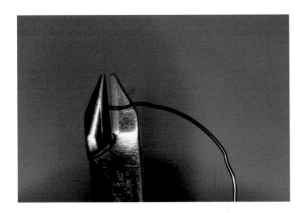

Figure 14.87. Also check the angle of adjustment loop, bend parallel to canine.

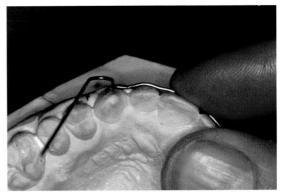

Figure 14.90. Check from occlusal; loop needs to be bent parallel to canine.

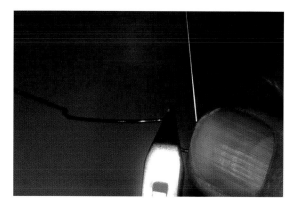

Figure 14.91. Place mesial side of adjustment loop into pliers, and with thumb, bend distal side of loop toward lingual. If wire was contacting the cast on the distal side, the bend would have to be made in the opposite direction.

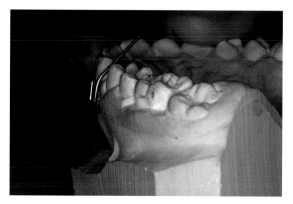

Figure 14.94. Check bend from distal buccal view.

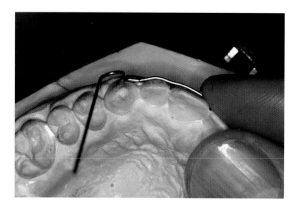

Figure 14.92. Check wire to cast again. Loop must not contact tissue and wire must still contact canine, lateral, and central.

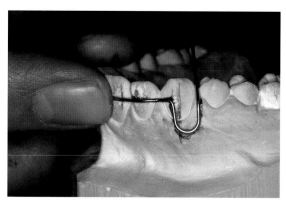

Figure 14.95. Check bend from facial view. Distal arm must align between canine and premolar.

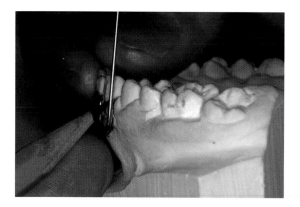

Figure 14.93. Mark where wire needs to bend toward occlusal embrasure.

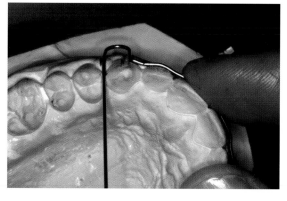

Figure 14.96. Check bend from occlusal view and mark for tight bend through the embrasure. Make a downward bend.

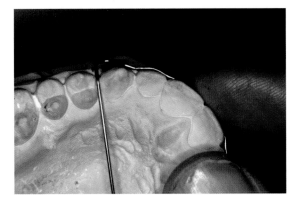

Figure 14.97. Check embrasure bend and mark wire for bend into palate. Bend wire tightly through embrasure.

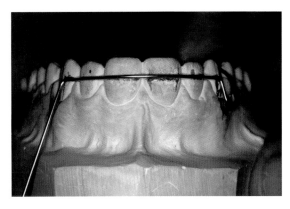

Figure 14.100. Place wire on cast, check horizontal plane, then bend the vertical 90-degree bend for the opposite adjustment loop.

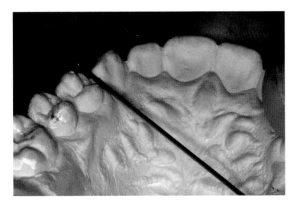

Figure 14.98. Check embrasure fit; wire needs to be 0.5 mm off tissue surface from embrasure to tip.

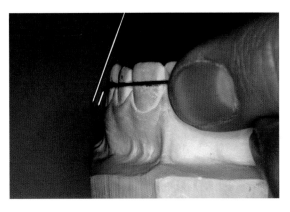

Figure 14.101. Bend adjustment loop and check against cast. If loop is too far away from tissue on the mesial, it must be bent toward the tissue to avoid lip irritation.

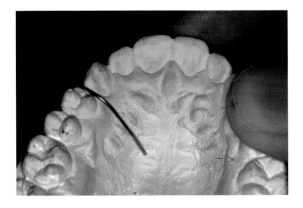

Figure 14.99. Cut wire arm 12 to 15 mm from embrasure contact.

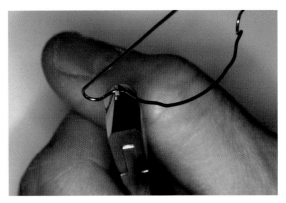

Figure 14.102. Place wire into pliers at 90-degree vertical bend.

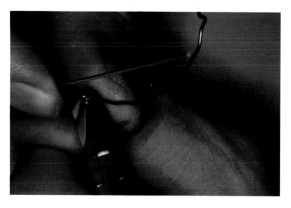

Figure 14.103. Bend tip of adjustment loop toward lingual with finger or thumb.

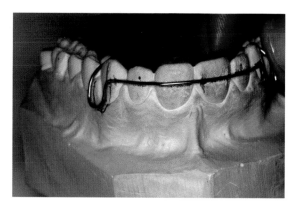

Figure 14.106. Check wire to horizontal plane line. Adjust to level if necessary.

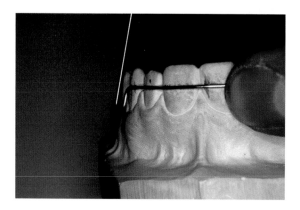

Figure 14.104. Check wire against cast. Adjustment loop must be close to but not touching gingival tissue.

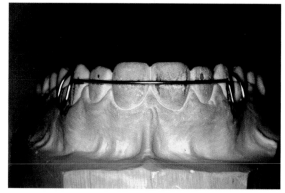

Figure 14.107. Bend wire arm down tightly through embrasure and 0.5 mm off palatal tissue. Cut to same length of opposite side arm.

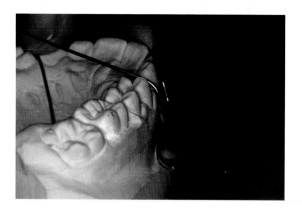

Figure 14.105. Bend distal arm of loop toward occlusal embrasure to contact between canine and premolar.

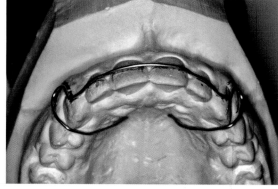

Figure 14.108. Check wire fit against all anterior teeth canine to canine.

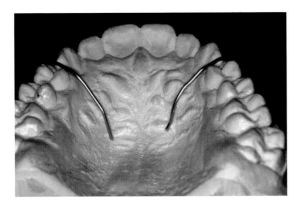

Figure 14.109. Check embrasure fit. Labial bow wire must be passive when complete.

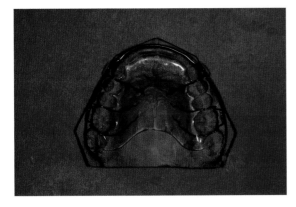

Figure 14.110. Labial bow in a completed standard maxillary Hawley retainer.

Ball Clasp

The ball clasp is commonly used on primary teeth with sufficient undercut created by two adjacent teeth. The ball clasp is a preformed stainless steel wire available in sizes 0.024 through 0.032 inch. The thinner wires are used to minimize occlusal

interference but are more easily distorted by the patient during removal and reinsertion of the appliance. The arrow clasp is similar to the ball clasp but is more often used on permanent teeth. Figure 14.111 shows a prescription for a maxillary retainer with labial bow and ball clasps. Figure 14.112 shows a completed ball clasp. Figures 14.113 through 14.124 illustrate the bending of a set of ball clasps.

On the cast, prepare the interdental papilla area by cutting 1 mm of stone from the interproximal space and simulate the margins of the two adjacent teeth. Place the desired wire ball end into the prepared space, approximately 1.5 mm below the contact of the two adjacent teeth. Mark the wire at the occlusal embrasure. Place the wire in the bird beak pliers at the ball head side of the mark and make a 100-degree bend around the tip of the conical beak of the pliers. Try the wire on the cast and mark the wire where it contacts the two teeth at the same position. Bend the wire tightly through the occlusal embrasure along the occlusal interproximal contacts. Mark and bend the wire toward the tissue surface and then upward at the lingual interdental papilla to prevent tissue contact. The wire should follow approximately 0.5 mm away from the tissue. On a maxillary cast, the wire should be about 10 to 12 mm in length from the lingual occlusal embrasure. Add acrylic retention bends at the end of the wire.

Retention bends can be loops, zigzag, or right-angle bends. The author prefers making zigzag bends with three-prong pliers in maxillary wires and right-angle bends on mandibular wires for acrylic retention. To make zigzag bends, start at the end of the wire and bend in the mesial direction. Rotate the pliers and create a second bend in a distal direction; rotate again to bend it a third time in the mesial direction. Be sure to bend in the same plane as the lateral palatal wall. To make right-angle bends on a mandibular clasp wire, always bend to the mesial if possible and leave a 5- to 6-mm length of wire mesial to the vertical section of wire. Zigzags can be made but are not necessary for mechanical retention. Figure 14.125 shows an arrow clasp.

Doctor	R. Maruosh	No. 1951	Date 10/12/06
Patient	Ivy Rose		No. 92206
Date Needed	10/28/06	Time	1:15

R

Please fabricate a Maxillary
Hawley with a labial bow
canine to canine and ball
clasps mesial to 1st molars

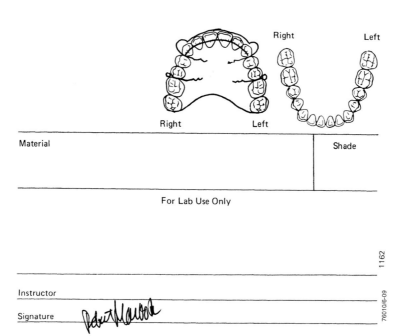

Right   Left

Right   Left

| Material | Shade |

For Lab Use Only

Instructor

Signature

1162

76010/6-09

Figure 14.111. Maxillary Hawley with ball clasps prescription.

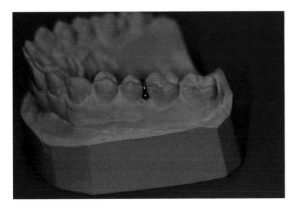

Figure 14.112. Maxillary ball clasps.

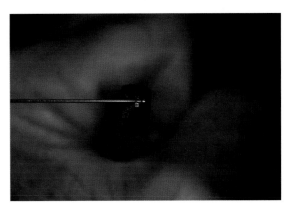

Figure 14.115. Place ball clasp into pliers with mark just outside pliers beak.

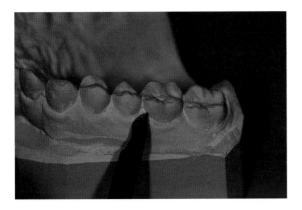

Figure 14.113. Prepare cast between teeth by removing about 1mm gingival tissue below contact.

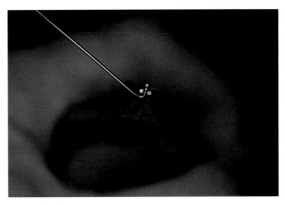

Figure 14.116. Make a 120-degree bend close to tip of bird beak pliers.

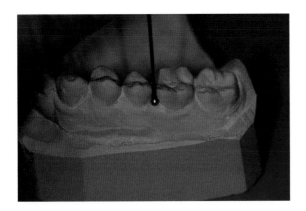

Figure 14.114. Place 0.032-inch wire ball clasp into gingival embrasure and mark the occlusal embrasure bend.

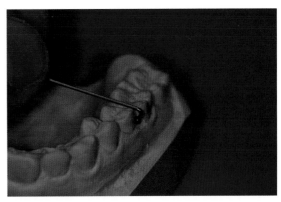

Figure 14.117. Place ball clasp into undercut. Mark point of contact on occlusal between bicuspid and molar.

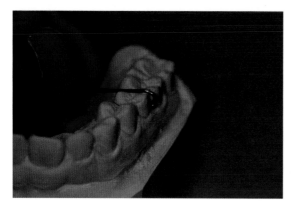

Figure 14.118. Bend wire tightly through occlusal embrasure.

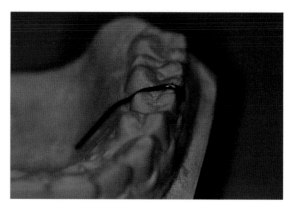

Figure 14.121. Bend wire to follow palatal tissue and 0.5 mm above tissue all the way to the tip.

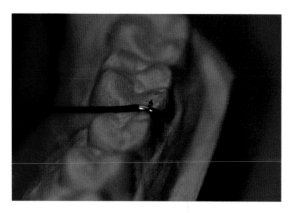

Figure 14.119. Mark ball clasp wire at lingual occlusal embrasure.

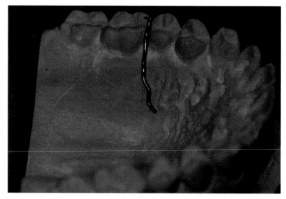

Figure 14.122. Place zigzag bends in a mesial direction for mechanical retention of the wire in the retainer acrylic.

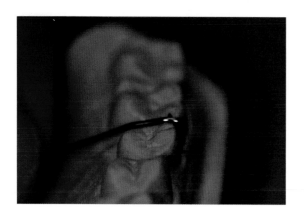

Figure 14.120. Bend wire down toward palate.

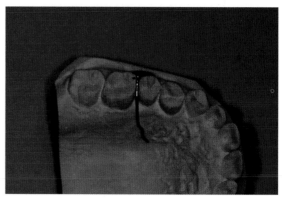

Figure 14.123. Occlusal view of a completed ball clasp.

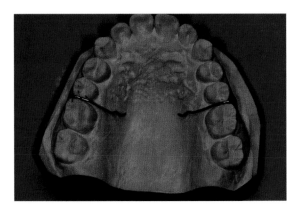

Figure 14.124. Two completed maxillary ball clasps.

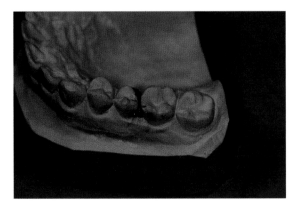

Figure 14.125. Maxillary arrow clasp. Arrow clasps are used mostly with adult patients.

C-Clasp

The circumferential clasp, or c-clasp, is used on posterior teeth and will not interfere with the occlusion when used on the most posterior teeth. It gives average retention but requires more adjustments. Begin by surveying the mesiobuccal and distobuccal undercuts on the tooth you wish to clasp. A c-clasp may be placed on a posterior tooth if the gingival tissue is just below the height of contour exposing 0.010 inch of mesiobuccal

undercut. With a 3½-inch length of 0.036-inch wire, hold the end of the wire 1.5mm from the tip of a bird beak pliers and make a small curved bend. Fit the bent tip of the wire into the mesiobuccal undercut. Mark the next bend at the last point of contact with the tooth. Make another bend at that point. Check the wire against the tooth again and then continue bending around to the distal of the tooth. After crossing the middle of the tooth, keep the wire at the height of contour of the tooth, out of the distobuccal undercut. Cross behind the distal of the tooth. On the lingual side keep the wire 0.5mm above the tissue. Direct the wire toward the mesial and cut the length about 15mm from the distolingual line angle. Make zigzag bends at the arm end for mechanical retention in the acrylic.

When a 0.032-inch round labial bow is soldered to the c clasp, the clasp is reinforced, making it less vulnerable to patient distortion.

Figure 14.126 shows a prescription for maxillary Hawley with c-clasps and anterior bite plate. Figure 14.127 shows a prescription for a maxillary labial bow soldered to c-clasps. Figure 14.128 shows a completed c-clasp. Figures 14.129 through 14.134 illustrate bending a c-clasp. Figure 14.135 shows a completed maxillary Hawley retainer with labial bow and c-clasps on second molars.

Adams Clasp

In 1949, Dr. C. P. Adams introduced the most important, best-designed clasp for orthodontic appliances (Adams 1984). Adams recommended 0.028-inch stainless wires for molars and 0.024-inch wires for canines. We recommend a slightly smaller 0.026-inch wire for the molars in the appliances described in this text. The clasp has a bridge on the buccal surface, which connects two arrowhead loops that engage undercuts on the mesiobuccal and distobuccal surfaces of the clasped tooth. Arms pass over the mesial and distal marginal ridges and down onto the lingual palate and lower flange, where they are embedded in an acrylic body.

College of Dentistry
The University of Iowa
Department of Orthodontics

Doctor T.E. South No. 71599 Date 10-12-07

Patient S.E. BLAHA No. 8355

Date Needed 10-19-07 Time 8:45am

℞

Please fabricate a maxillary Hawley with .032 rd ss labial bow and C-clasps on 1st Molars. .036 rd ss for clasps. Also anterior biteplate to separate posteriors.

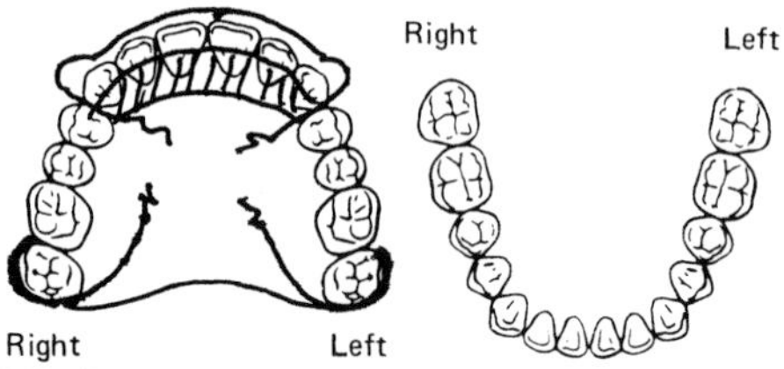
Right
Left
Right
Left

Material

Shade

For Lab Use Only

1162

Instructor Signature

76010/6-09

Figure 14.126. Prescription for a maxillary Hawley retainer with labial bow and c-clasps.

College of Dentistry
The University of Iowa
Department of Orthodontics

Doctor A. Able No. 712 Date 4-7-01

Patient KENDRA SMALL-BENN No. 80912

Date Needed 4-21-01 Time 4 pm

℞ Please fabricate a maxillary modified Hawley. .032 labial bow soldered to .036 c-clasps on 2nd molars.

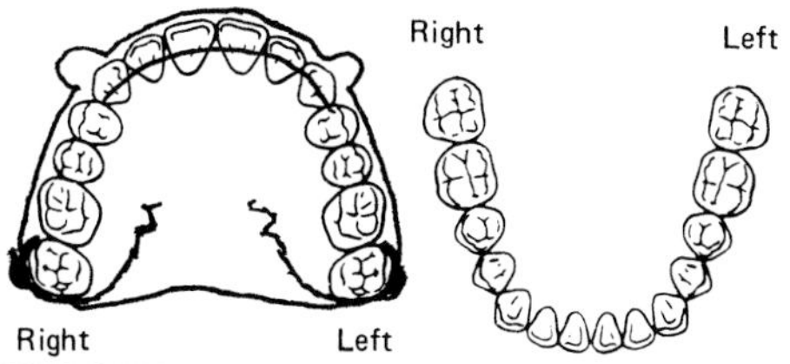

Right
Left
Right
Left

Material

Shade

For Lab Use Only

1162

Instructor

Signature

76010/6-09

Figure 14.127. Prescription for a maxillary modified Hawley with labial bow soldered to c-clasps on second molars.

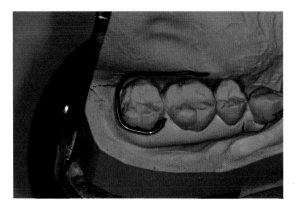

Figure 14.128. A c-clasp.

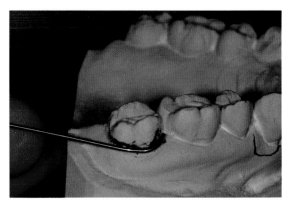

Figure 14.131. Make rounded bends to fit at height of contour from middle of tooth around to the distal.

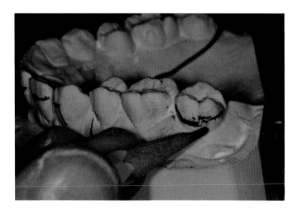

Figure 14.129. Draw a line at height of contour of molar to determine where clasp will engage undercut.

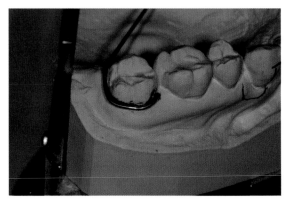

Figure 14.132. Continue to curve the wire around the distal side of tooth at the height of contour.

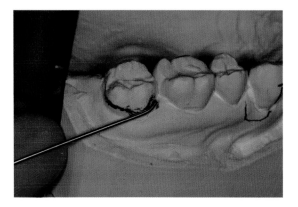

Figure 14.130. Place tip of 0.036-inch round wire into mesial undercut. Make a curved bend in end of the wire.

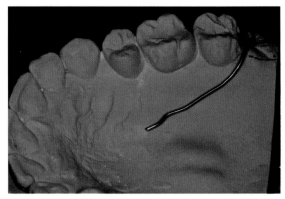

Figure 14.133. On the palatal side, curve the wire toward the anterior of palate and leave wire 0.5 mm off the tissue. Place zig-zag bends in the end and cut 12 to 15 mm in length from the distal lingual line angle.

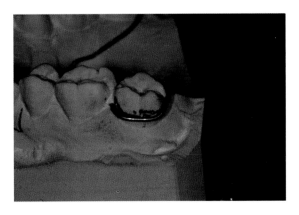

Figure 14.134. Bend a c-clasp for the opposite molar. Place the tip into the mesial undercut and remember to stay out of the distal undercut.

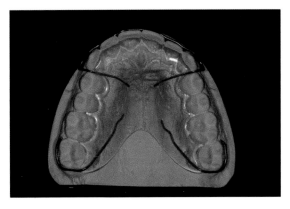

Figure 14.135. Completed standard Hawley retainer with labial bow and c-clasps on second molars.

The Adams clasp (Fig. 14.136) is a highly retentive clasp for use with maxillary and mandibular retainers, especially when springs are added to retainers to move individual teeth. Figure 14.110 shows a maxillary Hawley retainer with labial bow and Adams clasps.

Begin preparing the working cast by removing the gingival tissue between the teeth, so that you can fit the arrowheads of the clasp against the tooth, not the embrasure. Fitting them deep into the undercuts on some fully erupted teeth in adults can make placement and removal of the clasp and appliance very difficult.

Using a 3½-inch length of 0.026-inch wire, start by placing the wire near the tip of the beaks in bird beak pliers and make a 90-degree bend near the middle of the wire. Make another 90-degree bend at a point that is approximately two-thirds as long as the mesiodistal width of the tooth to be clasped. Place the beaks of the pliers 1mm away from the bridge and bend the wire in a 180-degree turn to form an arrowhead loop that is about 3mm long. Bend another arrowhead on the other side of the bridge. Next bend the arrowheads up toward the occlusal surface of the tooth and approximately 45 degrees to the bridge to fit the gingival contours of the tooth. Fit the clasp to the cast to determine whether the arrowheads fit properly against the tooth. Adjust mesial and distal angles up or down as necessary.

The next bend that takes the wire over the contact point from the arrowheads is extremely important and more difficult to make. Place the tip of the conical beak of the pliers inside the arrowhead loop. Rotate the wire so that the square beak is at the point where the straight arm begins to curve into the arrowhead loop. At this point make a bend 90 degrees from the bridge and toward the occlusal embrasure. Make the same bend on the opposite arrowhead. Place the clasp against the tooth with the bridge at a 45-degree angle above the tissue and check the last bends to see if they line up with the embrasures and contact between the adjacent teeth and the tooth being clasped. Adjust until you have arrowhead contacts and occlusal embrasure contacts. Now bend each arm tightly through the occlusal embrasures and then down toward the lingual tissue. Bend each arm so that it remains 0.5mm above the tissue while also bending in a mesial direction. For a maxillary retainer, cut wire arms 12mm from the point where they leave the occlusal embrasure. Place zigzag bends or other mechanical retention bends at the end of each arm. Adams clasps are to fit passively on the cast with the arrowheads in contact with the mesiobuccal and distobuccal undercuts and fit tightly through the embrasures.

Figure 14.137 shows a prescription for a Hawley retainer with a labial bow and Adams

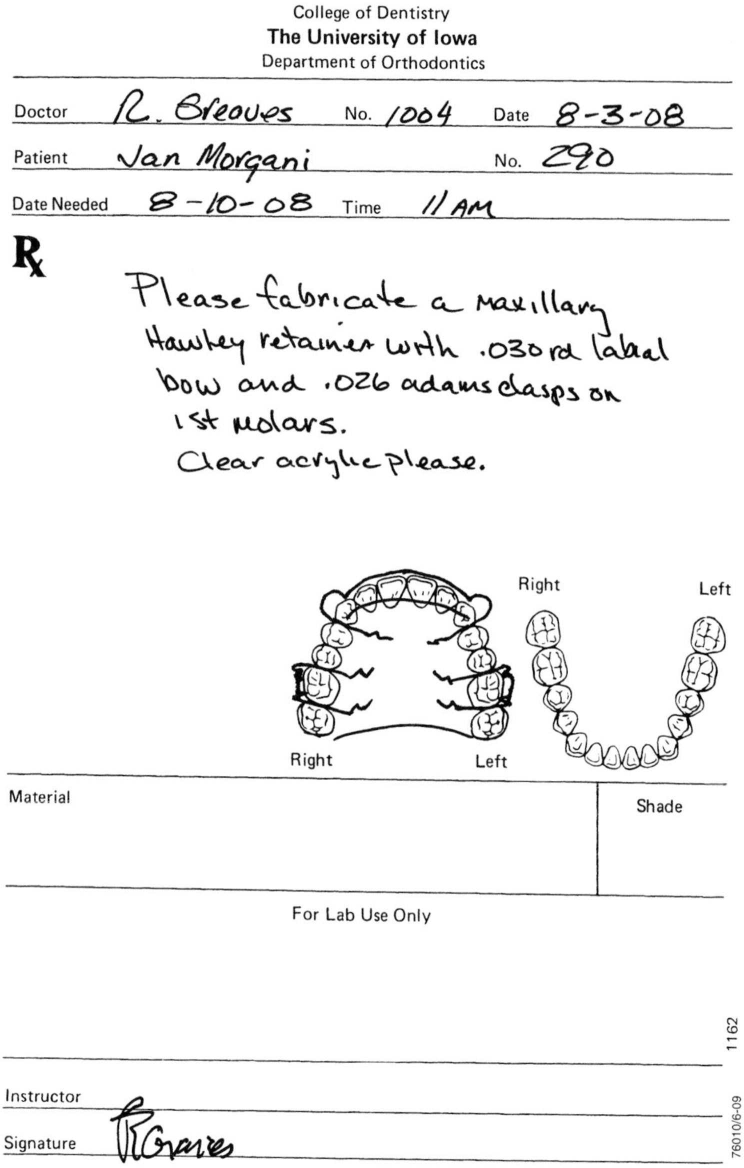

College of Dentistry
The University of Iowa
Department of Orthodontics

Doctor *R. Greoves* No. *1004* Date *8-3-08*

Patient *Van Morgani* No. *290*

Date Needed *8-10-08* Time *11 AM*

℞

*Please fabricate a maxillary
Hawley retainer with .030 rd labial
bow and .026 adams clasps on
1st molars.
Clear acrylic please.*

Right   Left

Right   Left

Material _____ Shade _____

_____

For Lab Use Only

Instructor _____

Signature *R. Greaves*

1162

76010/6-09

Figure 14.136. An Adams clasp.

clasps. Figure 14.136 shows an Adams clasps. Figure 14.138 shows the anatomy of an Adams clasp.

Figures 14.139 through 14.163 illustrate the bending of the Adams clasp. Figure 14.164 shows a completed maxillary Hawley retainer with Adams clasps on the first molars. Figure 14.165 shows a prescription for a modified Hawley retainer with a labial bow soldered to the Adams clasps. Figures 14.166 through 14.170 illustrate steps in the fabrication of a labial bow soldered to Adams clasps. Figure 14.171 shows a completed maxillary modified Hawley with the labial bow soldered to Adams clasps on the first molars.

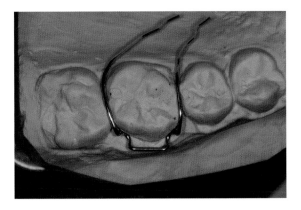

Figure 14.137. Maxillary Hawley retainer with labial bow and Adams clasps prescription.

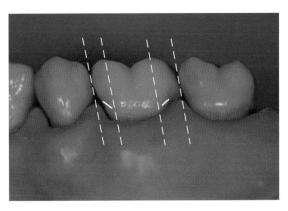

Figure 14.140. Tips of arrowheads on Adams clasp must contact tooth between cusp tips and mesial and distal surfaces of clasped tooth.

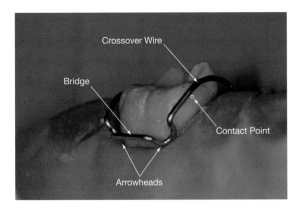

Figure 14.138. Anatomy of an Adams clasp.

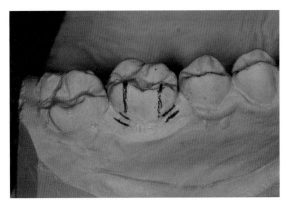

Figure 14.141. Mark width of cusp tips and then the mesial and distal undercuts.

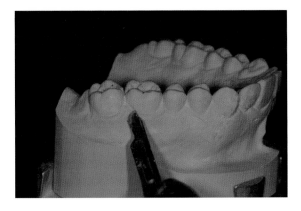

Figure 14.139. Prepare cast by removing 1 mm of gingival tissue at mesial and distal undercuts.

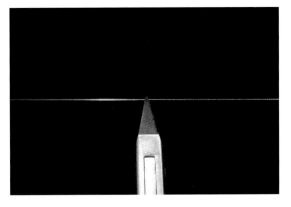

Figure 14.142. Use a 3½-inch length of 0.026-inch round wire. Hold the middle of the wire near tips of the bird beak pliers and make a 100-degree bend.

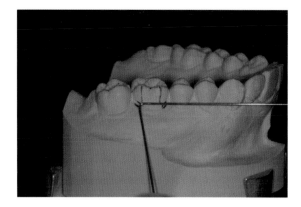

Figure 14.143. Place wire against the cast to determine Adams clasp bridge length. The bridge should be two-thirds the width of the facial surface. Mark wire for bend.

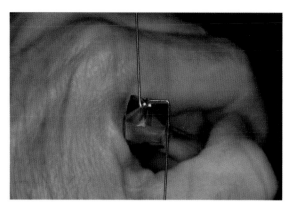

Figure 14.146. Completed 180-degree bend for arrowhead of Adams clasp.

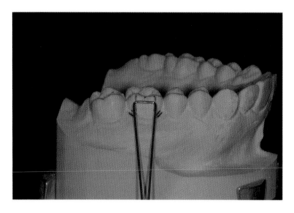

Figure 14.144. Make the second 100-degree bend to complete the bridge. Check the width of the bridge.

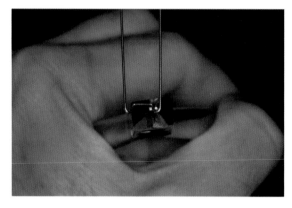

Figure 14.147. Make the same 180-degree bend on the opposite side of the Adams clasp bridge.

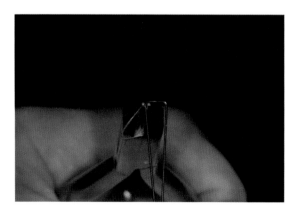

Figure 14.145. With wire close to tip of pliers and the square beak against bridge, bend wire 180 degrees around conical tip of pliers.

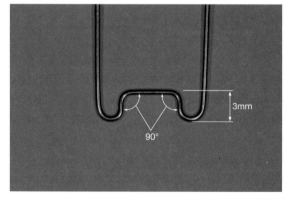

Figure 14.148. Arrowheads should be 3 mm in length from tips of arrowheads to the bridge. Maintain 90-degree bends at bridge.

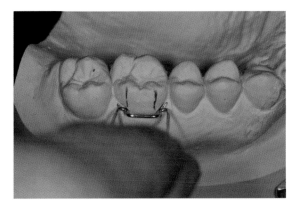

Figure 14.149. Check arrowhead tip width against tooth. Tips should contact tooth and bridge should be 1½ mm from the facial surface of the tooth.

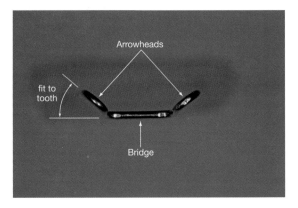

Figure 14.150. Arrowheads need to angle up toward occlusal embrasures.

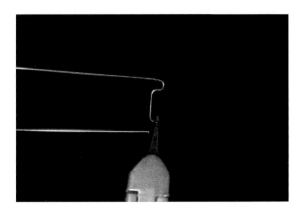

Figure 14.151. Hold across arrowhead and bend up 45 degrees.

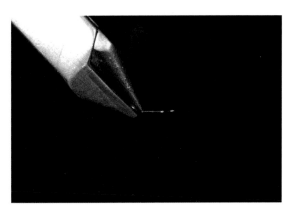

Figure 14.152. Completed 45-degree arrowhead bend. Make the same 45-degree bend on the opposite arrowhead.

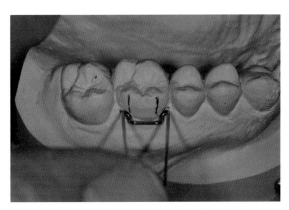

Figure 14.153. Adjust arrowheads to match undercut angles on cast.

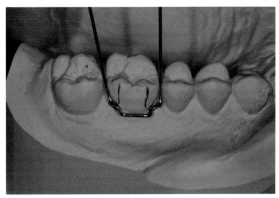

Figure 14.154. Next bends will take the wire from the arrowheads to the occlusal embrasure contacts.

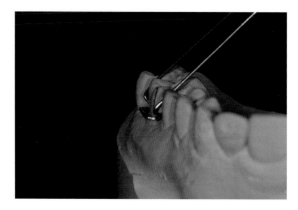

Figure 14.155. Place round beak inside arrowhead loop and bend a 90-degree bend across the square beak. Do the same on the opposite side of the clasp.

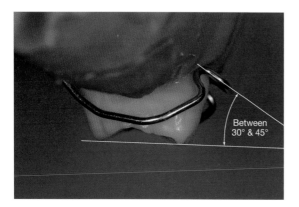

Figure 14.156. With the bridge at a 45-degree angle from the buccal surface, the mesial and distal arms need to be adjusted to touch the occlusal embrasures.

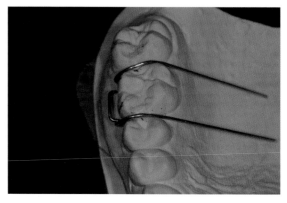

Figure 14.158. Bend the clasp crossover arms to fit tightly through the mesial and distal embrasures.

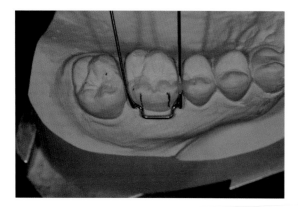

Figure 14.157. Align the arms through the occlusal embrasures. The bridge should be parallel to buccal surface.

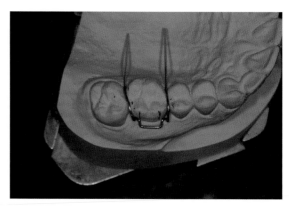

Figure 14.159. Clasp wire should sit passively with arrowheads in contact with tooth, bridge parallel to buccal surface, and bridge at a 45-degree angle to buccal surface.

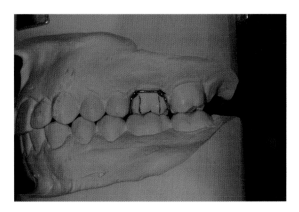

Figure 14.160. Clasp must fit tightly into mesial and distal occlusal embrasures to avoid occlusal interferences.

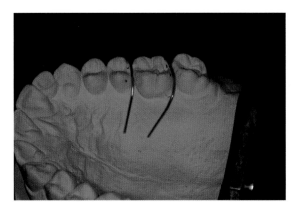

Figure 14.161. Crossover arms of the clasp need to go straight through occlusal embrasures then turn slightly to the mesial at the palatal tissue.

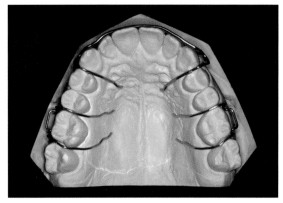

Figure 14.163. Completed wires for labial bow and Adams clasps on first molars for a standard maxillary Hawley retainer.

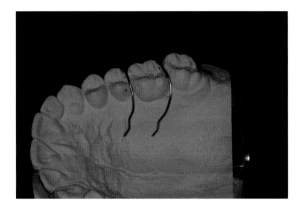

Figure 14.162. Place zigzag bends at the ends of each arm. The arms should be 12 to 15 mm in length from lingualembrasures and maintain a 0.5-mm space between palate and wire.

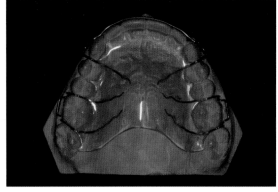

Figure 14.164. Completed standard maxillary Hawley retainer with Adams clasps.

College of Dentistry
The University of Iowa
Department of Orthodontics

Doctor R Greaves No. 1004 Date 8-20-7

Patient Alaina Lillian No. 149

Date Needed 8-27-7 Time 3pm

℞

Please fabricate a maxillary Modified Hawley retainer with .030 labial bow soldered to .026 adams clasps on 1st molars. Clear acrylic please

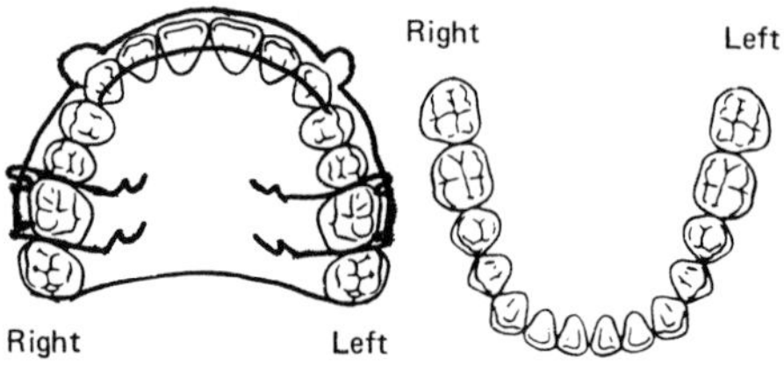

Right
Left
Right
Left

Material

Shade

For Lab Use Only

1162

Instructor

Signature R Greaves

76010/6-09

Figure 14.165. Maxillary modified Hawley retainer with labial bow soldered to Adams clasps on first molars prescription.

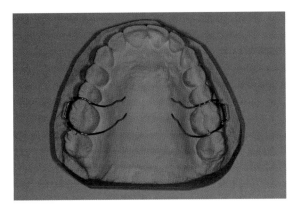

Figure 14.166. The 0.026 Adams clasps ready for labial bow bending for modified Hawley retainer.

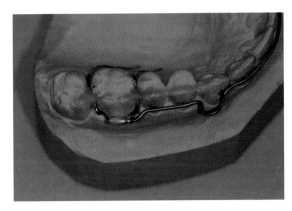

Figure 14.169. With wires off, cast flow solder completely around both labial bow and Adams clasp bridges. (See Figs. 14.198 through 14.200 for electric soldering.)

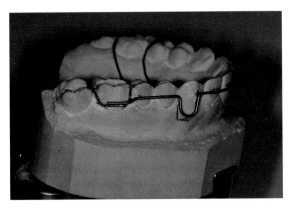

Figure 14.167. Bend the labial bow to fit canine to canine. Extend the wire back to the Adams clasps bridges. (See Figs. 14.196 and 14.197 for spot welding.)

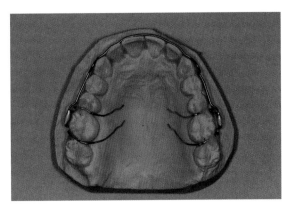

Figure 14.170. Maxillary modified Hawley labial bow soldered to Adams clasps on cast ready for acrylicing.

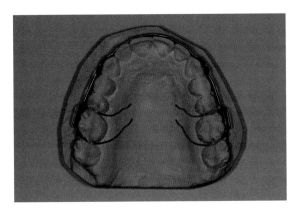

Figure 14.168. Labial bow should contact premolars, step out to the clasp bridges with bayonet bends, and cut 1 mm short of distal arrowhead loops. Spot weld the labial bow to the Adams clasps.

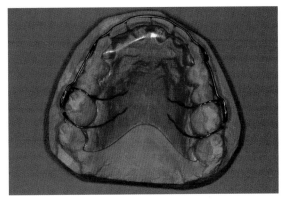

Figure 14.171. Completed maxillary modified Hawley labial bow soldered to Adams clasps retainer.

College of Dentistry
The University of Iowa
Department of Orthodontics

Doctor R Graves No. 1004 Date 8-13-07

Patient Grace Anne No. 187

Date Needed 8-20-07 Time 1:30 pm

℞

Please fabricate a Maxillary modified Hawley retainer with .032 labial bow soldered to .032 ReSta clasps on 1st Molars.

* Pink acrylic please.

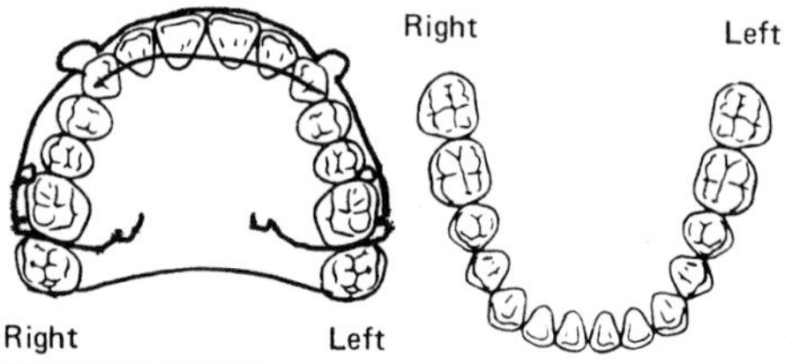

Right
Left
Right
Left

Material

Shade

For Lab Use Only

1162

Instructor

Signature R Graves

76010/6-09

Figure 14.172. Maxillary modified Hawley with a labial bow soldered to ReSta clasps on first molars' prescription.

ReSta Clasp

The ReSta ("res-tay") clasp (Staley and Reske 1987, 1989) is a very versatile retentive clasp that has been used in the Orthodontic Department at the College of Dentistry, University of Iowa since 1984. The ReSta clasp is used most often when an Adams clasp cannot be used because of occlusal interference on either the mesial or distal of the clasped posterior tooth. With a labial bow soldered to ReSta clasps, the clasps will solidly retain a removable appliance.

The ReSta clasp consists of a superior-quality ball clasp with a 0.032-inch stainless steel wire and a 0.065-inch ball. The ball will fit into the mesiobuccal or distobuccal undercut of a tooth, and an arrowhead loop is bent to fit into the opposite undercut, thus making contact with two buccal surface undercuts like an Adams clasp. In patients in whom interdental embrasure spaces do not allow any wires to cross the occlusion without causing an occlusal interference, many clinicians will request a wraparound labial bow that only crosses the occlusion distal to the most posterior teeth. However, the length of the labial bow makes such a design very flexible and easily distorted by the patient, is difficult for the clinician to adjust, and has questionable retention.

ReSta clasps may be placed on the most posterior teeth with a labial bow soldered to it to create an appliance with much more retention and adjustability than the wraparound retainer. The wraparound retainer designed with ReSta clasps on the most posterior molars is similar to a labial bow soldered to a c-clasp but has better retention and adjustment capabilities. If less flexibility of the labial bow is desired, the ReSta clasp may be moved more anteriorly and placed on a first molar or a premolar. The labial bow wire is then wrapped around the most posterior tooth to control excessive bow movement. Many varations of the ReSta clasp may be used to successfully retain removable appliances.

Figure 14.172 shows a prescription for a maxillary modified Hawley retainer with a labial bow soldered to a ReSta clasp. Figures 14.173 through 14.190 illustrate the bending of the ReSta clasp.

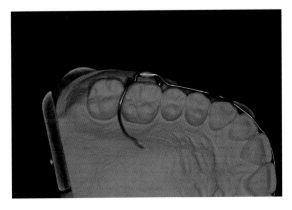

Figure 14.173. ReSta clasp with labial bow soldered. The ReSta clasp is a ball clasp for undercut contact on one end and an Adams clasp arrowhead for contact on the other end.

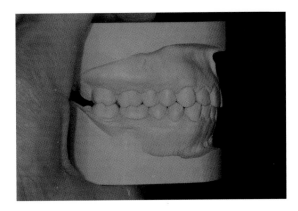

Figure 14.174. When an Adams clasp cannot be used because of a tight mesial embrasure, a ReSta clasp on the first molar can be a useful clasp.

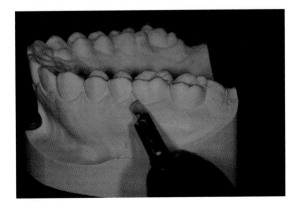

Figure 14.175. Prepare tissue undercuts for ReSta clasp fabrication.

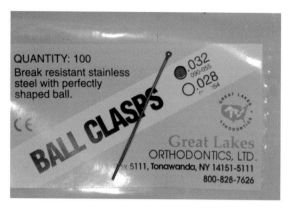

Figure 14.176. Use a superior quality 0.032-inch wire ball clasp.

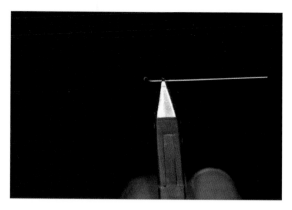

Figure 14.179. Place the ball clasp wire in pliers with the wire perpendicular to the pliers.

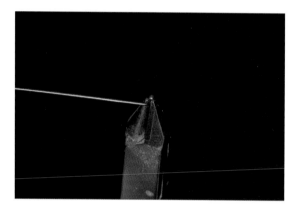

Figure 14.177. With ball clasp ball against pliers, make a curved 90-degree bend around conical beak.

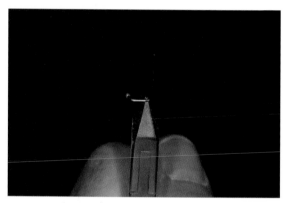

Figure 14.180. Make a 90-degree bend around the conical beak toward the tooth.

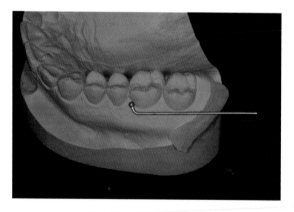

Figure 14.178. Mark the wire for a 90-degree bend toward distal undercut to start the arrowhead loop.

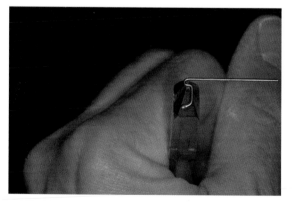

Figure 14.181. Place square beak against bridge of ReSta clasp and bend wire around the conical beak 180 degrees, creating an arrowhead.

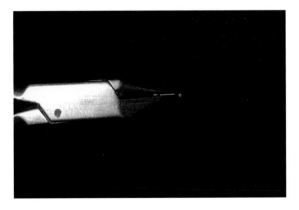

Figure 14.182. Hold wire across arrowhead and bend up 45 degrees.

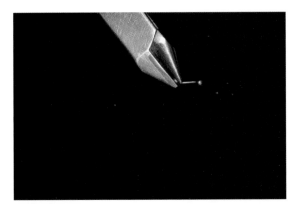

Figure 14.183. The 45-degree arrowhead bend.

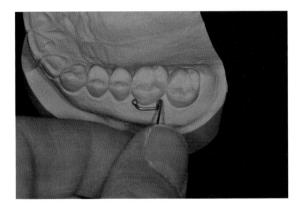

Figure 14.184. Place clasp to buccal surface of the tooth. Ball and arrowhead should fit into mesial and distal buccal undercuts. Bridge should be 1½ mm from and parallel to the buccal tooth surface.

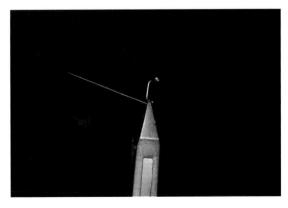

Figure 14.185. Place conical beak tip into arrowhead and bend wire 90 degrees from the bridge.

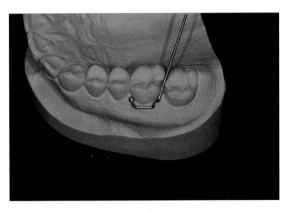

Figure 14.186. With the bridge 30 degrees up off tissue, crossover arm needs to fit between the teeth and contact at the occlusal embrasure.

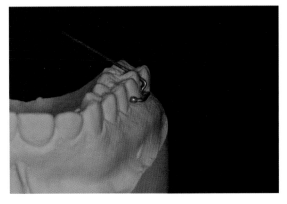

Figure 14.187. Mesial view of ReSta clasp. Mark the wire at occlusal contact and bend down tightly through the embrasure.

Figures 14.191 through 14.197 illustrate the bending and soldering of the labial bow to the ReSta clasp. Figure 14.198 shows a completed maxillary modified Hawley retainer with labial bow soldered to ReSta clasps on first molars. Figure 14.199 shows a completed maxillary modified Hawley with labial bow soldered to ReSta clasps on second molars. Figure 14.200 shows a prescription for a maxillary modified Hawley with labial bow soldered to ReSta clasps on second molars.

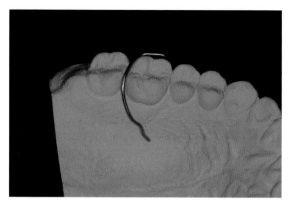

Figure 14.190. Bend wire toward mesial and place zigzag bends at end of the wire arm.

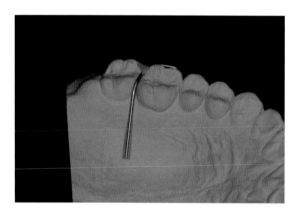

Figure 14.188. Cross wire tightly through embrasure and down toward the palatal tissue.

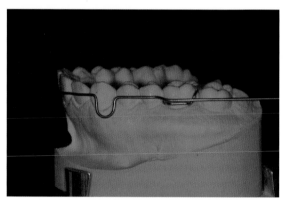

Figure 14.191. Bend ReSta clasp for opposite side. Bend a labial bow to fit the anterior teeth, contacting the premolars and fit passively to the ReSta clasp bridges. Cut the wire 1 mm mesial to the arrowhead loop.

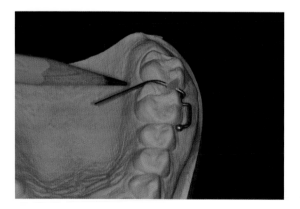

Figure 14.189. Mark wire to continue bending wire down with 0.5-mm space between wire and palatal tissue.

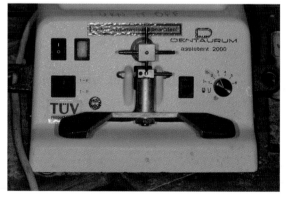

Figure 14.192. An electric soldering and spot welding machine.

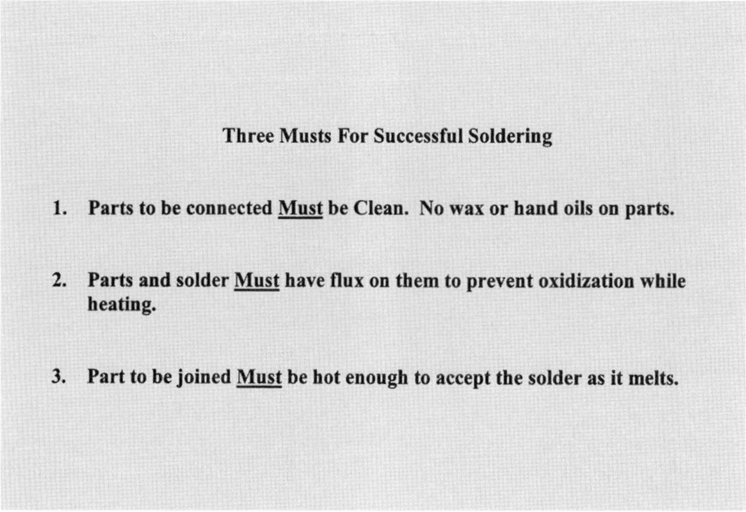

Three Musts For Successful Soldering

1. Parts to be connected <u>Must</u> be Clean. No wax or hand oils on parts.

2. Parts and solder <u>Must</u> have flux on them to prevent oxidization while heating.

3. Part to be joined <u>Must</u> be hot enough to accept the solder as it melts.

Figure 14.193. Three rules for all successful soldering operations.

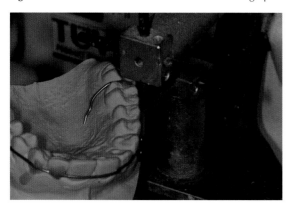

Figure 14.194. Spot weld the labial bow to ReSta clasps on both sides of the arch. Two spots per clasp should be sufficient.

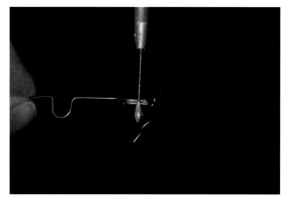

Figure 14.196. Flux is applied to both wires and the electrode solder ball.

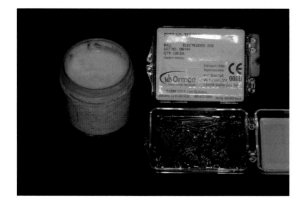

Figure 14.195. A good-quality floride flux (*left*) and a quality medium or large 0.032-inch ball soldering electrode (*right*) are used in the electric soldering machine.

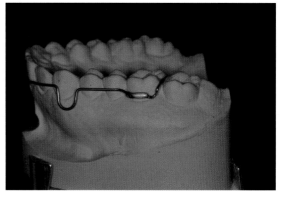

Figure 14.197. Completed solder joint. Be sure solder encircles both wires for maximum joint strength.

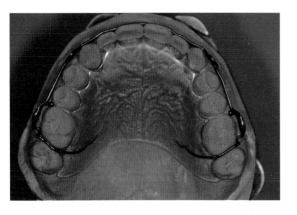

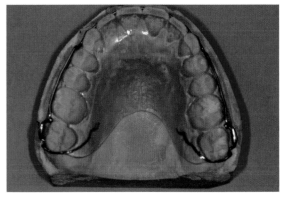

Figure 14.198. Completed maxillary modified Hawley retainer with a labial bow soldered to ReSta clasps on first molars.

Figure 14.199. Completed maxillary modified Hawley retainer with the labial bow soldered to ReSta clasps on second molars.

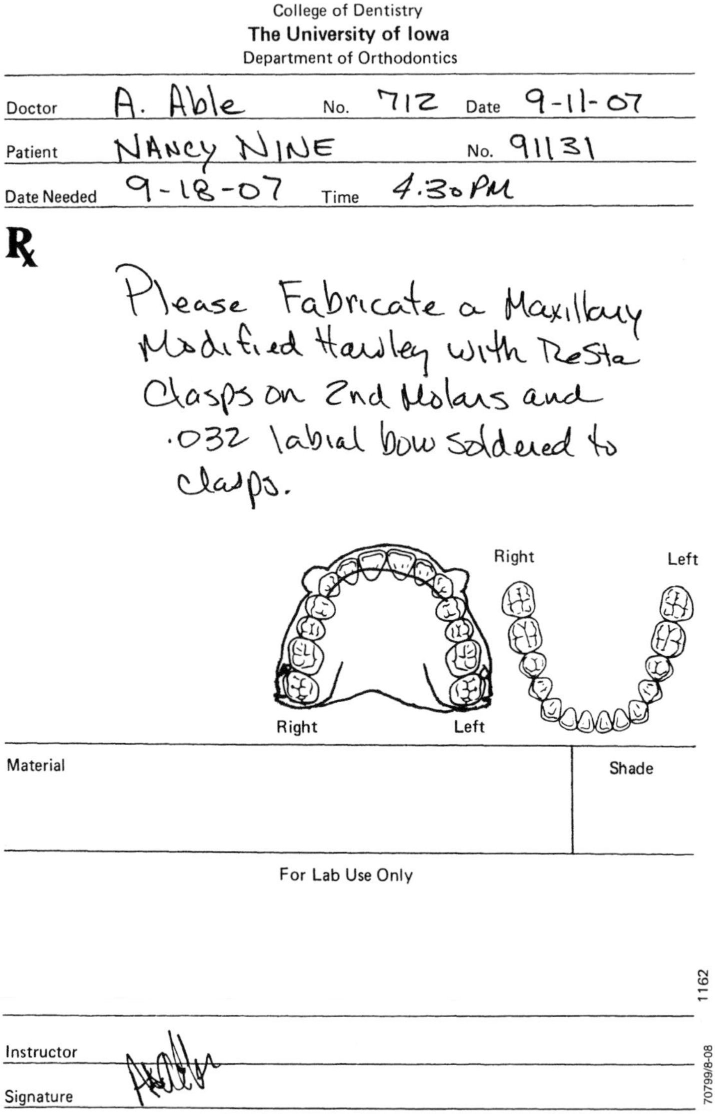

College of Dentistry
The University of Iowa
Department of Orthodontics

Doctor	A. Able	No. 712	Date	9-11-07
Patient	NANCY NINE		No.	91131
Date Needed	9-18-07	Time	4:30 PM	

Rx

Please Fabricate a Maxillary Modified Hawley with ReSta Clasps on 2nd Molars and .032 labial bow Soldered to clasps.

Right   Left

Right   Left

Material	Shade

For Lab Use Only

Instructor
Signature

Figure 14.200. Prescription for a maxillary modified Hawley retainer with labial bow soldered to ReSta clasps on second molars.

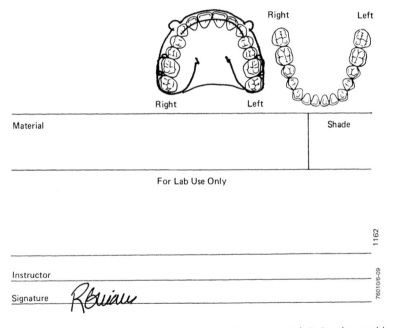

College of Dentistry
The University of Iowa
Department of Orthodontics

Doctor *R Greaves* No. *1004* Date *9-4-7*

Patient *Ron Thomae* No. *840*

Date Needed *9-11-7* Time *9 am*

℞

Please fabricate a Maxillary Modified Hawley retainer with .032 labial bow soldered to ReSta Clasps on 1st Molars then wraparound 2nd Molars. Clear acrylic please

Right   Left

Right   Left

Material   Shade

For Lab Use Only

Instructor

Signature *R Greaves*

Figure 14.201. Prescription for a maxillary modified wraparound Hawley retainer with ReSta clasps soldered at first molars.

Figure 14.201 shows a prescription for a wraparound labial bow soldered to ReSta clasps on first molars with the bow wraparound to the distal of the second molars. Figures 14.202 through 14.215 illustrate the bending of a labial bow and soldering the bow to the ReSta clasp. Figure 14.216 shows a completed maxillary modified Hawley retainer with soldered ReSta clasps on first molars and a wraparound labial bow to the distal of the second molars.

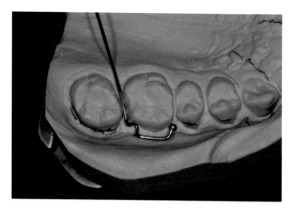

Figure 14.202. ReSta clasp prepared a for wraparound labial bow to be soldered to the bridge of the clasp.

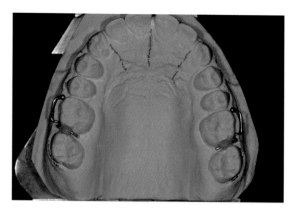

Figure 14.205. ReSta clasps on first molars ready for bending the wraparound labial bow.

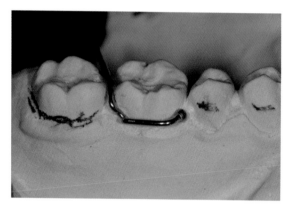

Figure 14.203. Retention arms of ReSta clasps can be cut off and the clasp waxed to occlusal embrasure while bending wraparound labial bow.

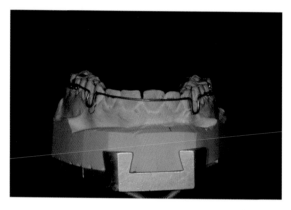

Figure 14.206. Anterior view of labial bow fitted over ReSta clasps on first molars.

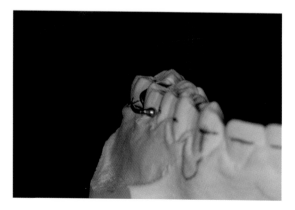

Figure 14.204. Mesial view of ReSta clasp. The bridge is slightly tilted up off the tissue.

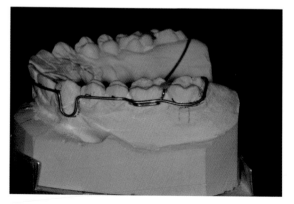

Figure 14.207. Wraparound labial bow passively sitting across the ReSta clasp and following the height of contour of the second molar, then crossing behind molar and finishing in the palate.

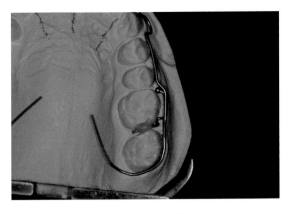

Figure 14.208. Occlusal view of labial bow soldered wrap-around wires before spot welding.

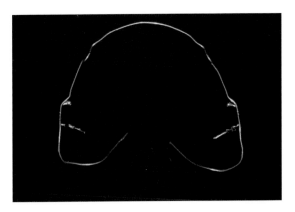

Figure 14.211. Carefully remove spot welded wires from the cast for soldering.

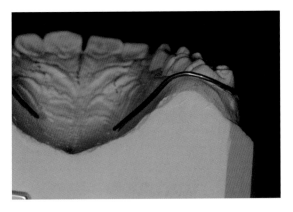

Figure 14.209. Wraparound labial wire fitted tightly around distal of second molar. Wire needs to remain 0.5 mm off the palatal tissue.

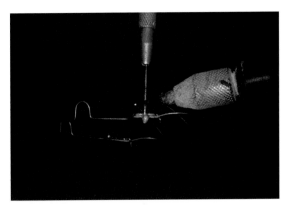

Figure 14.212. Flux wires and solder ball and apply heat with carbon electrode until solder flows around the labial bow and ReSta clasp wires.

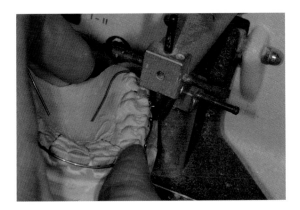

Figure 14.210. Spot weld the labial bow to ReSta clasps, two spots per clasps.

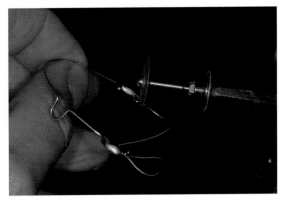

Figure 14.213. After soldering, remove the faux retention crossover arms at the arrowheads.

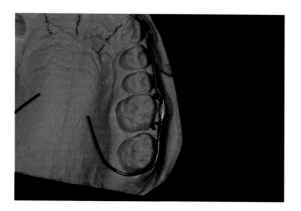

Figure 14.214. Soldered wire in pace on cast.

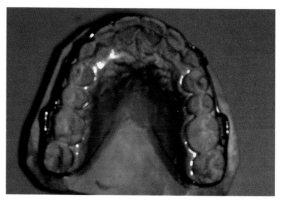

Figure 14.216. Completed maxillary modified Hawley wrap-around retainer with a labial bow soldered to ReSta clasps on first molars.

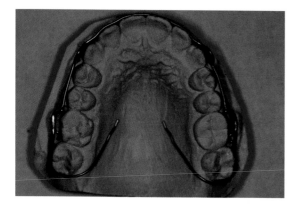

Figure 14.215. Zigzag bends at end of retention arms. Arms need to be 15 mm from distal lingual line angle of second molars. Wires are ready for acrylicing.

Mandibular Labial Bow

The mandibular labial bow is fabricated in a similar fashion to the maxillary labial bow. The bow follows the arch form at the middle third of the clinical crowns. Draw a horizontal line on the mandibular cast from the middle of the canine on one side to the middle of the canine on the other side. Draw adjustment loops of 4 to 6 mm in width and length near the midpoints of the canines and terminating in the acrylic in the lingual flange mesial to the first premolars.

A 7-inch length of 0.028- or 0.030-inch round stainless steel wire is bent into an ideal parabolic curve around a wire turret approximating the arch form. Bend the wire to contact mesial line angles to distal line angles on both centrals and

laterals and the mesial line angles to the midpoint on each canine. Care must be taken to intimately contact all anterior teeth to prevent rotations from occurring. Slight canine offsets are usually necessary to produce properly fitting mandibular labial bows. Bend adjustment loops and be certain each loop is slightly off the gingival tissue. Bend the distal aspect of the adjustment loop up toward the embrasures and be sure to follow the tissue closely up to the embrasure in order to prevent occlusal interferences with teeth in the opposing arch. Bend the wire tightly through the embrasures and maintain 0.5-mm space between wire and tissue on the lingual side of the arch. Make right angle bends toward the midline of the cast 2 to 3 mm below the point of contact through the occlusal embrasures. Bend the wire to overlap or at least meet at the midline to reinforce the lower horseshoe-shaped acrylic. Now bend occlusal rests with scrap pieces of 0.030- or 0.032-inch round stainless steel wire on first molars. Be sure rests do not interfere with opposing maxillary lingual stamp cusps when casts are in centric occlusion.

Figure 14.217 shows a prescription for a mandibular Hawley retainer with a labial bow and occlusal rests. Figures 14.218 through 14.241 illustrate the bending of the mandibular labial bow and occlusal rests. Figure 14.242 shows a completed mandibular Hawley retainer with labial bow and occlusal rests.

College of Dentistry
The University of Iowa
Department of Orthodontics

Doctor R Greaves No. 1004 Date 8-10-08

Patient Janelle Marie No. 299

Date Needed 8-17-8 Time 3:45 PM

℞

Please fabricate a mandibular Hawley retainer with .030 rd labial bow and .032 occlusal rests.

* Pink acrylic please.

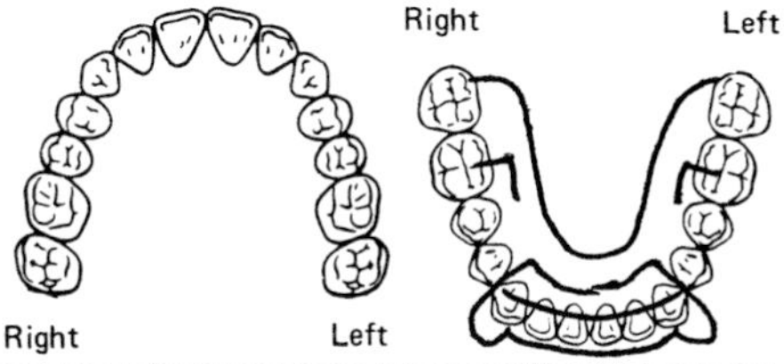

Right
Left
Right
Left

Material

Shade

For Lab Use Only

1162

Instructor

Signature R Greaves

76010/6-09

Figure 14.217. Prescription for a standard mandibular Hawley retainer with labial bow and occlusal rests.

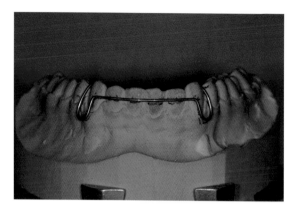

Figure 14.218. Mandibular labial bow.

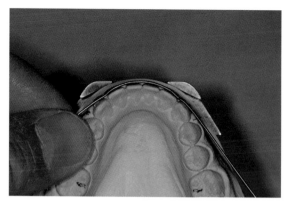

Figure 14.221. Adjust to contact line angle to line angle on the centrals, laterals, and mesial half of the canines. Mark the vertical bend of one adjustment loop 1 mm mesial to the middle of the canine.

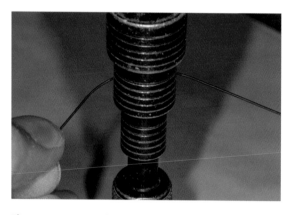

Figure 14.219. Bend a 7-inch length of 0.030-inch wire around a wire turret to create a perfect parabolic curve.

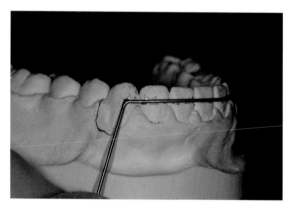

Figure 14.222. Draw 5- to 6-mm adjustment loops on cast. Bend 80-degree mesial arm of the adjustment loop. Remember to bend the loop out away from tissue contact.

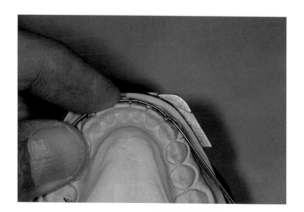

Figure 14.220. Open or close the curve to fit across centrals. Bend the wire to contact across laterals. Mark and bend the canine offsets.

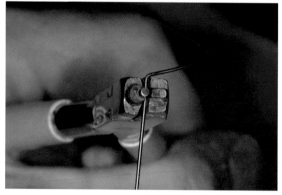

Figure 14.223. Bend adjustment loop. The loop is shown being bent around the large rounded beak of the Hawley loop pliers.

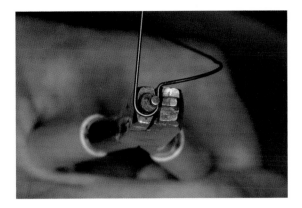

Figure 14.224. Completed adjustment loop bend.

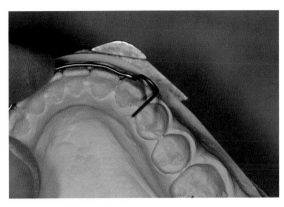

Figure 14.227. View from occlusal. Loop must parallel the canine and be slightly off the tissue.

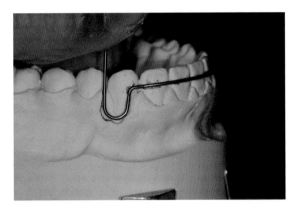

Figure 14.225. Loop may be opened or closed to fit the distal arm of the loop between canine and premolar embrasure.

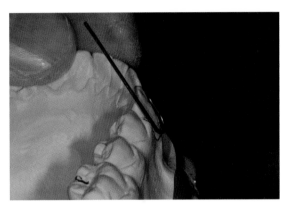

Figure 14.228. Distal view before bend toward the occlusal embrasure.

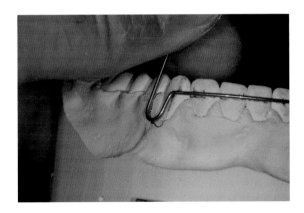

Figure 14.226. Bend distal arm of loop following the tissue and toward the occlusal embrasure.

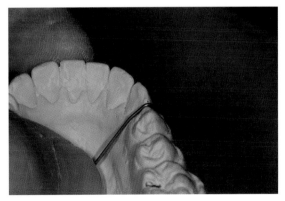

Figure 14.229. Make bends over the embrasure onto the lingual of the cast. Wire on the lingual needs to be 0.5 to 1 mm off the tissue to end of the wire.

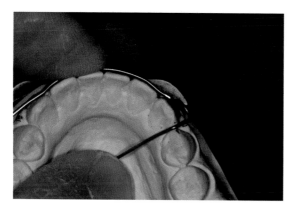

Figure 14.230. Occlusal view of the wire fitted tightly through the occlusal embrasure.

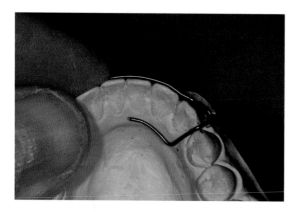

Figure 14.231. Wire is bent mesially off the tissue and cut at the midline.

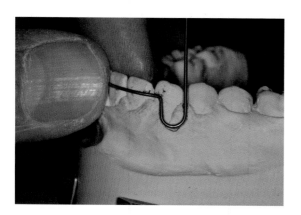

Figure 14.232. Adjustment loop is made on the opposite side.

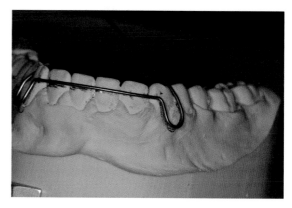

Figure 14.233. Distal arm of adjustment loop is bent toward the occlusal embrasure.

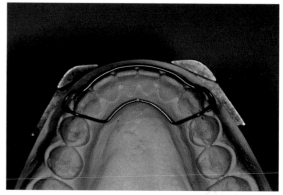

Figure 14.234. Wire bends are completed when the labial bow fits passively on cast with wire in contact facially with all six anterior teeth, fits tightly through the embrasures, and is 0.5 to 1 mm off the lingual side tissue.

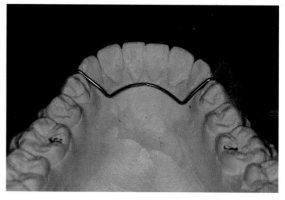

Figure 14.235. To help strengthen acrylic on the mandibular retainer, the labial bow wire should meet or cross at the midline. The wire is positioned just below the gingival margins and above the tongue attachment.

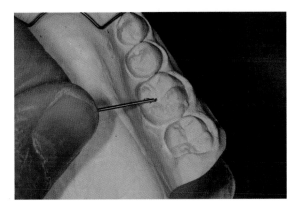

Figure 14.236. Occlusal rests are fabricated with 0.030- or 0.032-inch scrap wire.

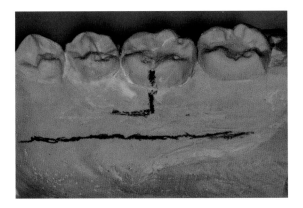

Figure 14.237. Bottom line indicates the approximate lingual flange of acrylic, 8 to 10 mm below the gingival margins. The right-angle retention bend is halfway between the gingival margin of the molar and the flange edge.

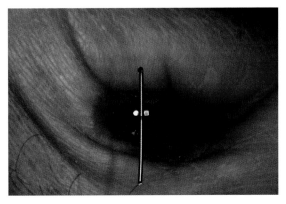

Figure 14.239. Mark and make a right-angle retention bend toward anterior of the cast.

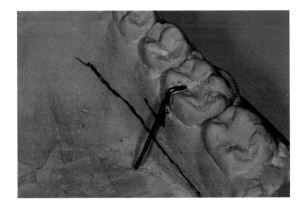

Figure 14.238. Right-angle bend is made at the line angle of the occlusal lingual central grove and the lingual surface of the tooth.

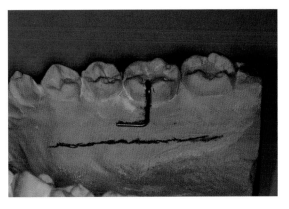

Figure 14.240. Retention arm is cut at 5 to 7 mm and needs to be 0.5 to 1 mm off the lingual tissue. Make the opposite side rest in the same manner.

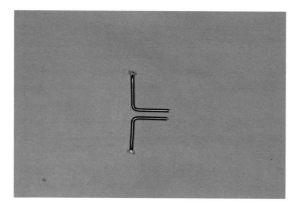

Figure 14.241. Mirror image left and right occlusal rests are ready to be included in the mandibular retainer.

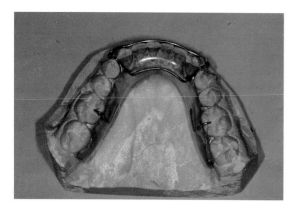

Figure 14.242. Complete standard mandibular Hawley retainer.

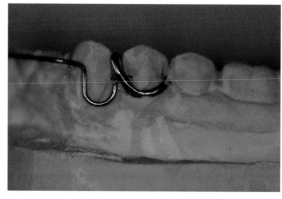

Figure 14.243. For a mandibular retainer with limited undercuts on the lingual of posterior teeth, a c-clasp may be soldered to the distal of the labial bow adjustment loop.

Figure 14.243 shows a mandibular Hawley retainer with a c-clasp soldered to the distal of the labial bow adjustment loop and engaging the distal undercut of the first premolar for retention. This design is used when the lingual surfaces of the posterior teeth are vertically short or the undercuts below the gingival margins are not exposed.

Figure 14.244 shows a prescription for a mandibular Hawley retainer with c-clasps soldered to the distal of the adjustment loop of a labial bow.

College of Dentistry
The University of Iowa
Department of Orthodontics

Doctor	A. Able	No. 712 Date 9-18-06
Patient	Grover Munster	No. 73230
Date Needed	10-1-06	Time 3 PM

℞

Please fabricate a mandibular Hawley with .030 Labial bow with .030 C-Clasp soldered to distal of adjustment loops. And rests on 1st molars Lingual of posterior teeth are short. No undercuts for retention and no space for clasping.

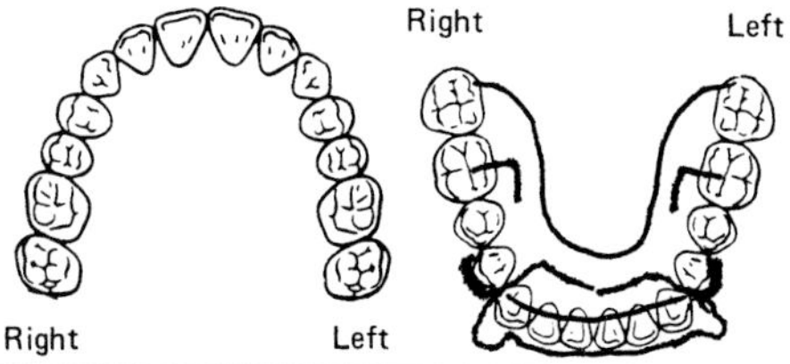

Right   Left

Right   Left

Material   Shade

For Lab Use Only

Instructor

Signature

1162

76010/6-09

Figure 14.244. Mandibular Hawley retainer with c–clasps soldered to the distal of the labial bow loops prescription.

Acrylicing Retainers

On completion of wire-bending tasks, an acrylic base is formed that will hold the wires securely. Three types of materials are used for orthodontic retainers: (1) cold-cure methylmethacrylate, (2) light-cure acrylic, and (3) thermoformed acrylics. The cold-cure acrylics are the most common, but the light-cure and thermoformed are especially useful for individuals with allergies to methylmethacrylate (Willison and Waruhnek, 2004).

Cold-cure acrylics consist of a two-part mix of liquid (monomer) and powder (polymer) methylmethacrylate. When mixed, the two become a solid acrylic. There are two methods to adapt this material to the cast. The first method is the "salt and pepper" system of dispensing the "salt" polymer to the cast and then dripping the "pepper" monomer to be absorbed by the powder. This dispensing of polymer and monomer continues in thin layers until the desired thickness is achieved. The second method is to mix 1 part liquid to 2 parts polymer. After mixing, polymerization begins and the acrylic resin passes through a doughy state when the acrylic is finger adapted to the cast.

Care must be taken when handling these materials. Monomer fumes should be controlled by ventilation and gloves used for individuals with skin sensitivity. Prior to attaching the labial bow, clasps, or springs to the cast, a small amount of liquid separator is brushed on the lingual, palatal, and occlusal surfaces of the cast and allowed to dry. With a wax spatula and Bunsen burner, secure the wires to the facial surface of the cast with small amounts of base plate wax. Check wires for fit, especially how tightly they fit through occlusal embrasures. NOW IS THE TIME TO MAKE **SURE** WIRES ARE CORRECTLY FITTED! Figures 14.245 through 14.260 illustrate the steps involved in preparing the casts for acrylicing a retainer. Figures 14.261 through 14.271 illustrate steps involving the "salt and Pepper" method of applying acrylic for maxillary and mandibular retainers.

Immediately after applying acrylic to the appliance, place the cast into a warm, humid pressure pot under 20 psi for 10 to 15 minutes to increase the density and durability of the acrylic base as it hardens. After the appliance goes into the pressure curing pot, acrylic can be applied to another appliance. Place the second appliance immediately into the pressure pot and cure it for 10 to 15 minutes. After the acrylic has cured, remove the second cast from the pressure pot.

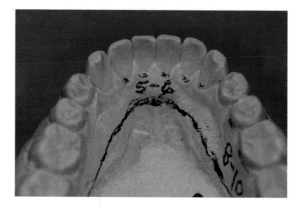

Figure 14.245. Anterior lingual flange will normally be 5 to 6 mm below the gingival margins of the teeth.

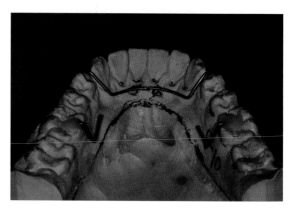

Figure 14.246. Mandibular labial bow retention arms should be 3 to 4 mm above the proposed lingual flange.

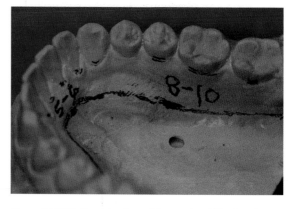

Figure 14.247. Posterior lingual flange should be 8 to 10 mm below the gingival margins of the teeth.

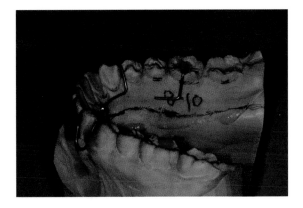

Figure 14.248. Wires need to be 3 to 4 mm above flanges in case the flange needs to be shortened for patient comfort.

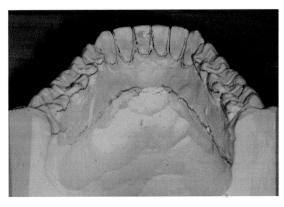

Figure 14.251. Excessive lingual undercuts of the teeth must also be blocked out. Draw a line at the height of contour of the posterior teeth to determine if blockout is needed.

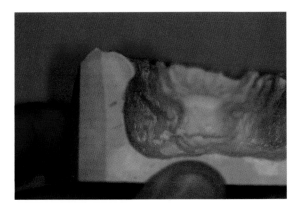

Figure 14.249. Large undesirable undercuts need to be blocked out with wax.

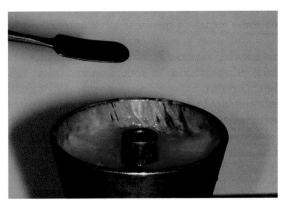

Figure 14.252. Soften base plate wax with a Bunsen burner.

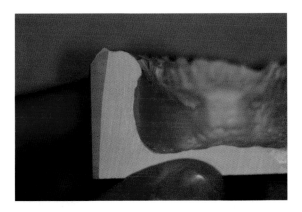

Figure 14.250. Wax blockout of large tissue undercuts.

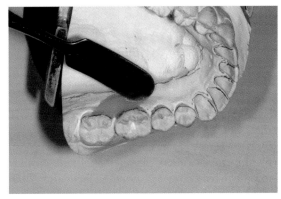

Figure 14.253. Apply wax to the cast filling tissue and tooth undercuts to the height of contour.

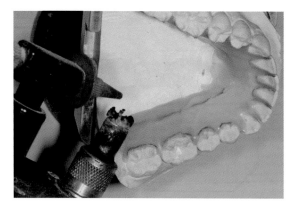

Figure 14.254. Smooth wax by flaming with an alcohol torch.

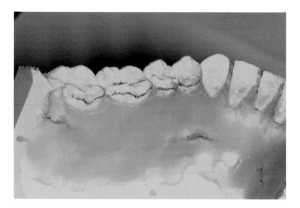

Figure 14.257. Completed tissue undercut blockout.

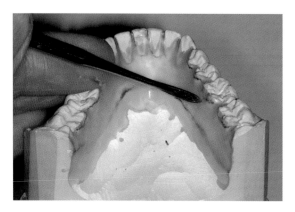

Figure 14.255. With a pointed wax spatula, remove wax 1½ mm below tooth height of contour on each posterior tooth.

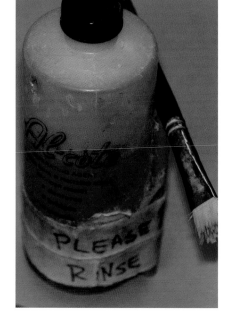

Figure 14.258. Paint casts with a thin layer of a tin foil substitute separator.

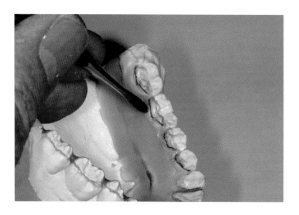

Figure 14.256. Wax removed below height of contour simulating the normal lingual gingival tissue position.

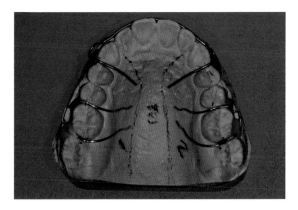

Figure 14.259. After separator has dried, wax wires securely to the cast. At the facial occlusal embrasures, maxillary cast is shown with numbers indicating the order of areas to be acryliced.

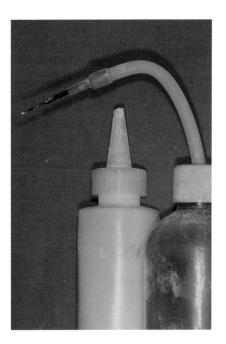

Figure 14.261. "Salt and pepper" technique acrylic powder dispensing bottle (*left*) and liquid dispensing bottle (*right*). The wire tip on liquid bottle allows drop-by-drop control.

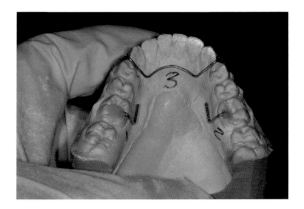

Figure 14.260. Wax labial bow and occlusal rests securely to mandibular cast. Numbers indicate the order for acrylicing the retainer.

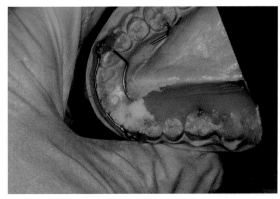

Figure 14.262. Tilt the cast so acrylic can be applied from occlusal lingual line angle of teeth to floor of cast in thin layers until the acrylic body is 2 to 2½ mm thick.

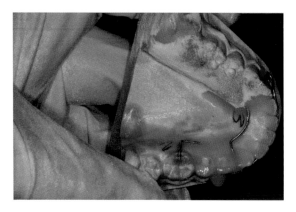

Figure 14.263. Finish first side with extra powder to "freeze" acrylic in position while applying acrylic to the opposite side.

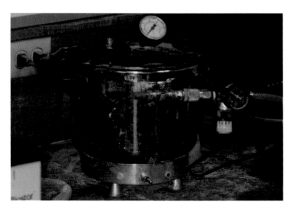

Figure 14.266. Immediately place acryliced cast into a heated pressure pot set to 18 to 20 lb pressure. Cure for 10 to 15 minutes.

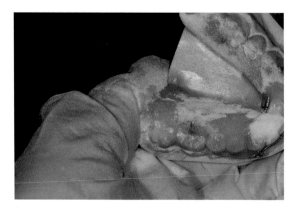

Figure 14.264. Apply extra dusting of powder to "freeze" second side. Try to complete acrylicing in 5 minutes or less to improve the acrylic density.

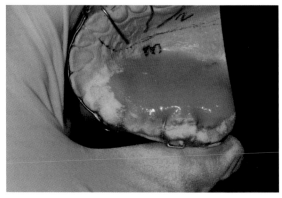

Figure 14.267. Tilt the maxillary cast and apply acrylic in thin layers until the retainer body is 2 to 2½ mm thick. Dust with powder.

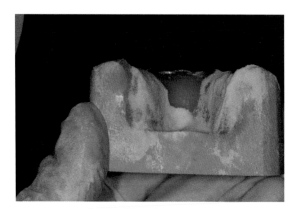

Figure 14.265. Finish by acrylicing the anterior to the incisal edges of the teeth and dust with powder.

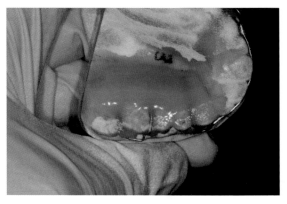

Figure 14.268. Apply acrylic to the opposite side of palate and dust with powder.

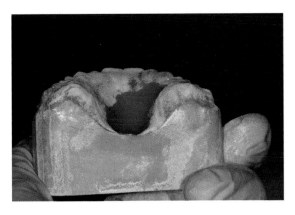

Figure 14.269. Complete acrylicing by connecting the acrylic in middle and anterior sections.

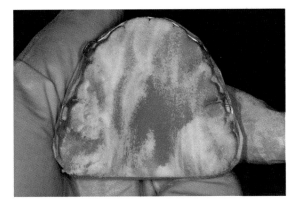

Figure 14.270. Complete acrylicing by dusting with powder to help minimize settling of acrylic toward middle of the palate.

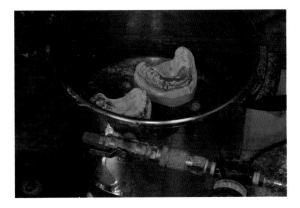

Figure 14.271. Immediately place acryliced cast into the pressure pot and apply pressure for 10 to 15 minutes. The pressure pot has a raised platform with 1 inch of water below the platform.

Acrylic Finishing and Polishing

The final phase of retainer fabrication involves the trimming to proper size and thickness to achieve the strongest and most comfortable and stabile appliance possible, which also resists calculus and plaque build-up.

After removing the retainers from the pressure curing pot, remove wax from the wires, and with a plaster knife, carefully slip the knife under the posterior edges and pry the acrylic up from each distal corner. This is easily accomplished while casts are still warm from curing. If casts have been set aside for a while and have cooled, place casts in a bowl of warm water for a few minutes to rehydrate the casts to help with separation of the acrylic from the cast.

Retainer trimming or finishing can be divided into three parts: (1) rough trimming, (2) final trimming, and (3) polishing. Rough trimming refers to cutting the retainer to the basic shape, followed by thinning and smoothing excessive bulkiness. Final trimming refers to detailed acrylic trimming of the anterior acrylic, posterior trimming around the teeth, and the posterior edge. Polishing is the final phase in which the retainer is smoothed and brought to a highly shined state.

Figures 14.272 through 14.302 illustrate steps to finish and polish retainers. Trimming, thinning, and finishing can be accomplished using a dental handpiece, a bench lathe, or both. This author prefers to use both the dental handpiece and bench lathe for reducing bulk and finishing the edges of the retainer.

Start the trimming process with a ball nose Kutzal bur in a handpiece, rough trimming the posterior border of the maxillary retainer, thinning the palate to 2-mm thickness, and reducing the acrylic over the teeth and anterior lingual areas to the middle of the lingual surfaces of the teeth. On the mandibular retainer, reduce the length distal to the last tooth on each side of the arch; shorten lingual flanges to 6 to 8 mm in the posterior and 5 to 6 mm in the anterior region. Thin the flanges to 2.5 mm and reduce the acrylic over the anterior lingual area to the middle of the teeth.

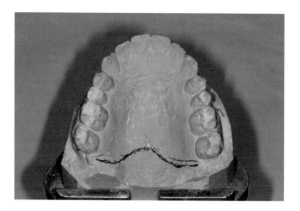

Figure 14.272. A maxillary cast with the acryliced retainer removed. Mark the desired posterior length of the retainer. A horseshoe design may be necessary if the patient is prone to gagging.

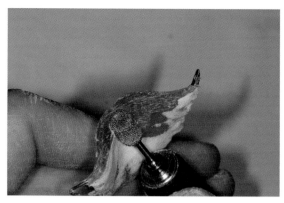

Figure 14.275. Remove the retainer and rough trim acrylic to approximately 2 mm in thickness.

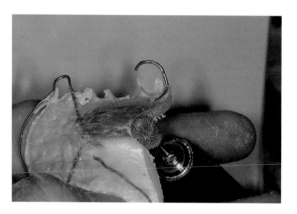

Figure 14.273. Kutzall bur is used to rough trim the posterior border.

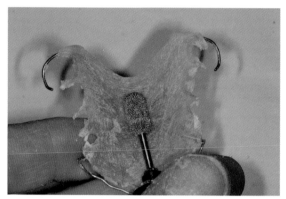

Figure 14.276. Remove bulk across and into palatal vault of the retainer.

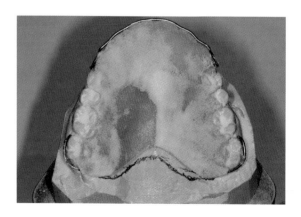

Figure 14.274. Posterior border roughly trimmed.

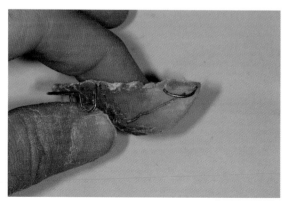

Figure 14.277. Check thickness with a finger into the palate.

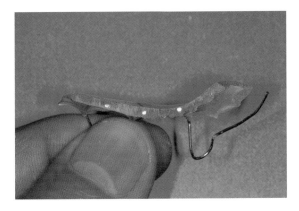

Figure 14.278. A cross section of a retainer shows ½-mm acrylic below the wire, ½-mm acrylic above the wire, and a wire of ¾ mm (0.030 inch), which means the minimum thickness possible is 1¾ mm.

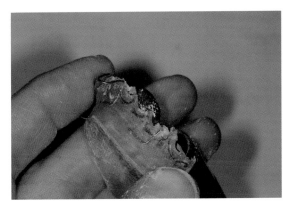

Figure 14.281. Switch to a smooth cutting tapered acrylic bur and scallop around posterior teeth.

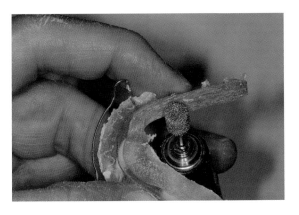

Figure 14.279. Bulk trim the mandibular retainer thinning to about 2½ mm.

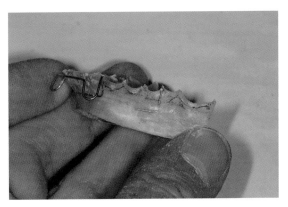

Figure 14.282. Leave 1½ mm of acrylic above the gingival margins, shown with a pencil line at margin.

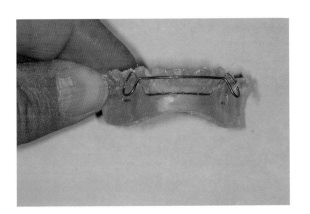

Figure 14.280. Rough trim the lingual flange.

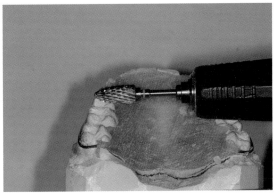

Figure 14.283. Always maintain hand piece across horizontal plane while scalloping and trimming.

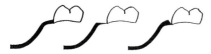

Correct   Incorrect   Incorrect

Figure 14.284. Trim retainers maintaining 1½ to 2 mm thickness to the lingual surface of posterior teeth. Drawing shows the correct thickness (*left*) at tooth contact. Incorrect thickness (*middle*) is too thin at tooth contact. Incorrect thickness (*right*) has only point contact and a V-shaped gap. Both incorrectly trimmed examples tend to break easily.

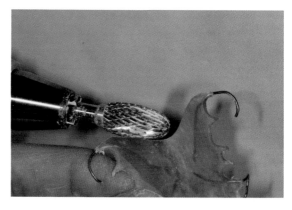

Figure 14.287. Use the large bur to smoothly trim the posterior border of maxillary retainer and the lingual flanges of the mandibular retainer.

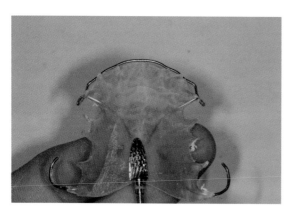

Figure 14.285. Remove all marks left by the bulk trimming bur and thin where necessary.

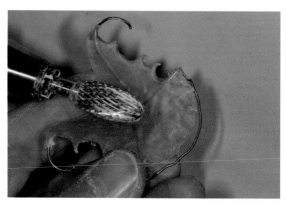

Figure 14.288. Smooth the entire tongue side of the maxillary and flanges of mandibular retainers and finalize thickness reduction with the lathe bur. The small acrylic bur tends to leave small divots in the acrylic.

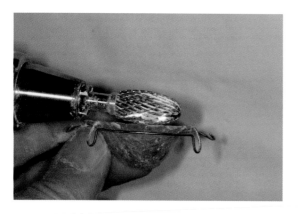

Figure 14.286. Use a large egg-shaped bur on a bench lathe to trim anterior acrylic parallel to the labial bow.

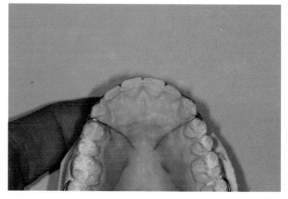

Figure 14.289. Finish the anterior acrylic to desired height, usually above the cingulums and out of contact with mandibular incisors.

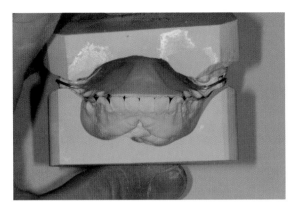

Figure 14.290. With the maxillary retainer on the cast, hand articulate and adjust retainer for desired contact. This photograph shows no contact of mandibular teeth to the maxillary retainer.

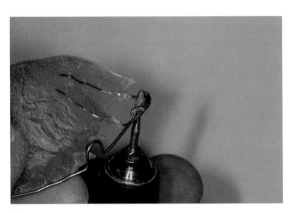

Figure 14.291. If your retainer has a labial bow soldered to clasps, trim the bulk solder with a green stone or tapered bur.

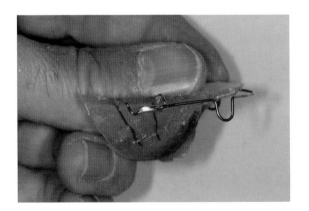

Figure 14.292. Do not expose wires. Solder should still wrap around both labial bow and clasp bridge wires.

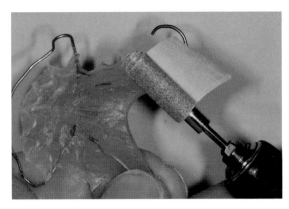

Figure 14.293. Complete finishing with a sandpaper mandrel and 150 grit sandpaper in a slow hand piece. Smooth tissue side edge *only* on the maxillary and mandibular retainers.

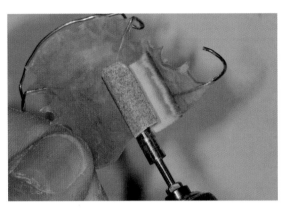

Figure 14.294. Smooth edge and entire tongue side of maxillary and mandibular retainers.

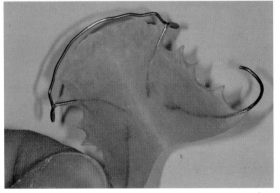

Figure 14.295. Sandpaper leaves a smooth matte appearance across any previously trimmed surface, including the posterior border of the maxillary and the lingual flanges of the mandibular retainers.

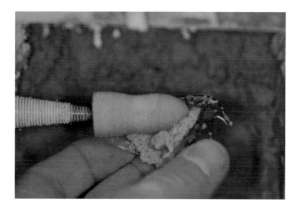

Figure 14.296. Completion of the finishing steps requires pumicing on a bench lathe—first a damp felt cone on high speed moves pumice into palate and across entire tongue side of retainer.

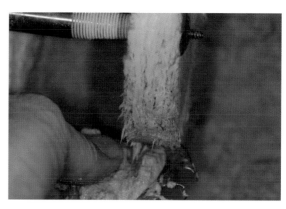

Figure 14.299. Next pumice with a muslin buff wheel on slow speed. Move retainer in all directions to remove scratches left by the sandpaper. Do not forget the edges!

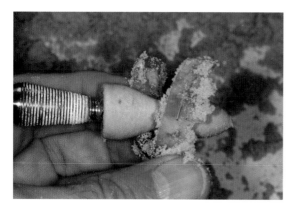

Figure 14.297. Felt cone also is used to smooth tongue side of the mandibular retainer, especially the narrow anterior region.

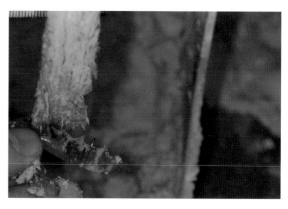

Figure 14.300. Be careful of occlusal rests and flexible wires so they do not catch on the muslin buff wheel.

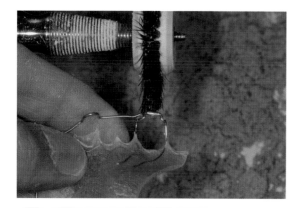

Figure 14.298. Solder joints are finished with a brush wheel and pumice on high speed. This will remove any heat stains and leave a matte appearance.

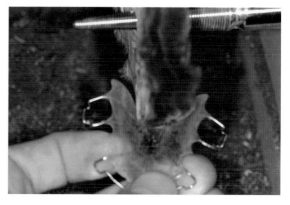

Figure 14.301. Use a dedicated muslin buff with tripoli compound on slow speed to polish tongue side surfaces and borders of retainers.

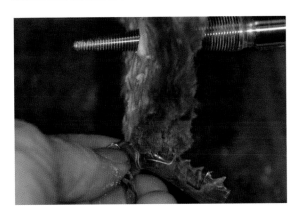

Figure 14.302. Use another dedicated muslin buff with acrylic high-shine compound of slow speed for a dazzling polish of retainers. Also lightly polish wires.

Next use a smooth cutting tapered carbide acrylic bur on both maxillary and mandibular retainers to remove all grooves and smooth the acrylic on the tongue side surfaces only. Look at the retainers from the tissue side; while holding the handpiece parallel to the occlusal plane, scallop around the posterior teeth. Be sure to leave approximately 1.5 mm of acrylic above the gingival margins of the teeth. This should leave acrylic in the lingual undercuts of the teeth from the height of contour on each posterior tooth to the gingival margin. Clinicians at the University of Iowa like to use a "high trim" finish, where the anterior acrylic of the maxillary appliance covers the cingulum of the teeth. Trim the anterior acrylic parallel to the labial bow while looking at the appliance from the anterior view. The wire is usually slightly below the height of the acrylic. At this point, the author likes to use a large ½-inch egg or tapered acrylic bur on a bench lathe to finish thinning the palate and flanges on the retainers and to smooth the posterior edge on the maxillary and flange edges on the mandibular retainers. The large bur is shaped like the palate and will smooth the palate and the anterior lingual flange of the mandibular retainer nicely in these areas. The smaller acrylic finishing bur tends to leave small divots and irregularities in the edges of the acrylic.

Fit the maxillary retainer on the cast, and hand articulate it with the mandibular cast. If the clinician wants the mandibular incisors to contact the maxillary retainer and open the bite in the posterior, reduce the maxillary anterior acrylic to the desired separation of the posterior teeth while trying to maintain incisal edge contacts from canine to canine. This active bite plate should be approximately 5 mm wide.

If the clinician wants a passive bite plate, reduce the anterior acrylic on the maxillary retainer until there is maximum posterior tooth contact while keeping the mandibular anterior teeth in contact with the maxillary anterior acrylic. This passive bite plate should be approximately 5 mm wide. If the clinician wants no contact of the mandibular incisors with the anterior acrylic of the maxillary retainer, reduce the acrylic to remove all contacts of mandibular anterior teeth to the acrylic of the maxillary appliance. Then the author uses a dental handpiece with a 150 grit sandpaper mandrel. Slightly bevel the tissue side edge and tongue side posterior edge of the maxillary retainer. Smooth the tongue side of the maxillary retainer to remove all bur scratches. Slightly bevel the tissue side edge and tongue side edge of the flange on the mandibular retainer. Completely sand all tongue side surfaces to reduce all scratches left by burs. Acrylic tongue side surfaces should now have a matte appearance and feel smooth to the touch of a finger or thumb.

Polishing the appliances starts with a damp felt cone and damp coarse pumice on high speed on a bench lathe. A blunt ¾-inch felt cone is great for getting deep into the palate on the maxillary appliance and the anterior lingual area on the mandibular appliance. Use a lot of pumice while continuously moving and altering directions of the appliance across the cone. Next a 4-inch lead center 28-ply muslin wheel is used with wet pumice on slow speed to smooth all tongue side surfaces and edges that had been trimmed and sanded. Always use lots of pumice, keep the appliances moving, and vary directions while pumicing to prevent heating the acrylic and possibly warping the appliance. Also try to protect wires with your thumbs while pumicing to prevent accidentally catching wires with the spinning muslin wheels and damaging the wires and acrylic. Especially be careful with mandibular retainers with occlusal rests and maxillary and mandibular wraparound design appliances that tend to get caught in the spinning muslin wheels. Rinse the pumice from the retainers. Inspect dry appliances. All previously bur ground and sanded surfaces should have uniform matte smooth surfaces and edges.

On a bench lathe, use a 4-inch 30-ply muslin wheel that is dedicated to tripoli polishing compound and polish all tongue side surfaces and edges at slow speed. The author likes to go one step further by using an acrylic high-shine compound on another dedicated 4-inch 30-ply muslin wheel at slow speed, bringing the retainers to a high luster.

Figure 14.303 shows a set of maxillary and mandibular Hawley retainers. The retainer is then cleaned in a cool ultrasonic cleaner and/or brushed with soap and water. Check retainers on the model for fit and adjust wires if necessary. Adjustments usually consist of tightening the labial bow on the mesial arm of the adjustment loops with three-prong pliers. Figure 14.304 shows the location for the adjustment to tighten

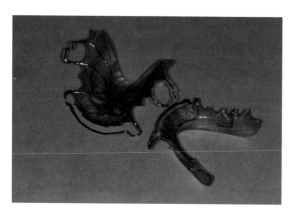

Figure 14.303. Completed set of standard Hawley retainers.

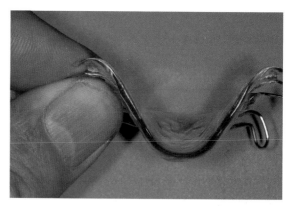

Figure 14.305. A 2-mm-thick finished and polished maxillary Hawley retrainer.

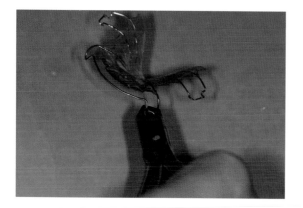

Figure 14.304. With a three-prong pliers, lightly tighten labial bow adjustment loops toward the facial surface of the teeth. Adjust clasps toward the gingival direction if necessary.

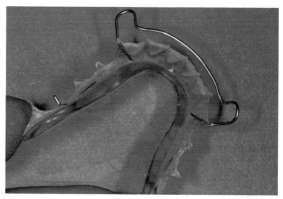

Figure 14.306. A 2½-mm-thick finished and polished mandibular Hawley retainer.

the labial bow. Clasps usually need to be tightened through the occlusal embrasures and buccal embrasures with bird beak pliers.

Figure 14.305 shows the ideal thickness for a finished maxillary Hawley retainer. Figure 14.306 shows the ideal thickness for a finished mandibular Hawley retainer.

Complete the fabrication process by disinfecting appliances for 10 minutes with a suitable disinfectant following accepted practices (NADL 1986).

REFERENCES

Adams, C. P. 1984. The design, construction and use of removable orthodontic appliances. 5th ed. Bristol, England: John Wright & Sons Ltd.

Hawley, C. A. 1919. A removable retainer. Int. J. Orthod. 2:291–298.

Kesling, H. D. 1946. Coordinating the predetermined pattern and tooth positioner with conventional treatment. Am. J. Orthod. 32:285–293.

NADL (National Association of Dental Laboratories). 1986. Infection control compliance manual. Washington, DC: NADL.

Sheridan, J. J., et al. 1993. Essix retainer fabrication and supervision for permanent retention. J. Clin. Orthod. 27:37–45.

Staley, R. N., and Reske, N. T. 1987. A one-arm wrought wire clasp that engages two buccal surface undercuts. Quint. Dent. Technol. 11(2): 123–127.

Staley, R. N., and Reske, N. T. 1989. A new clasp for orthodontic retainers, the Resta Clasp. Oral Health 79:19–22.

Willison, B. D., and Waruhnek, S. P. 2004. Practical guide to orthodontic appliances: a comprehensive resource from theory to fabrication. Buffalo: Great Lakes Orthodontics, Ltd.

Orthodontic Materials

15

Introduction

Orthodontists and orthodontic technicians use a variety of materials, equipment, and procedures as they treat patients and construct appliances. Only a brief survey of some materials will be included in this chapter. For an excellent in depth coverage of the topic, we recommend the book written by Brantley and Eliades (2001).

Orthodontic Wires

Four basic types of wires are used by orthodontists: (1) austenitic stainless steel, (2) cobalt-chromium-nickel, (3) beta-titanium, and (4) nickel-titanium. The wires have different uses during orthodontic treatment based on their physical properties (Table 15.1).

Stainless Steel Wires

The 18-8 stainless steel wires are composed of iron (73.75%), chromium (18%), nickel (8%), and carbon (0.25%). The 18-8 alloys are strong

Essentials of Orthodontics: Diagnosis and Treatment
by Robert N. Staley and Neil T. Reske
© 2011 Blackwell Publishing Ltd.

and ductile at room temperature. They resist tarnish and corrosion because of the presence of chromium. A thin, transparent layer of chromic oxide, known as a passavating film forms on the surface of the wire and prevents corrosion. If the oxide layer is disturbed by mechanical or chemical actions the wire can corrode. The nicks and rough places left on a wire after it is bent with pliers may produce localized electric couples that allow corrosion cells to form in the presence of an electrolyte solution such as saliva. If bits of carbon steel are incorporated into the surface of a stainless steel wire that comes into contact with carbon steel pliers, cutters, or burs, the embedded carbon steel becomes a couple that starts the process of corrosion. Chlorine cleansers attack 18-8 steels and cause corrosion. Acetic and lactic acids do not attack the passavating film and can be used in the cleaning of Hawley retainers containing stainless steel wires.

Sensitization

Depending on their carbon content, the 18-8 alloys lose resistance to corrosion when heated from 400°C to 900°C (Fig. 15.1). The formation of chromium carbide at the grain boundaries causes the alloy to lose its resistance to corrosion. Chromium carbide most rapidly forms at 650°C and begins to decompose above that

Table 15.1. Physical Properties of Major Orthodontic Wire Types[1]

Wire Alloy	Composition	Modulus of Elasticity	Yield Strength (MPa)*	Springback
Austenitic Stainless Steel	17–20% Cr 8–12% Ni 0.15% C Balance Fe	160–180	1100–1500	0.00600–0.0094 (AR) 0.00650–0.0099 (HT)
Cobalt-chromium-Nickel	40% Co, 20% Cr, 15% Ni, 15.8% Fe, 7% Mo, 2% Mn, 0.15% C, 0.04% Be	160–190	830–1000	0.0045–0.0065 (AR) 0.0054–0.0074 (HT)
Beta-titanium	77.8% Ti, 11.3% Mo, 6.6% Zr, 4.3% Sn	62–69	690–970	0.0094–0.011
Nickel-titanium	55% Ni, 45% Ti	34	210–410	0.0058–0.016

*Values correspond to 0.1% permanent tensile strain.
AR, as received; HT, heat-treated conditions.
[1]Brantley et al. 1997; Brantley 2001.

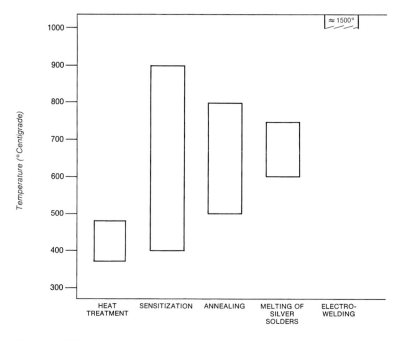

Figure 15.1. Effects of heat on 18-8 stainless steel.

temperature. The loss of chromium from the alloy that occurs with heat is known as **sensitization**. The corrosion along the grain boundaries where chromium carbide forms weakens the structure of the wire. Stainless steel can be stabilized against the formation of chromium carbide by adding an element such as titanium that precipitates as carbide in preference to chromium.

Very few of the stainless steel wires used by orthodontists are stabilized.

Cold Working

As a stainless steel wire is bent, tensile strength increases and ductility decreases (Fig. 15.2). Greatly strain-hardened wires are brittle and

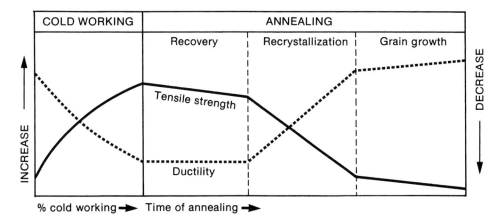

Figure 15.2. How cold working, recovery heat treatment, and annealing affect the tensile strength and ductility of stainless steel wires. (Redrawn from Richman 1967.)

break more easily. Put as few bends in a wire as possible, so that it will function without breaking. Wires continue to work harden as they move teeth, are adjusted, and altered during mastication.

Recovery Heat Treatment

The physical properties of cold-worked, strain-hardened stainless steel wires can be improved significantly with recovery heat treatment. When 18-8 steel wires are heated at moderately low temperatures of 370°C to 400°C after cold working (bending), the heat removes residual stresses, stabilizes the shape of the wire, and increases its elasticity, yield strength, and resilience (Fig. 15.2). Recovery heat treatment in a welder or oven should last from 1 to 2 minutes. The wire will turn to a light straw color. Sensitization occurs above 400°C; the wire darkens to dark brown at 500°C and a dark bluish brown at 600°C.

Annealing

If 18-8 stainless steel is heated above 500°C, the metal will begin to anneal and lose its elasticity and resilience (Fig. 15.2). Between 700°C and 800°C, a stainless steel wire becomes fully annealed. Annealing eliminates strain hardening and distorted grains associated with cold working. Orthodontic ligature wires are made from annealed stainless steel because ductility is important for that use. Figure 15.2 illustrates the relationships between tensile strength and ductility during cold working, recovery heat treatment, and annealing. The ends of an arch wire may be annealed and bent at the distal ends of the molar tubes to keep the wire from migrating mesially out of one of the tubes between appointments. A wire is annealed with an open flame or by passing an electric current through it using attachments on a welding machine. Arch wires, clasps, labial bows, and finger springs are not annealed, because these parts of an appliance must have tensile strength and elasticity.

Cobalt-Chromium-Nickel Wires

The cobalt-chromium-nickel wires were developed in the 1950s (see Table 15.1). They come in four levels of resilience: (1) blue, soft; (2) yellow, ductile; (3) green, semiresilient; and (4) red, resilient. The wires are protected from corrosion by a film of chromium oxide that forms on the exterior of the wires, similar to the 18-8 stainless steel wires. The softer wires can be bent easily and after bending can be heat treated to greatly increase their resilience and yield strengths. Heat treatment with an electric welder for 1 or 2 minutes or an oven for 10 minutes is effective at 500°C. The performance of cobalt-chromium-nickel and stainless steel wires is similar.

Beta-Titanium Wires

Beta-titanium wires were developed by Burstone and Goldberg (1980). The developers recognized that this alloy could deliver lower forces than the stainless steel and cobalt-chromium-nickel alloys and thus be more compatible with periodontal and alveolar bone tissues during orthodontic treatment. Compared to stainless steel, the modulus of elasticity of beta-titanium is favorably lower, about 40% of stainless steel, yield strength is less, about 60% of stainless steel, but their spring back that increases working range is much better than stainless steel (see Table 15.1). Beta-titanium wires can be easily bent. The beta-titanium wires should not be heat treated by the orthodontist, but they can be welded. These wires have a surface roughness that is associated with arch wire-bracket sliding friction.

Nickel-Titanium Wires

The nickel-titanium alloy wires were developed at the Naval Ordinance Laboratory by Buehler, Gilfrich, and Riley (1963). Andreasen and associates (1971, 1972, 1978) developed the alloy for use in orthodontic treatment. The nitinol wires have a very low modulus of elasticity and high flexibility, very low yield strengths, and wide elastic working range (see Table 15.1). Nickel-titatanium arch wires have two major phases: austenitic and martensitic (Brantley and Eliades 2001). The martensitic stabilized alloys do not have shape memory or superelasticity, an example of which is Nitinol Classic (3M Unitek Orthodontic Products, Monrovia, CA). The martensitic-active alloys achieve shape memory

through a thermoelastic effect. As the wire warms to mouth temperature, the deformed martensitic phase is transformed into the austenitic phase that moves teeth toward the intended shape of the wire. Neo Sentalloy (GAC International, Islandia, NY) is an example of a thermoelastic shape memory nickel-titanium wire. The austenitic-active alloys are transformed through stress into the martensitic phase. These alloys are super elastic wires; one example is Nitinol SE (3M Unitek Orthodontic Products). Further details about these unique wires are discussed by Brantley and Eliades (2001) and Khier, Brantley, and Fournelle (1991).

Physical Properties of Orthodontic Wires

Light and continuous forces move teeth optimally. An understanding of the properties of wires helps a clinician to choose the best type and size of wire for each phase of treatment. A light force may be ineffective and a heavy force may cause unwanted trauma to the tooth, periodontal ligament, and alveolar bone.

Wires have three properties of interest: strength, stiffness/springiness, and range. Each property is represented in a stress-strain curve: (1) the proportional limit, (2) the yield point (yield strength), and (3) the ultimate yield strength (Fig. 15.3). The point on the stress-strain curve that a beam first deforms is called the **elastic** or **proportional limit**. The point on the curve when a force deforms the beam 0.1% is called the **yield point** (Fig. 15.3). Ultimate tensile strength represents the highest load the wire can sustain before it goes on to failure (breaks) with higher loads. The ultimate tensile strength also represents the highest force the wire can deliver to a tooth.

The slope of the linear part of the stress-strain curve is called the modulus of elasticity. The modulus of elasticity describes the stiffness or springiness of a wire. As the springiness (elasticity) of a wire increases, the slope of the stress-strain curve becomes more horizontal, and vice versa (Fig. 15.3).

Range represents the distance a wire will bend elastically before it deforms permanently (Fig. 15.3). Spring back represents the distance a wire will return partially between the proportional limit and point of ultimate tensile strength on the stress-strain curve (Fig. 15.3).

The three major properties of wires have a relationship: the strength of a wire equals its stiffness times its range.

Resilience is the area under the stress-strain curve between the origin and proportional limit that represents the energy stored in the wire. Formability is the amount that a wire can be permanently deformed without breaking and is represented by the area under the curve between yield point and failure point (Fig. 15.3).

Figure 15.4 is taken from a 3M Orthodontic Products catalogue and it shows truncated stress-strain curves for stainless steel, cobalt-chrome-nickel, beta titanium, and nickel titanium wires that are sold by the company. A clinician will use the lighter force wires for initial alignment of teeth and gradually work up to larger wires to finish moving the tooth.

Changing the diameter of a cylindrical wire or the cross sectional area of a rectangular wire affects the strength, stiffness/springiness, and range of the wire (Thurow 1966). Doubling the diameter of a cylindrical wire increases its strength eight times, reduces its springiness (elasticity) to one-sixteenth of the original value, and

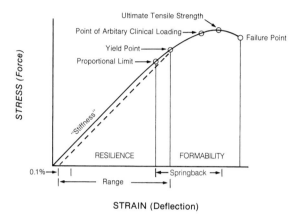

Figure 15.3. Stress-strain curve for an orthodontic wire. (Redrawn after Proffit, 1986.)

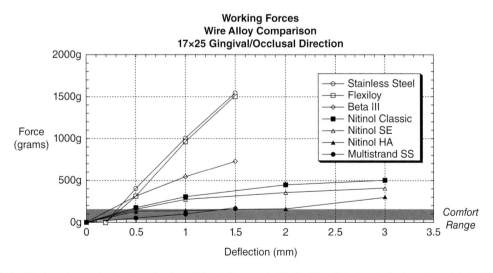

Figure 15.4. Working forces for basic arch wires: (1) stainless steel, (2) Flexilloy [blue], cobalt-chromium-nickel, (3) Beta III, beta titanium, (4) Nitinol Classic, martensitic, (5) Nitinol SE, super-elastic, (6) Nitinol HA, heat activated, and Multistrand SS. (From a recent catalogue, courtesy of 3M Unitek Orthodontic Products, Monrovia, CA.)

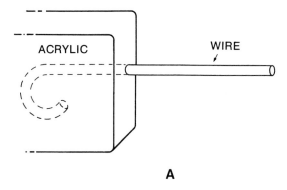

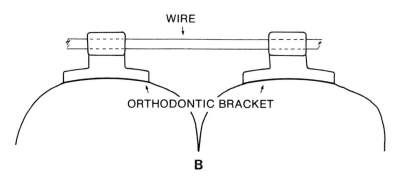

Figure 15.5. Orthodontic wire as (**A**) a cantilever beam, a finger spring mounted in acrylic, and (**B**) a supported beam, an arch wire in the edgewise appliance.

reduces its range to one-half of the original value. These changes affect both cantilever beams (finger springs) and supported beams or arch wires in the edgewise appliance (Fig. 15.5). When a cantilever beam is doubled in length, its strength is reduced by one half, its springiness is increased eight times, and its range is increased four times (Thurow 1966).

Wire Sizes

Wire sizes commonly used in orthodontic treatment are listed in Table 15.2. The dimensions of wires in the United States are given in

Table 15.2. Wire Size Conversion

Inch	Millimeter
0.014	0.35
0.016	0.4
0.018	0.45
0.020	0.5
0.024	0.6
0.026	0.65
0.028	0.7
0.030	0.75
0.036	0.9

thousandths of an inch. Other countries use the metric system. A mil is $\frac{1}{1000}$th of 1 inch; hence a 0.018 cylindrical wire can be described as an 18-mil wire.

Electric Welding

Special settings on welding machines are recommended by the manufacturers of beta-titanium arch wires. The following comments about welding pertain to stainless steel wires and bands. Stainless steel tubes and brackets are usually joined to bands with resistance spot welding. Electric welders have a transformer that produces a low voltage and high flow of current (300 to 1000 amperes) between the copper electrodes. The large electric current is forced to flow through a limited area at the electrode tips, and resistance to the current in the stainless steel generates heat that melts and fuses the steel parts held between the electrodes (Fig. 15.6). The steel parts to be welded are held together under pressure to achieve a successful weld. The heat generated depends on the amount of current and the time it flows through the electrodes. Too much recrystallization of the steel weakens the weld joint. An increase in the area of a weld strengthens the weld joint. In a good weld, the electrode makes a slight indentation on the metal surface. Excessive heat that discolors and splatters the metal surrounding the weld joint weakens the weld. The overheated annealed steel is weak and subject to corrosion that may eventually lead to failure of the weld.

The current in welding machines does not pose a shock hazard. The copper electrodes have low resistance to the current and thus do not get hot during welding. The electrode tips must be kept clean and flat to produce an optimum weld joint.

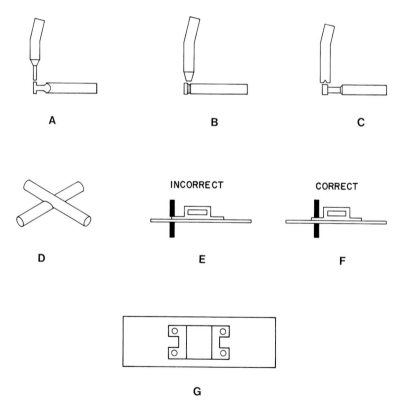

Figure 15.6. Electric welding: (**A**) electrodes for welding an attachment on a band, (**B**) electrodes for welding one wire to another wire, (**C**) electrodes for welding wires to bands, (**D**) the weld between two wires, (**E**) incorrect position of electrodes, (**F**) correct position of electrodes, and (**G**) a vertical tube welded on a band.

Most welders have a turret design that gives the welder several combinations of electrode types (Fig. 15.6, A–C). Small electrode tips are used to weld attachments to bands (Fig. 15.6A). In the welding of an attachment to a band, position the electrode tips properly on the welding flange (Fig. 15.6E is incorrect; Fig, 15.5F is correct). The blunt upper and grooved lower electrodes weld wires together (Fig. 15.6B). When two wires are welded together at right angles to one another, they fuse together but retain their outer surfaces when using the grooved electrode (Fig. 15.6, B and D). The notched upper and knob lower electrodes weld wires to bands (Fig. 15.6C).

Flame Soldering

Silver solders have low melting-point temperatures, making them suitable for joining stainless steel parts together. The melting points of silver solder range from 600°C to 750°C (Fig. 15.1). These temperatures sensitize and anneal stainless steel. Bands of sensitized and annealed stainless steel surround all solder joints. Choose solders that melt near 600°C. The silver solders are alloys of silver, copper, zinc, tin, and indium that corrode in an oral environment. These solders are acceptable for short-term use in the mouth. Smoothing and polishing the solder and stainless steel around a solder joint improves corrosion resistance, and hardens the annealed stainless steel by cold working it. When polishing the solder, avoid exposing the underlying wire, because exposure considerably weakens the solder joint.

Silver solder is available in several forms including wires, bars, and pastes. Use small-diameter solder wires or paste solder to solder small stainless steel wires to large wires. Paste solders contain a mixture of finely ground silver solder, flux, and a cleaning agent. Use larger-diameter solder wires and bar solders to join together large stainless steel wires and join large wires to stainless steel bands. The making of a band and loop space maintainer and lower lingual holding arch are examples of large wires soldered to a band.

Flux is essential for successful soldering of stainless steel. The flux contains a fluoride compound that dissolves the chromium oxide passivating film. The potassium fluoride enables the flux to wet the surfaces of the metals that will be soldered together.

The metal surfaces must be clean before flux is applied to them. A layer of black oxidation products can build up on the parts to be joined during soldering. Solder will not flow onto such surfaces. If oxidation products accumulate, they must be removed from the surfaces of the metals to be soldered in order to achieve a successful solder joint.

A thin needle-like gas-air flame is an excellent source of heat for soldering. The wires to be joined are held 3 mm (⅛ inch) from the tip of the blue cone in the reducing zone of the flame. The solidus-liquidus range of silver solders is small so that solders harden promptly when removed from heat, a necessity for free hand soldering. Before soldering, the wires to be joined are lightly tack welded together. If the stainless steel wires cannot be easily tack welded together, a soldering jig can be used to hold the wires in position. Coat the parts to be soldered with flux. Heat the larger wire first. Solder against a black background to see the color of the heated stainless steel parts. The steel parts to be soldered should not exceed a dull red color. After the flux fuses, add solder until it flows completely around the joint. After the solder flows around the wires, remove the wires from the heat quickly and quench them in room temperature water. Use as little heat as possible for as short a time as possible.

Electric Soldering

The heat generated by an electric welding machine is used to solder stainless steel parts together. The carbon tip and copper ball electrodes are used to solder a wire to a band (Fig. 15.7A). The soldering of a band and loop space maintainer

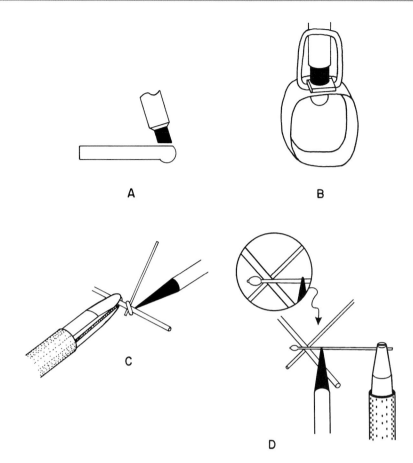

Figure 15.7. Electric soldering: (**A**) carbon tip and copper ball electrodes used to solder a heavy wire to a band, (**B**) the soldering of a wire to a band as in a band and loop space maintainer, (**C**) soldering of two wires together, and (**D**) the use of a brass wire soldering intermediary electrode to solder two wires together.

is illustrated in Figure 15.7B. Begin the process by first lightly tack welding the wire to the band. Then place the band and tack welded wire assembly between the soldering electrodes (Fig. 15.7B). Cover the surfaces to be soldered with flux. Cut and form the bar solder into a V-shape to fit over the wire (Fig. 15.7B). The clean carbon tip presses down on the solder. Initiate the flow of electric current and discontinue the current flow after the solder melts and flows over the wire and band.

A welding machine has an auxiliary soldering cable and clamp jaw electrodes to solder wires to wires and wires to bands imbedded in a stone working cast (Fig. 15.7, C and D). When possible, tack weld wires together before soldering (Fig. 15.7C). A tack weld holds the wires together and increases the flow of heat between them. Avoid creating a heavy weld that burns and oxidizes the wires. The clamp jaw holds the larger wire about 1.5 mm from the solder joint. A piece of wire solder is wrapped around the joint (Fig. 15.7C). Apply flux to the solder and wires and place the carbon tip auxiliary electrode either on the larger wire or on the solder (Fig. 15.7C). After the solder completely flows around the wires, withdraw the carbon tip promptly. If you choose to put the carbon tip electrode on the larger wire, do not remove the tip from the wire until after the solder sets. If you put the carbon tip electrode in direct contact with the solder, remove the tip before the solder sets.

A brass wire with a globule of solder on its end can be used as an electrode with the clamp jaw and carbon tip auxiliary (Fig. 15.7D). This method of soldering reduces the heat absorbed by the stainless steel wires being soldered together. Apply flux to the solder and wires to be joined. Keep the brass soldering electrode in contact with the largest wire to be soldered. Keep the solder globule near the wire joint and the carbon tip (heat source) on the opposite side of the wire joint (Fig. 15.7D). Solder flows toward the heat source. As the solder flows, slide the wires through the solder and pass the wires over the brass electrode to pull solder to the opposite side of the wires, keeping the brass electrode and wires in contact (Fig. 15.7D). Use only light pressure on the carbon electrode while applying heat to the brass electrode. If the carbon electrode breaks the brass electrode, the brass is being overheated. Adjust the welding machine setting downward, and use the lower setting for future soldering. Withdraw the joined wires from the brass wire before the solder sets. Both wires should be covered with solder.

Clean flux from the carbon electrode after each use. The flux can be washed off the carbon tip with water.

REFERENCES

Andreasen, G. F., and Hilleman, T. B. 1971. An evaluation of cobalt substituted nitinol wire for use in orthodontics. J. Am. Dent. Assoc. 82:1373–1375.

Andreasen, G. F., and Brady, P. R. 1972. A use hypothesis for 55 nitinol wire for orthodontics. Angle Orthod. 42:172–177.

Andreasen, G. F., and Morrow, R. E. 1978. Laboratory and clinical analyses of Nitinol wire. Am. J. Orthod. 73:142–151.

Brantley, W. A. 2001. Orthodontic wires. In Orthodontic Materials, Scientific and Clinical Aspects. Brantley, W. A. and Eliades, T. eds. Stuttgart: Thieme.

Brantley, W. A., Webb, C. S., Soto, U., Cai, Z., and McCoy, B. P. 1997. X-ray diffraction analyses of Copper Ni-Ti orthodontic wires. J. Dent. Res. 76:(IADR abstracts)401.

Brantley, W. A., and Eliades, T. 2001. Orthodontic materials. Scientific and clinical aspects. Stuttgart: Georg Thieme Verlag.

Buehler, W. J., Gilfrich, J. V., and Riley, R. C. 1963. Effect of low-temperature phase changes on the mechanical properties of alloys near the composition of TiNi. J. Appl. Physiol. 34:1475–1477.

Burstone, C. J., and Goldberg, A. J. 1980. Beta titanium: a new orthodontic alloy. Am. J. Orthod. 77:121–132.

Khier, S. E., Brantley, W. A., and Fournelle, R. A. 1991. Bending properties of super-elastic and non-super-elastic nickel-titanium orthodontic wires. Am. J. Orthod. Dentofac. Orthop. 99:310–318.

Proffit, W. R. 1986. Contemporary Orthodontics. St. Louis: The C. V. Mosby Company.

Richman, M. H. 1967. Introduction to the science of metals. Waltham, MA: Blaisdell Publishing Company.

Thurow, R. C. 1966. Edgewise orthodontics. 2nd ed. St. Louis: The C. V. Mosby Company.

Index

Essentials of Orthodontics: Diagnosis and Treatment
by Robert N. Staley and Neil T. Reske
© 2011 Blackwell Publishing Ltd.